DISEASED RELATIONS

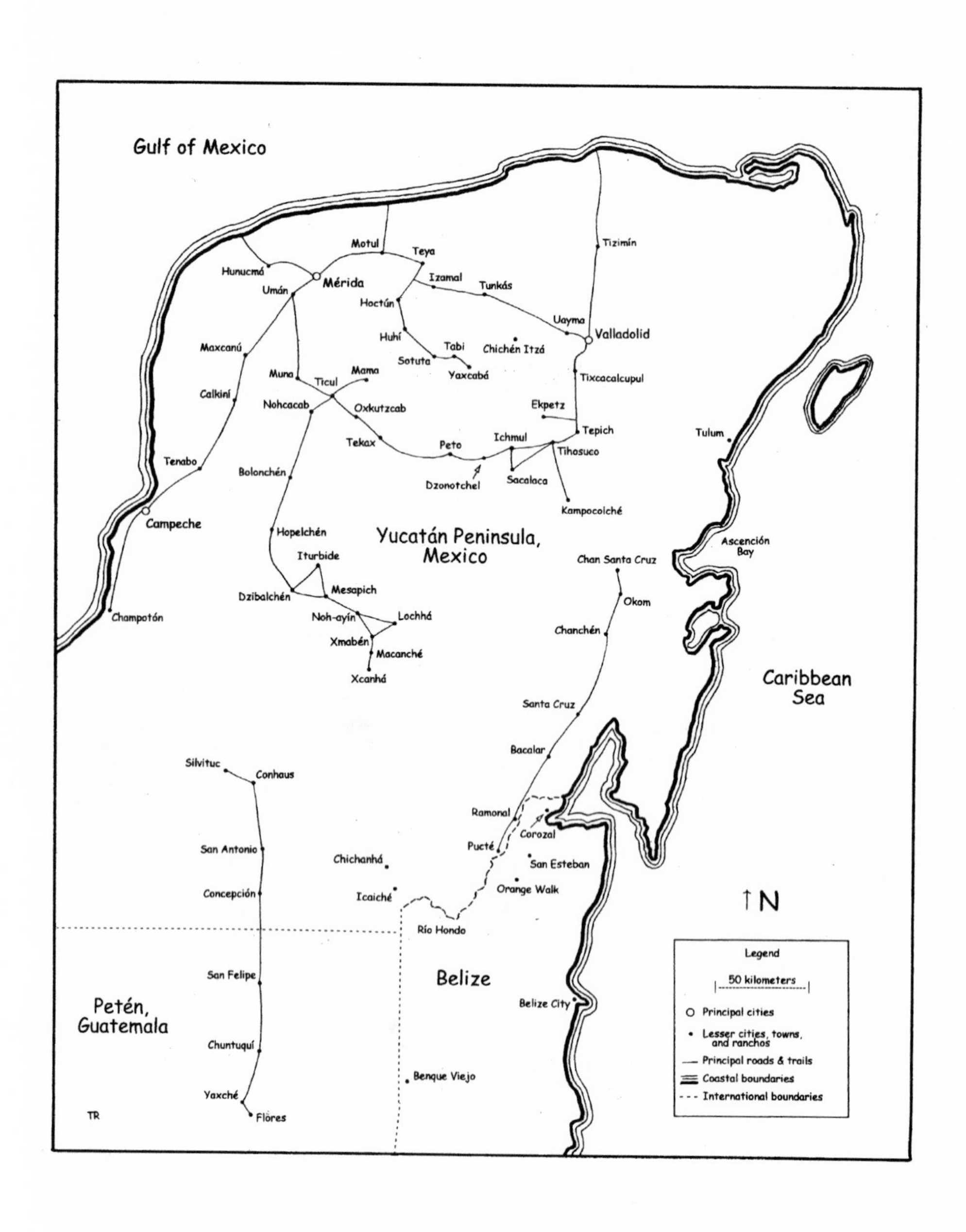
Gulf of Mexico
Motul
Teya
Hunucmá
Mérida
Umán
Izamal
Tunkás
Tizimín
Hoctún
Uayma
Valladolid
Maxcanú
Huhí
Tabi
Chichén Itzá
Sotuta
Yaxcabá
Muna
Ticul
Mama
Tixcacalcupul
Calkiní
Nohcacab
Oxkutzcab
Ekpetz
Tepich
Tulum
Ichmul
Tekax
Peto
Tihosuco
Tenabo
Bolonchén
Dzonotchel
Sacalaca
Kampocolché
Campeche
Hopelchén
Yucatán Peninsula, Mexico
Ascención Bay
Iturbide
Chan Santa Cruz
Mesapich
Dzibalchén
Okom
Noh-ayín
Lochhá
Champotón
Chanchén
Xmabén
Macanché
Xcanhá
Caribbean Sea
Santa Cruz
Bacalar
Silvituc
Conhaus
Ramonal
Corozal
Pucté
San Antonio
Chichanhá
San Esteban
Icaiché
Orange Walk
Concepción
N
Río Hondo
Legend
50 kilometers
Belize
San Felipe
Belize City
Principal cities
Petén, Guatemala
Lesser cities, towns, and ranchos
Principal roads & trails
Chuntuquí
Coastal boundaries
Benque Viejo
International boundaries
Yaxché
TR
Flores

DISEASED RELATIONS

EPIDEMICS, PUBLIC HEALTH, AND STATE-BUILDING IN YUCATÁN, MEXICO, 1847–1924

HEATHER McCREA

University of New Mexico Press | Albuquerque

Printed in the United States of America
15 14 13 12 11 10 1 2 3 4 5 6

LIBRARY OF CONGRESS CATALOGING-IN-PUBLICATION DATA

McCrea, Heather L.
Diseased relations : epidemics, public health, and state-building in Yucatán, Mexico, 1847–1924 / Heather McCrea.
p. cm.
Includes bibliographical references and index.
ISBN 978-0-8263-4898-2 (pbk. : alk. paper)
1. Public health—Mexico—Yucatán (State) 2. Epidemics—Mexico—Yucatán (State) 3. Medical policy—Mexico—Yucatán (State) I. Title.
[DNLM: 1. Disease Outbreaks—history—Mexico. 2. Disease Outbreaks—prevention & control—Mexico. 3. History, 19th Century—Mexico. 4. History, 20th Century—Mexico. 5. Indians, North American—history—Mexico. 6. Social Medicine—history—Mexico. 7. State Government—Mexico. WA 11 DM4]
RA452.Y83M43 2010
362.10972'65—dc22
2010039360

In memory of Dean C. and Hazel I. Burns

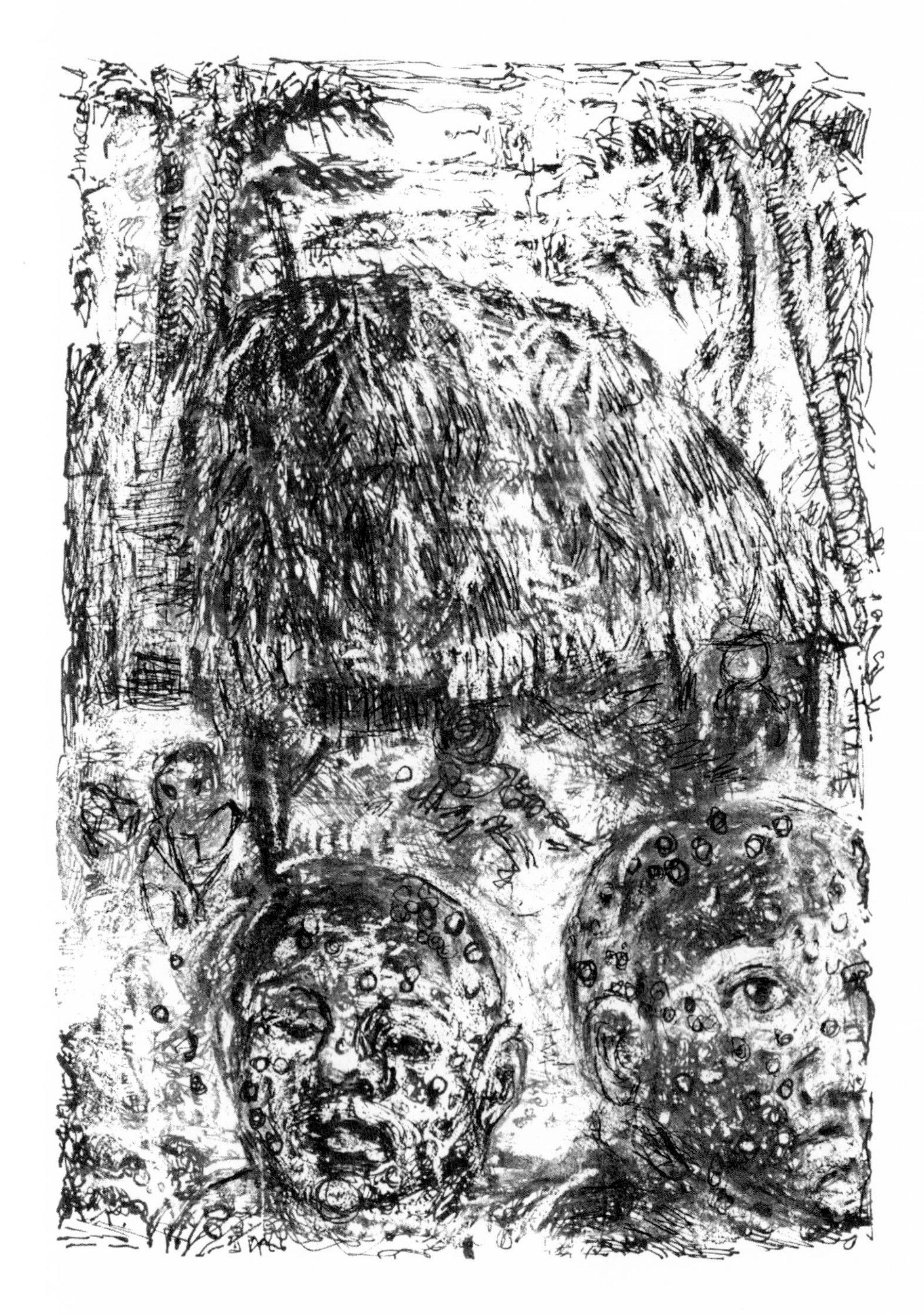

CONTENTS

LIST OF ILLUSTRATIONS

ACKNOWLEDGMENTS

THIS BOOK COULD not have been possible without the support and assistance of a number of individuals and institutions.

As an undergraduate at the University of Kansas, I took classes with Elizabeth Kuznesof, Anton Rosenthal, Robert Smith, and John Hoopes. My interest in Latin America and indigenous studies began with their classes. I have enjoyed their continued support. Since returning to the state of Kansas as an assistant professor of history at Kansas State University in 2006, the University of Kansas's Latin American and environmental studies faculty have invited me to present my work. Chapters 4 and 6 have benefitted from the insights provided at the Hall Center for the Humanities talks and Latin American Studies Center *merienda* colloquium.

During my graduate training at Stony Brook University, I had the privilege to study with Brooke Larson, Barbara Weinstein, Nancy Tomes, and Paul Gootenberg. As my thesis adviser, Brooke Larson patiently oversaw the development of this project. My interest in public health and the history of medicine began when Nancy Tomes presented her work at a History Department colloquium. Barbara Weinstein always offered sound professional advice. Eric Goode and Barbara offered many a great meal and conversation during my graduate years. Paul Gootenberg made archive work in Mexico City possible, ensuring that I understood how to maneuver the intricacies of conducting research at the Archivo General de la Nación. I owe a special debt to Allen Wells, who has offered valuable commentary on my work as a fellow Yucatecologist.

I also gratefully acknowledge the support of the Fulbright-Robles Foundation for supporting my field research for one year in Mérida, Yucatán.

My research in Yucatán would not have been possible without the assistance of the director of the Archivo General del Estado de Yucatán (AGEY), Dra. Piedad Peniche Rivero. I am deeply indebted to archivists and friends at the AGEY: Elías Teyer Carmona, Jorge Canto Alcocer, Candy Flota Garcia, Andrea Vergoda Medina, Cinthia Vanessa Fernández Vergara, and all the others who have made me and my family feel welcome every time we visited. Additionally, I had the assistance of two invaluable *ayudantes* (assistants): Wendi Aracelly Cob and Leni Malveda. In Mérida, Miguel Güemez Pineda and Lupe Graniel, Luisa Sosa, Olga Uc Doriega, Marcia Good, Brian Maust, and Tonio Castels Talens all made me feel welcome in their homes and offered unwavering support. Learning Yucatec Maya would not have been possible without instruction under Miguel Güemez Pineda and Hilaria Más Colli. At Universidad Autónoma de Yucatán–Centro de Investigaciones Regionales, Othon Baños Ramirez, Alejandra García Quintanilla, and the late Hernán Menendez all offered comments and practical advice during my field research.

I would also like to thank the exceptionally knowledgeable staffs at the Hemeroteca José María Piño Suárez, Biblioteca Menéndez, Archivo Histórico de Archidiócesis de Yucatán (in particular Padre Camargo for granting permission to consult church records), Centro de Apoyo de Investigacion Histórica de Yucatán, and the Biblioteca Crescencio Carrillo y Ancona. The Doctors Laviada opened their personal archives in Mérida, allowing me to review valuable information.

A number of fellow Yucatecólogos also offered assistance and advice, including Paul Eiss, Ben Fallaw, Wolfgang Gabbert, Christopher Gil, Gilbert Joseph, Matthew Restall, and Peter Sigal.

The staffs at archives in Campeche (Archivo General del Estado de Campeche) and in the national archives of Belize at Belmopan were welcoming and helpful. In the United States, archivists at the Williams Center for Research in New Orleans, Tulane University's Latin American Library, and the American Antiquarian Society; Christian Kelleher at the University of Texas at Austin's Nettie Lee Benson Latin American Library; and Bethany J. Antos and Tom Rosenbaum at the Rockefeller Foundation Archives provided invaluable assistance. The Rockefeller Foundation also graciously provided funds for me to travel to their masterfully organized archives. Thank you also to the Rockefeller Foundation for granting permission to reproduce the photograph in chapter 6.

In Mexico City archivists and staff at the Archivo General de la Nación, the Archivo Histórico de la Secretaría de Salud (formerly the Archivo Histórico de Salud y Salubridad y Asistencia), the Centro de Estudios de Historia de México de Condumex, and the Archivo Histórico de la Facultad de Medicina at the Universidad Nacional Autónoma de México all provided expert guidance.

At California State University at Fullerton, I received funding that made research for chapters 5 and 6 possible from the Faculty Development Center. A number of good friends and colleagues in California saw me through the transformation of my dissertation into a manuscript, including Gordon Bakken, the Bartz family, Gail Brunelle, Touraj Daryaee, Kristine Dennehey, Christine Hetrick Eubank, Nicholas Eubank, Reyes Fidalgo, Nancy Fitch, Natalie Fousekis, Cora Granata, William W. Haddad, Maria Figueroa, Volker Janssen, Robert McLain, Mindy Mechanic, Sandra Pérez-Linggi, Catherine A. Reinhardt, and Philippe Zacair.

I would like to thank Jamie Rodriguez and the outside reader at *Mexican Studies/Estudios Mexicanos* for comments on my article "On Sacred Ground: The Church and Burial Rites in Nineteenth-Century Yucatán" (vol. 23, no. 1, 2007), of which parts appear in chapter 3. I would like to thank University of Oklahoma Press for granting permission to print the map of Yucatán that appears in the introduction.

At Kansas State University, I would like to thank the Chapman Center for Rural History, Big XII Fellowship, and the Office of Research and Grants for their generosity. Colleagues in the Department of History at KSU have provided consistent encouragement. In particular, James Sherow offered invaluable advice as a faculty mentor, and David Stone read and commented on draft chapters of the manuscript.

Susan Gauss, Jenise DePinto, Christine Cleaton, Eustacia Wilson, and Scott Wilson supplied a foolproof support mechanism throughout graduate school and friendship. I have been fortunate to discuss all or part of my research with the following friends and colleagues: Claudia Agostoni, Magally Alegre Henderson, Annalyda Alveraz-Caldero, Warwick Anderson, Noberto Barreto-Velázquez, Katherine Bliss, Louise Breen, Charles Briggs, Christopher Boyer, Steve Bunker, Lina del Castillo, Sandra Chism, Marcos Cueto, Gregory T. Cushman, Judy Davis, Michael Ducey, Chris Endy, Sterling Evans, Martha Few, Jamie Gentry, Eduardo Gonzalez, Albert Hamscher, John Hart, Paul Hart, Derek Hoff, Lane Ikenberry, Michelle Janette, Bonnie Lynn-Sherow, Victor M. Macías-González, John Maschino, Miriam Melton-Villanueva, Kristin Michel, Martín Monsalve, Kristin Mulready-Stone, Jolecyn Olcott,

Peter Parides, Pablo Piccato, Alexandra Puerto, Liliana Rodriguez, Laura Sainz, Mark Saka, Nicole Sanders, Myrna I. Santiago, David Sartorius, Lise Sedrez, John Soluri, Gabriela Soto Laveaga, David Sowell, Joel Q. G. Spencer, Donald Stevens, Alexandra Tolin-Schultz, Zeb Tortorici, Brett Troyan, David Vail, Rosanna Vail, Joel Vessels, Adam Warren, Robert Wilcox, Derek Williams, Andrew Wood, Angus Wright, Sue Zschoche, and Ann Zuwalski.

Terry Rugeley deserves a special note of thanks. He never let me forget "the book first," and without him it most assuredly would not have materialized.

Roger Gathman provided critical assistance with revisions in the final stages of this manuscript project. Clark Whitehorn proffered practical advice and guidance—a necessity for a first-time author. Sarah Soliz's careful editing and eye for detail also considerably improved the book.

Fuego, Tierra, Chongo, Río, Cuco, Cali, Adriana, and Soda all offered their own unique brand of support.

Richard Leslie and Amy Young nurtured my interests, questioned my methods, and allowed me to crash—repeatedly—at their Brooklyn apartment. Thanks also to my brother, Blair McCrea, and my father, Wyatt McCrea.

Thanks to my in-laws, Michael and Irene Krysko, for their unwavering support.

My mother, Judith Burns McCrea, is a professor of art at the University of Kansas and the artist who created the line drawings based on the historical narratives contained within this book. My mother has been my source of professional inspiration. Her unconditional love and support is woven into every fiber of this book. I would also like to thank Lucero Gilbert (Mick) García of Oracle, Arizona.

Finally, but by no means less important, my colleague, fellow historian, best friend, and husband, Michael Krysko, read and commented on countless drafts of this manuscript. Without his consistent love, support, and dedication to the telling of a good story, this book would not have been possible. Our daughter, Liliana Zacil, entered our world as my dissertation writing began. Now at eleven years old she is ready for it to be done. So, Ms. Lili, this one is for you, darling.

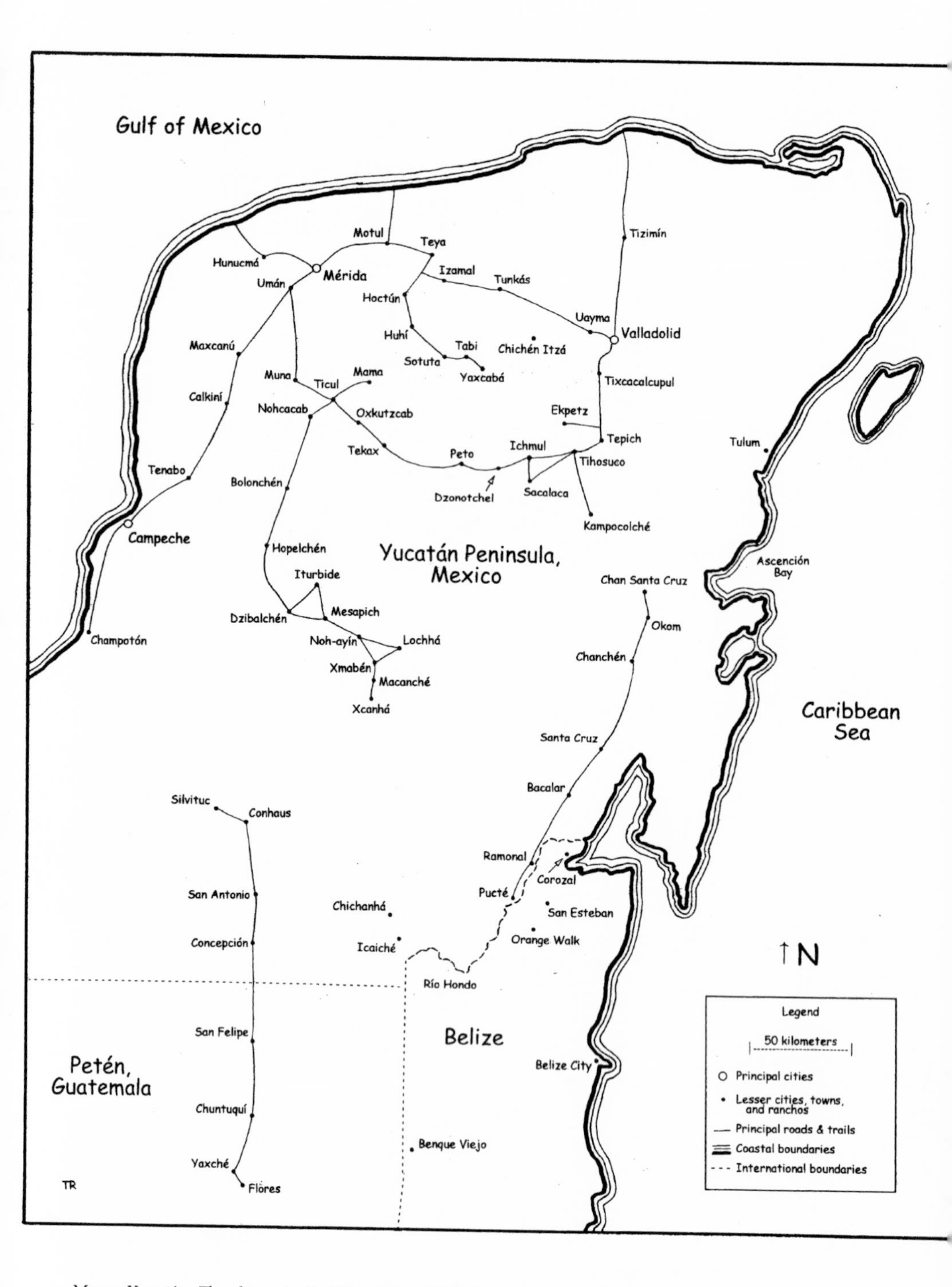

Map 1: Yucatán. Thank you to the University of Oklahoma Press for permission to reprint this map from Terry Rugeley's *Maya Wars: Ethnographic Accounts from Nineteenth-Century Yucatán*. Norman: University of Oklahoma Press, 2001, p. 2.

CHAPTER ONE

INTRODUCTION

Region, Ethnography, and Medicine in Yucatán, Mexico

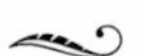

THIS BOOK EXAMINES THE CONSTRUCTION of modern Mexico through the lens of public health and disease. Nineteenth- and early twentieth-century Mexicans endured crushing epidemics while the political and social order around them changed drastically. As in other nineteenth-century states, the federal and state governments took on more and more responsibility for public health policies as it became apparent that individual health was often the effect of collective measures surrounding hygiene and sanitation. However, inside the programs designed to promote health, the state was also extending its reach far into the private sphere. In a peripheral state like Yucatán, with its mostly rural, indigenous Maya population and its small creole elite, public health issues were folded into a larger ideology, pitting "civilization" against "barbarism." The Yucatán state, throughout the period covered by this book, was intent on redefining and exerting control over public spaces, regulating the system of raising and selling foodstuffs, creating a system of mass vaccinations, eradicating pests, and controlling drinking water; all these projects were carried out in the name of the "welfare" of the people. Yet, as we shall see, this state activity was overdetermined by other agendas, most notably that of subjecting a population to the norms of a modern Mexico-in-process.

The time frame of my study extends from 1821, when Mexico gained independence from Spain, up to the postrevolutionary period in the early twentieth century, when the state took on many of the features that we recognize today. Public health programs and discourse were an inescapable presence in the lives of Mexico's citizens and were held out as a modernizing force legitimating the state's governance. The core of this work focuses on relationships between humans and their shared environments through an examination of people's interactions with emergent public health initiatives. By mapping pivotal shifts in public health policy and the implementation of disease prevention campaigns, I reveal a buried narrative of state-building, citizenship, and insurrection. Collectively, these interactions point toward the formation of a distinct regional Mexican identity born out of the matrix of devastating disease epidemics, civil insurrection, revolution, and modern medicine.

Mexico's southern Yucatán Peninsula, with its tropical ecology, is a particularly interesting case study because of the region's political, cultural, and geographical marginalization from the center of the Mexican republic. Yucatán experienced a strong separatist movement; underwent one of the longest wars in Latin America, the so-called Caste War; and, after the American Civil War, became the lynchpin of the great U.S. agricultural boom due to the farming of sisal (or henequen), a native plant that was used for making the twine that bound harvested grains. In the nineteenth century, it went from being one of the poorest of Mexican states to one of the richest—although a small elite largely appropriated the export wealth. For these reasons, the trajectory of Yucatán's history cannot be reduced to the history of Mexico; rather, it shares features with the circum-Caribbean network between Cuba, British Honduras (Belize), and New Orleans, as well as with Mexico.

Yucatán's tropical environment includes a wide range of animal and plant species endemic to the tropical rain forests. The peninsula contains no internal tributaries, but cenotes (natural sinkholes that collect rainwater) dot the sparse limestone terrain, providing much-needed water stores for inhabitants. Henequen, or sisal, became a major crop in northern Yucatán in the nineteenth century, partly because of the climactic conditions and partly because the thin soil was ideal for the growth of the cactuslike plant.[1] Sugarcane production had been encouraged after independence, as well as livestock farming, and maize was grown mainly for domestic consumption. These physical characteristics formed the microenvironment in which a set of diseases "inherent" to Yucatán would impinge on inhabitants and foreigners alike as the process of modernization went forward. Herein the stage was set upon which tensions between center and periphery, church and state, and Maya and creoles were clearly woven into the policies, rhetoric, and sociocultural fabric of an emerging nation-state.

After independence, the ruling creole elite made their first order of business to "civilize" the Yucatecan environment, both natural and human. Due to its position on the Gulf and its relative isolation from the mainland (communication with which was mainly by boat until, in the twentieth century, railroad connections were finally established), Yucatán was peculiarly susceptible to a number of tropical diseases and epidemics spread by shipping. As we will see, these included smallpox, cholera, malaria, yellow fever, and typhoid—all of which exacted a fearsome toll from the population. In the nineteenth century, the geography of disease was often overlaid by the symbolism of race, hence the idea, for instance, that the tropics were not "good" for white people. Yucatán, as Mexico's most tropical state, suffered from this stigma. Throughout our time frame, the policy-making elite was well aware of Yucatán's reputation as a "sick" zone for the civilized European or American and sought to counteract it by creating a modern, hygienic state with good drinking water, good sewage services, and good hospitals and by enforcing sanitary codes in the name of "civilization" over "barbarity." These strategies gradually developed in the nineteenth century and, reconfigured by the Revolution of 1910's ideological populism, expanded to include, at least theoretically, the entire populace in the early twentieth century.

Thus, the narrative I trace in this book is distinct from the heroic, popular narrative of disease control in the tropics that has been predominantly represented in the United States. In Paul De Kruif's *The Microbe Hunters*, a popular science book written in 1926, the subtitle for the chapter on Walter Reed, the scientist most associated in the United States with the battle against yellow fever, is "In the Interests of Science—And for Humanity!"[2] This succinctly encodes what one might call the official legend of public health. Vast changes in human-ecological interaction have often been seen solely from the seemingly unimpeachable view toward making humans healthier, in conjunction with another equally triumphant narrative that recounts the progress of medical science in its struggle both to understand disease and to battle against public ignorance. In this more complex story, I do not seek to demystify the motives of the great figures of public health but, instead, to show how the development of public health is really embedded in interventions that collectively changed the dynamic interchange between the indigenous Maya peasantry, mestizos, creole elites, statesmen, foreigners, and medical practitioners in Yucatán, which included some of the most violent episodes in nineteenth-century Mexican history, specifically Yucatán's civil Caste War beginning in 1847 and ending in 1902. This was followed by Yucatán's distinctly socialist experience with the Mexican Revolution beginning in 1915, which ended in violence in 1924 when Yucatán's socialist governor, Felipe Carrillo Puerto, was murdered.

In contrasting arcs of violent upheaval with overlapping waves of disease, I bring key debates into focus, debates that I argue are central to the formation of a modern nation-state. In the nineteenth century, citizenship was articulated in terms of civilization versus barbarism, with the former possessed by the creole elites and the latter inherent to indigenous cultures. Through this lens the elites interpreted and responded to the insurrectionary activities of the Maya *cruzob* Caste War rebels. At the turn of the twentieth century, civilizing campaigns dovetailed with the revolutionary campaign calling for the overthrow of the nepotism, graft, and corruption characteristic of the reign of President Porfirio Díaz, who ruled Mexico between 1877 and 1880 and from 1884 to 1911. The Mexican Revolution of 1910 was a notoriously decentralized event, with different leaders in different parts of the republic fighting for different agendas. Not surprisingly, these leaders, among them Francisco Madero, Emiliano Zapata, Pancho Villa, Plutarco Calles, Venustiano Carranza, and Alvaro Obregón, then fought among themselves. The Yucatán Peninsula remained somewhat removed from the unrest until 1915, when controversy over a state governor's election threw the region into a unique version of the national revolution. Yucatán's revolutionary experience was driven by grassroots demands for improved public services, including better schools, medicines, and physicians and tighter regulation of public refuse, drunkenness, roaming animals, and prostitution.

These demands for progressive governance occurred just as the biomedical science of the late nineteenth century went through a pivotal, if not revolutionary, shift in medical theory and practice. After the mid-1880s, Dr. Robert Koch, building on Louis Pasteur's germ theory and John Snow's discovery of the connection between cholera and polluted water, discovered the cholera bacillus, which gave rise to theories implicating microscopic "germs" as the ultimate causative agents of disease.[3] The advances in biological and hygiene sciences of the mid- to late nineteenth and early twentieth centuries provided policy makers with a powerful tool to penetrate ever more deeply into the private lives of populations. The resulting public health policies, meant to suppress vectors of disease and immunize vulnerable populations, were key developments in creating a Mexican presence in a population that, until then, had either been resistant to federal control or mostly ignored by the state. Medical history in this book is thus presented not from the narrow perspective of medical problems formulated and resolved, but as a social instrument through which Mexican modernity, nation-building, and identity were, in part, forged.

The groundwork for this book is built on the narratives of public health administrators, statesmen, doctors—both foreign and regional—medical students, patients, indigenous and mestizo peasants, workers, and rebels, as well as local leaders and revolutionaries who struggled to lead healthful lives in spite of violent clashes and policies that often contradicted long-held customs and rituals. Decisions regarding who would be vaccinated for smallpox and yellow fever and who would not were not made in a political vacuum; nor were decisions regarding safe ways to grow and process foodstuffs, nor decisions involving the construction of a medical infrastructure of physicians, clinics, and pharmaceuticals, which created different levels of access to health care. Politics, as well, determined the regularity and thoroughness of sanitation services. This book analyzes the evolution of these policies in an effort to uncover important clues about state formation, particularly during regional civilizing campaigns to "tame" indigenous populations and revolutionary and civil insurrections.

Overshadowing the campaigns to combat smallpox, measles, cholera, yellow fever, and malaria is a background history of sociopolitical violence. In this context of violent upheavals, public health initiatives were often pursued with the dual objective of containing contagion and controlling human populations, and they were often resisted by those populations who perceived that dual purpose. The educated elite saw this resistance as an expression of "superstition," a perspective canonized in the heroic, positivist narrative of medical history. The creation of a hygienic and disease-free environment that included animals, insects, plants, and humans frequently overlapped with broader state initiatives to civilize indigenous populations, control violence, entice foreign investment, and implement modernizing projects.

From the Maya perspective, the meaning of *citizen* went through many transformations during the Caste War on up through the final days of Yucatán's socialist revolution in the mid-1920s. The Maya initially sought to distinguish themselves amid a myriad of colonial and postcolonial categories such as *batab*, hidalgo, *pacíficos, indio*, cruzob, or *bárbaro*. What the Maya peasant, pacífico, or indio wanted from the state and how they envisioned their communities determined their interaction with state representatives and medical professionals. For them, the services of the medical professionals were not and could not be merely technical, for in accepting them the Maya were inevitably accepting massive changes to their way of life. More often than not these exchanges were indirect and positioned them in uncharted terrain wherein they strove to integrate emergent public health policy and legislation within their existing sociocultural frameworks.[4] A structure for understanding the Maya peasantry and their abuse and subordination during disease epidemics can be constructed by drawing upon James Scott's notion of the divide between the great (urban) and little (peasant) tradition and his concept of "negotiated subordination."[5]

Michael Taussig's studies of peasant economies in Colombia are also useful in constructing an analytical framework for understanding Maya communities as part of a larger arc encompassing those who have "unequal access to means of production" and in providing a stable framework for uncovering the history of marginalized, subordinated peoples whose voices are difficult to access. Most of these histories do not have their own archives or press and did not produce a great deal of printed matter. Nonetheless, in order to understand the history I am outlining, these histories must be articulated.[6]

Barrington Moore cuts to the heart of how the governance of public health can seem maximally oppressive, rather than optimally safe, in Scott's *The Moral Economy of the Peasant*. In discussing exploitation as an incitement to rebellion, Moore states, "The timing of changes in the life of the peasantry, including the number of people simultaneously affected, are crucial factors in their own right. I suspect that they are more important than the material changes in food, shelter, clothing, except for very sudden and big ones . . . what infuriates peasants (and not just peasants) is a new and sudden imposition or demand that strikes many people at once and that is a break with accepted rules and customs."[7] The diseased landscape outlined in this book provides a series of backdrops for unraveling the history of the Maya and their relationship with the state, the church, landowners, physicians, and public health officials. These diseased moments are rife with the chaos and fear wrought by waves of devastating violence and illness, during which the struggle intensified between those who sought to enforce regulations or apply new ones—officers of the state, doctors, village officials—and those affected populations who tended to ignore conventions and regulations as the incertitude of illnesses, the illnesses and deaths of significant family members, and the holes ripped in the usual social networks enveloped every aspect of their lives, from the material need for food and shelter to the more immaterial desire to feel safe and valued.

The major historical, ecological, and social settings of nineteenth- and early twentieth-century Yucatán, Mexico, are littered with the victims of devastating disease epidemics. In the decades following Mexico's independence from Spain, Mexicans experienced the mortality and pain wrought by the constant re-emergence of European "Old World diseases" such as smallpox, measles, and the plague. These occurrences of Old World diseases were then intensified by virulent outbreaks of new diseases such as cholera, various manifestations of tuberculosis and lung-related illnesses, and syphilis, as well as "tropical" maladies such as yellow fever, malaria, and hookworm. These epidemics are conceptualized as diseased "moments" in the following chapters, offering insights into processes of state-building and identity formation as Yucatán's troubled relations with the Mexican nation worsened in the nineteenth century and growing tensions between the indigenous Maya and creole elites of the peninsula escalated into violence manifested in the Caste War. Similar to Charles Rosenberg's work on cholera in nineteenth-century New York City, this book explores cholera epidemics, as well as other diseases and illnesses, as a means of analyzing state and society tensions over a wide span of time.[8]

However, my use of diseased "moments" differs from Rosenberg's on a number of levels. By examining diseases other than cholera, such as smallpox and diseases of the "tropics," I have been able to track the shifts in public health policy and campaigns more closely, noting the influential role each epidemic played in shaping policy and practice. And by focusing on a non-Western region, I have been able to trace how Western-influenced medicine and therapeutics resonated with non-Western peoples. The following chapters illustrate how Yucatecans and the Maya reconfigured, and in some cases rejected, elements of Western medicine in this tropical periphery. Finally, this study expands on Rosenberg's class-based analysis with an examination of how racial and ethnic tensions and miscommunications may have exacerbated disease prevention campaigns and undermined the state's legitimacy in the Indian periphery.

A Brief History of Yucatán, 1821–1924

This section provides a brief overview of the tangled history of disease and the politics of Yucatán from independence in 1821 to the end of socialist rule in Yucatán in 1924. As I have pointed out, political history is usually recounted separately from medical history, as though the politics of a region unfolds independently of the health and well-being of the region's inhabitants. This misplaced disciplinary exclusionism is particularly distorting when applied to a tropical periphery state such as Yucatán, whose very image in the rest of the world was, for so long, the product of its reputation for disease. Yucatecan history is a notoriously complex history, rich in factions, coups, wealth, poverty, displacement, and violence. I cannot possibly do justice to its every intricacy here; rather, I will attempt a simple outline.

The first era of Yucatán's history, from independence to the end of the war with America in 1848, was dominated by the question of Yucatán's relationship to Mexico. Like other Central American states, the Yucatán Peninsula, consisting of what are now the states of Campeche, Yucatán, and Quintana Roo, did have the makings of an independent polity. The peninsula was connected to the rest of Mexico by only one major harbor, Campeche, and it had not undergone any military struggle, unlike the rest of Mexico. In 1821, after the Spanish were defeated in Mexico, the Spanish governor had simply resigned, thus ending Spanish rule. "In an evil hour," as John Lloyd Stephens put it, Yucatán representatives had been sent to Mexico City to deliberate forming a nation.[9]

As a landscape of disease, Yucatán, as we will see in chapter 2, still suffered chronic epidemics of smallpox, the biggest killer of colonial times. Sketching out the trajectory of smallpox prevention campaigns, from their commencement in the early 1800s to the 1880s, illustrates how significant a threat smallpox was; its eradication was to be one of the positive signs that independence had brought a better, more modern way of life. I show how vaccination campaigns, designed to protect the public, served as a political platform to marginalize the indigenous Maya as passive and unwilling to accept vaccines. Elites' marginalization of the Maya as acutely antimodern and uncivilized did not address the reality of epidemiological consequences and medical practices in the field. Ultimately, physicians tried to do something to save the Maya from smallpox attacks, but the multiple obstacles they encountered did nothing to facilitate a more evenhanded implementation of smallpox prevention throughout the region. In the end, the Maya remained largely skeptical of state-sponsored medicine and continued to rely on their own therapeutics.

Intersecting with state efforts to combat smallpox and cholera epidemics at midcentury was a number of serious conflicts between Yucatán and the newly formed Mexican republic. In Yucatán, two main factions formed: the liberal centralists and the conservative federalists. Within the peninsula, the strain between Campeche and Mérida was colored by these factions, with Campeche generally associated with centralism and Mérida with federalism.[10] The principles behind these factions were, however, very plastic. In general, they were masks under which groups organized and mobilized around regional and personal interests.

The two major politicians of this period were Santiago Méndez Ibarra and Miguel Barbachano y Tarrazo. Méndez's power base was in Campeche, where he was known as a successful merchant. He served as governor on three separate occasions between 1840 and 1857. Barbachano, a Liberal, was a wealthy merchant who had been educated abroad and had been involved in regional politics since 1840, when he served as Méndez's vice governor. When Mexican president Antonio López de Santa Anna sent federal troops to Yucatán in 1842 to try to force its reentry into the republic, Méndez and Barbachano strategized to overpower federal troops. By 1843, a treaty had been signed under which Yucatán was supposed to reunite with the Mexican nation, but when Santa Anna failed to honor the terms of the agreement, Yucatán seceded again in 1845.[11]

Miguel Barbachano, who had also participated in the brokering of the 1843 treaty with Mexico, was elected as military leader and provisional governor of Yucatán under the promise of bringing honor back to the region. Barbachano served as military head—effectively governing the region—on five separate occasions between 1841 and 1853. In 1846 as provisional head of Yucatán, Barbachano decided to forge yet another alliance with the Mexican republic.[12] Campechanos, however, had other plans. Taking advantage of the disorder wrought by the Mexican-American War between 1846 and 1848, elites led by one of Méndez's political party members, Campeche native Domingo Barret, rebelled against Barbachano's Mérida-based government. The Campeche-driven revolt was bent on wresting power from Barbachano and securing Yucatán's independence from Mexico.[13] Barret's revolt briefly placed the Campechano elites in power and led to another secession of Yucatán from Mexico in May of 1847. However, Maya rebels, who had been armed by the Yucatán government, began their own rebellion—the start of the Caste War in 1847—that spanned the century. This determined the political course of Yucatán history over the rest of the century.[14] The separation of 1847 endured only for a year until Barbachano's troops once again assumed power in Mérida, which they held until 1853. But the impetus for independence among the elite was not lost, only refocused on the internal split between the power centers of Mérida and Campeche. In 1858 Campeche declared its independence from Yucatán.

This backdrop of violent conflicts between Yucatán and Mexico, Mérida and Campeche, and the creole elite and Maya rebels is important as the context for the cholera epidemic of the 1850s, which I will discuss under the guise of cemetery management in chapter 3 (which delves into the struggle for power between the church and state during the critical decades following the Reforma [1856–57]). The second wave of epidemic cholera paralleled the height of Caste War violence between 1847 and 1855. Citizens struggled to deal with the grief of losing loved ones even as the state was placing new regulations on burials. Often these laws were designed to hasten the burial of cholera victims, putting the laws in conflict with regional burial rituals and processions sacred to families. This intrusion into a sacred and private realm frustrated the citizenry, who found themselves caught in the middle of a power struggle between church and state officials.

Tensions between church and state grew concurrently with the acute disaffection between creole elites and Maya peasants, which culminated when the Maya, armed by Yucatán's creole elite for both the war against the United States and the internal struggles between factions in the peninsula, turned those weapons on the state structure. This conflict, it turned out, was to last much longer than anybody at the time could have foreseen. On the one hand, this weakened the resistance of the elite to the central government, as the elite needed allies in the war. On the other hand, it also encouraged the British to the south, in Belize, to advance their interests in Yucatán—along with the Americans to the north.[15]

The stronghold of the Conservative Party in Yucatán made the state a bastion of resistance against the growing Liberal agenda that ultimately culminated in the forging of the 1857 Constitution, which specifically addressed the role of the church and the autonomous power of the states. Contained in the 1857 Constitution was restrictive legislation that curtailed the income, as well as the social and political power, of the church and forced the clergy to redefine their relationship with parishioners. Liberals themselves were caught between a faction that promoted centralization of state power versus one that, more traditionally, advocated the increase of the power of the states. It was in the interstices of this conflict that Conservatives saw their opportunity.

Liberal disaffection with communal property underlay Reforma legislation. Liberal belief in free trade, including breaking up the traditional customs and rights of the commons, encouraged the breakup and sale of church properties, civil corporate lands, and those owned by pueblos.[16] In particular, the Ley Lerdo of 1856 provoked resistance throughout Mexico with the abolition of communal tenure that allowed many Indian villages to divide up large blocks of land into individual plots for their residents.[17] Mexican philosopher and Liberal statesman José María Luis Mora (1794–1850) rationalized that communal land ownership posed a significant obstacle to Mexico's progress. Ignorance, resistance, and apathy were attributed, more than anything else, to the "laziness" engendered by communal property.[18]

In the wake of direct national attacks on the church by the Liberals during the 1850s, Yucatán's reluctance to subject the church to the program of property expropriation and constitutional clerics irked national leaders and subsequently propelled the peninsula into the political periphery. At the same time, we must recall the status of the indigenous peoples in Yucatán. Almost all of the Maya who inhabited the Yucatán Peninsula in the 1850s were monolingual, making negotiations with rebel factions somewhat difficult. In the eyes of many Yucatecan statesmen, priests who understood the Yucatec Mayan dialect and were able to negotiate with rebel Maya became a real necessity.[19]

Assuredly, the nature of relations between church, state, and the Maya changed as a result of the Caste War, but disease also trailed behind the troops, lingered in rebel strongholds, and spread rapidly among civilians. In the 1850s, epidemic cholera reached the Yucatán Peninsula, following its spread through Canada and the United States. Chapter 4 moves into the violent upheaval caused by the changes introduced into the disease landscape by the Caste War. As military squadrons and rebel cells mobilized and made contact with villages in the interior, they became vectors of disease, as well as virtually immobilizing public health campaigns and inculcating panic. The political establishment responded by merging the regional and national civilizing agendas, of which the army was the public face among the Maya, with public health projects. Goals to advance the assimilation of the indigenous Maya dovetailed with missions to clean, sanitize, and regulate daily life. Policy makers and the medical community envisioned a kind of bourgeois prosperity at the end of their program, one in which, through a synchronized strategy of interventions, disease would be controlled and violence by the lower class suppressed. Undoubtedly, violence from the Caste War, combined with power struggles between Campechano and Méridano elites and disruptions from the Mexican-American War, made bringing tranquility to the region an almost impossible feat. There was little hope then for controlling unseen "miasmas" and enforcing quarantines if the peninsula's residents were constantly at odds with local officials, subject to troop and rebel invasions, and cut off from assistance.

Not until President Porfirio Díaz in the 1880s sent troops equipped with modern weapons under the leadership of General Bravo to Yucatán, while restoring relations with England, did the tide decisively turn against the Maya rebels.[20] During Díaz's thirty-five-year dictatorship from 1876 to 1911, Mexico entered the age of modernity.[21] The mantra of the Porfiriato, "order and progress," served as the banner of the administration, while full and willing participation in Porfirian modernization operated to demarcate the civilized from the savage, the modern from the traditional, the citizen from the rebel, the natural from the unnatural, and, ultimately, the accumulated power of modern Mexico from the vestiges of colonial New Spain.[22] During the Porfiriato, sweeping modernizing campaigns that included the construction of monuments, boulevards, opera houses, new wings on the hospital for tropical medicine, and state-of-the-art laboratories were aimed at transforming this regional "backwater" into a modern, prosperous jewel for the Mexican republic. In 1906 when President Díaz came to Yucatán, he announced that Yucatán had completed its transformation.[23]

Modernizing campaigns of the Porfiriato also produced gross misrepresentations of the extent to which Mexican society was benefiting from Porfirian programs in a hyperbolic push to expand export economies and entice foreign investment and colonization. The collection of such reports for President Porfirio Díaz promoted the construction of an image of Mexico that was far from the much starker reality of enormous wealth disparities and an inability to generate endogenous capital—thus creating structural dependence on American and European capital. The legacy of these fallacies was embodied in rural revolt, perpetual complaints regarding filth and unsanitary conditions, famine, crop failure, and disease.

It was also during the Porfirian period that the henequen plantations experienced their largest expansion in Yucatán, and the trade in henequen endowed the creole elite with a hitherto unknown opulence.[24] Díaz also arranged for the exploitation of Yucatán's other natural resources, including timber, all of which required massive encroachment on land traditionally belonging to the Maya.[25] Forging a solid power block, the region's *henequeneros* brokered relationships with U.S. companies and political elites. These alliances effectively constituted a trade monopoly replete with price fixing, labor exploitation, and deep levels of political and economic graft.

Export henequen haciendas returned the Maya to colonial-era work conditions, a story exploited by the American yellow journalist John Kenneth Turner in his sensationalistic book *Barbarous Mexico* published in 1910.[26] Chapter 5 explores this watershed moment in Yucatecan history wherein the boom in Yucatán's exports, the end of the Caste War in 1902, and diseases converged. It was during this period that one of the most tragic events in Mexican/Yucatecan history occurred, as Yaquis from the north were deported to fulfill labor needs in Yucatán and as a measure aimed at pacifying Mexico's northern states. The deportations were marked by loss of life, broken up families, cultural dissolution, and the spread of disease within the dispersed population, mostly yellow fever and malaria.

Porfirio Díaz's infamy as a hard-line "carrot and stick" politician who deported Indians from their native territories to other parts of the country in order to work the fields like slaves certainly brought public redress when Turner's work was published in 1910. In fact, Turner's *Barbarous Mexico* likely stood out as a stark contrast to earlier depictions of Díaz as a benevolent dictator and family man with a deep passion for his country. Two years before Turner published his book on the excesses of the elites and the grinding poverty of the poor in Mexico, U.S. reporter James Creelman interviewed President Díaz for *Pearson's Magazine*. In the 1908 interview, Creelman described Díaz as "an astonishing man" who also vowed to retire from politics and not run in the next national election.[27] Two years later, Francisco Madero, the well-educated son of landowners from the northern state of Coahuila, declared his candidacy for the presidency of Mexico under a new anti-re-electionist party.[28] Díaz promptly reneged on his promise and jailed Madero right before the 1910 elections. Madero lost the election, garnering only 2 percent of the vote from his jail cell in San Luis Potosí.[29] After the election Madero managed to escape to Texas and drafted the Plan de San Luis de Potosí wherein he declared the elections void and declared himself as provisional president of Mexico.[30] Madero's call for an armed revolution met with the eruption of revolts throughout northern Mexico by November of 1910. Less than one year after the fighting began, the revolutionaries overwhelmed Díaz's army.

Also contributing to Díaz's downfall were his ideological stubbornness and his undermining of powerful *científico* elites (scientists or intellectuals who adopted French positivist philosopher Auguste Comte's "scientific" views of society) who dominated the Mexican cabinet.[31] In May of 1911, sensing an imminent end to his term as president, General Porfirio Díaz fled the country for the warmer climate of the Spanish riviera.[32]

To a lesser degree, shock waves from national instability reverberated in the southeast, most notably during the period between 1911 and 1913 when revolutionary president Francisco Madero—officially elected to office in 1912—occupied Mexico's presidential chair. During this period five different men governed Yucatán, some only lasting a couple of months.[33] Madero's time in office was brief; he was overthrown in a coup orchestrated by Porfirian-era general Victoriano Huerta in 1913. Huerta then ordered both Francisco Madero and his brother Gustavo jailed. Shortly after their incarceration, in February of 1913, both were shot and killed.[34] Revolutionary leaders like Constitutionalist Party leader Venustiano Carranza denounced the Huerta presidency.[35] With Madero martyred, violence escalated among revolutionary factions under Carranza and Alvaro Obregón in the central valley, Pancho Villa in the north, and Emiliano Zapata in the south. Throughout the revolution, Mexico experienced multiple waves of overlapping epidemics and illnesses including influenza, tuberculosis, yellow fever, malaria, syphilis, and rabies. The assassination of Madero, a democratically elected president, compelled U.S. president Woodrow Wilson to take action against Huerta. In 1914 Wilson ordered the U.S. Marines to invade Mexico by way of Veracruz and force Huerta out of office. Later that same year, under the combined pressures of the revolutionary violence and the U.S. occupation, Huerta abandoned the presidency.[36]

Interim president Carranza sent in his own military leaders in 1914 to dramatically reform Yucatán's "slavelike" system of debt peonage and implement his radical reforms. Carranza's reforms included massive restructuring of labor, agrarian, education, and public health systems.[37] In Yucatán, socialist revolutionary discourse facilitated the implementation of this repertoire of public works projects, placing the importance of community above that of the individual and subsequently allowing the arms of the state to reach into the private sphere in the name of the revolution.[38]

The revolution arrived late to Yucatán. Years after the national revolution began in 1910, Yucatán's decidedly socialist revolution began in 1915 with the arrival of Carranza loyalist General Salvador Alvarado and all but ended with Governor Felipe Carrillo Puerto's assassination in 1924. The penultimate chapter of this book examines Yucatán's unique experience with the Mexican Revolution concurrent with waves of yellow fever and malaria. In an effort to rid the region of yellow fever and malaria, the Rockefeller Foundation's International Health Board (IHB) sent doctors to Yucatán during the region's socialist revolution. In doing so, the IHB found structured socialist resistance leagues (*ligas de resistencia*) that facilitated the successful completion of their agenda.

Herein we see the intimate relationship that is forged between public health and politics. In fact, each chapter in this book utilizes disease epidemics such as smallpox, cholera, and yellow fever and efforts by the state and its residents to cope with these maladies as windows into the workings of sociopolitical phenomena such as civilizing and modernizing efforts, insurgency, and revolution. Specific disease prevention campaigns are analyzed not simply in relation to their mechanism and goals, but to their larger cultural and political meanings. In effect, I am exploring the political unconscious of Yucatán's disease moments, which loom large in its nineteenth- and twentieth-century history.

Yucatán's Diseased Ethno-topography

A history of public health straddles politics and medicine. It is easy to fall into the unconscious assumption that the history of medicine, at least, is straightforward. As we shall see, however, what might have been seen in 1850 as an "advance" by the official medical establishment would be seen in 1900 as a regression. Inasmuch as medicine is not a science that is confined to the laboratory, but a combination of techniques for curing or preventing disease, controlling populations, and symbolizing "civilization" against indigenous "barbarity," this introduction will conclude with a survey of the human geography of Yucatán from the "enlightened" European and North American perspective of the nineteenth century.

Among the challenges faced by public health modernizers and local politicians alike were Yucatán's harsh climate and topography. Southeastern Mexico, and in particular the Gulf Coast and the Yucatán Peninsula, qualify as tropical zones. In the nineteenth century, travelers, businessmen, and archaeologists would distinguish between the "drier and more healthful" climate of the Yucatán and the wetter regions to the south, like Chiapas. The 1911 *Encyclopedia Britannica* assured its readers that the climate was "healthy, though enervating." Ellsworth Huntington, an American geographer, devoted a chapter to Yucatán in his book about the climate of America, writing,

> Climactically, as well as in other ways, Yucatán is relatively simple. It lies in the trade wind belt from 19 to 21 degrees north of the equator. In winter the brisk winds from the ocean pass over the land without giving up much moisture. . . . Further south, however, or where the hills begin to rise, the rainfall increases rapidly, and showers are frequent. . . . In summer, as might be expected in this latitude, the zone of equatorial rains exerts its accustomed influence and gives rise to heavy tropical showers.[39]

But the hopeful references to the healthfulness of Yucatán by geographers and travelers were contradicted by other sources, who saw a disease-ridden tropical region.[40] In 1863 the bishop of Yucatán, Crescencio Carrillo y Ancona, wrote of his homeland that "during the rainy season waters pool in different public places, evaporating into infectious gasses under the rays of the sun, causing no shortage of illnesses."[41] The ecology and climate of the peninsula link the region more to its tropical Caribbean neighbors to the south and across the Gulf of Mexico than to the Mexican mainland.[42]

But its proximity and importance for the United States made it a key target for testing experimental "tropical" medicines and therapeutics.[43] Yucatán participated in the diseased "moments" that occurred within a Caribbean nexus. Its public health profile was not too different from that of Veracruz, Mexico's other major outlet to the Caribbean, but was much different than, say, Mexico City's. In order to obtain smallpox vaccine, medicines, doctors, and other forms of aid, regional bosses (*jefes políticos*) and administrators looked to their Caribbean neighbors and the southern United States for assistance. Thus, Yucatán was more oriented toward Havana, Central America, and the infrastructure of tropical medicine institutes that sprang up in the metropoles of the imperial powers (London, New York, Paris) than toward the Mexican medical establishment.

The cultural geography of Yucatán was perceived by the creole elite as the source of its "backwardness." Of course, to the hegemonic European powers, Mexico was itself a retrograde and "uncivilized" Latin American nation. Foreigners marveled at the lack of sophistication with which everyday activities proceeded in Mexico and condescended to what they felt was the lack of a work ethic among the people, attitudes that show up not only in private communications and popular works, but in more serious works of geography, ethnography, and science.[44]

Thus, the disease prevention campaigns that were mounted in Mexico's southern Yucatán Peninsula offer a unique set of conditions for understanding the environment that brought together institutional science and the dynamics of power and dominance, conquest and subjugation, which was the leitmotif of nineteenth-century global history. The Porfirian científicos saw Yucatán, with its perennial revolts, its exploitable labor force, and its tropical natural resources, as a stark and shaming contrast to the national agenda—and yet, due to the henequen trade, Yucatán was also Mexico's richest state by the time of the revolution. Yucatán was thus, from the beginning, an outlier state, and the relationship between the state and the federal authority was such that Yucatán's political elite often looked elsewhere for support. One of the subthemes in this work will be the connection between this "marginalized" Mexican region and its inhabitants and the tropical environments and populations of the circum-Caribbean.

The geopolitical repositioning of Yucatán was not just a matter of ecological similarities. When, after the American Civil War, Yucatán's henequen plantations became essential suppliers of the twine that powered the U.S. agricultural revolution, the economic and social structure of the peninsula was changed.[45]

This change to the production of an essential organic commodity within a plantation system using low-wage manual labor paralleled other Caribbean economic developments, for instance, the boom in bananas or coffee in the late nineteenth century.[46] Thus, there is good reason to see Yucatán in terms of the Caribbean paradigm. Indeed, development and control of, for example, yellow fever–bearing mosquitoes in Havana had a direct impact on Yucatán's own experience with disease control in the Caribbean, and exchanges of professional advice between these regions were much more valued by local elites than conversations with public health experts in Mexico City. In addition, an informal trans-Caribbean network of exchange emerged at midcentury through which medical advice, workers, and supplies were channeled into the peninsula. The Yucatecan newspaper *El Siglo XIX* regularly reprinted helpful therapeutic advice from Havana's *Diario de la Mariana*, which "produced good results during [Havana's] last invasion of Asiatic cholera."[47] The material network of assistance (which could also operate as the vector for the spread of pandemics) extended to New Orleans and Great Britain's colonies in the Caribbean, including the neighboring colony of British Honduras (Belize).[48] In fact, Yucatán remained geographically isolated from the rest of Mexico, to which it was not connected by rail until the twentieth century.

Contact by sea took place principally through the peninsula's major port at the time of independence, Campeche, which served as a stop for ship traffic from Veracruz. Mérida's port, Progreso, was inaugurated in 1870, taking the place of the obsolete facilities of the old port of Sisal. Even after Porfirio Díaz's sweeping modernization campaign in the late nineteenth century, Yucatán, which had more internal railroad mileage than any other Mexican state, did not have a railroad connection to the mainland. Instead, the rails were devoted to facilitating the movement of exports from the interior to ports.[49] Almost all of the railways that crisscrossed Yucatán were the result of carefully crafted relations between henequen elites and foreign entrepreneurs.[50]

Thus, in many ways Yucatán had more in common with Caribbean trading partners, particularly Cuba, Jamaica, Belize, and the port city of New Orleans, than with Mexico. This perspective, of course, animated the early secessionist movement. And even though that movement failed, the geographic facts still remained—which is why this study highlights Yucatán's circum-Caribbean relations and the way in which prevailing imperial ideologies classified the entire region in terms of widespread tropes concerning the tropics, which stressed isolation, dirtiness and unhealthiness, and the idle temperament of the natives. This set of circumstances made it difficult, in the nineteenth-century view, for European whites to bring "civilization" to the area because the whites were as likely to be struck down by disease or to be infected by the temperament and "go bad."

As we will see, public health officials and medical professionals in Yucatán began to create their own unique blend of diagnosis and treatment specifically tailored to their region's conditions, taking advantage of the models generated by similar environments in Cuba, British Honduras, and New Orleans. The elite rightly saw that they needed to construct a system of health care and prevention more suited to the human geography of Yucatán than was realized by a distant national government intent on imposing its own program of modernization.

Civilization versus Barbarism: The Clash of Attitudes

So far, I have shown the reasons for Yucatán's alienation from the Mexican mainstream in terms consonant with those of the creole elite. Of course, that elite was only a small part of the population. The majority consisted of the indigenous Maya. The relationship between the creole ruling class and the Maya made up one of the strands in the cultural distinctiveness of Yucatán and imposed itself upon the long history of strained relations between the peninsula and the rest of the Mexican nation, culminating in the endgame of the Caste War, when Díaz's forces, as a reward for helping the Yucatán state, in 1902 broke off the southeast portion of the peninsula and made it a separate state, Quintana Roo.[51] The distinction between Yucatán and Mexico goes back to the postconquest period, when Franciscan missionaries were chosen by the Spanish Crown to subdue and Christianize the Maya. While New Spain's economy was based on central Mexico's silver mines, the Yucatán Peninsula's apparent lack of exploitable natural resources challenged colonial authorities to consider other options for royal revenue. The large Maya population offered a substantial resource for the Spanish Crown and clergy in the form of taxation, tribute, and labor.[52] The colonial basis of this unique relationship between Crown authorities and Maya "Indians" underscores the legacy of Maya-creole tensions throughout Yucatán and, moreover, created an enclave-like culture that separated Yucatán's elite from the Mexican elite.

A reexamination of the role of "Indian" participation and agency in some ethnographic scholarship uncovers some of the deeply buried narratives of the subaltern during the sixteenth-century reconquest of the Maya.[53] Building on these studies, we can craft a useful model for engagement with "other" narratives by integrating knowledge gleaned from regional scholarship focusing on local struggles, class tensions, the emergence of political economies, and grassroots rebellions. From the conquest to the turn of the twentieth century, Yucatán's Maya-creole relations were doubly determined, on the one hand by the national debates concerning the role of the "Indian" in Mexican society—generally constructed according to the Liberal principle that sought to "free" Indians from the church and mobilize them as free labor—and on the other hand by dynamics internal to the peninsula, where the ideological binary of civilization versus barbarism held sway.

Of course, the self-image of a culture will find an echo in subsequent histories of that culture. The nineteenth-century creole ideology was often absorbed and reproduced in the micro-ethnographic studies on the Yucatán that were published in the 1940s up through the 1970s. To some degree, the authors of these studies concurred with the historical assumption that the Yucatán was socially, culturally, and politically "backward." Unwittingly, anthropologists contributed to the image of the backwardness of the peninsula by focusing on the cultural tenacity of the indigenous Maya and their prolonged debt servitude.[54] In particular, Howard Cline's work was influential in promoting this image. In the thirty-nine years since Cline's book was published, a body of scholarship has emerged to address some of Cline's suggestions for further study.[55]

Nelson Reed followed Cline's lead in his monograph *The Caste War of Yucatán*, the first full-scale treatment of this episode in English. Reed expanded on Cline's theory of "regionalism" by demonstrating how ethnic factions, coupled with an unstable power structure, caused the outbreak of the Caste War.[56] While Reed's work has remained one of the most widely read regional histories of the Yucatán, his work primarily fashioned the Caste War through the eyes of nineteenth-century Yucatecan authors.[57] Recent scholarly work on Yucatán has moved beyond micro-historical research to consciously link rebellion, revolution, and the Yucatán's export boom in henequen to broader historical themes.[58] This book draws heavily on these regional studies, wherein broader issues concerning nation-building, modernity, citizenship, rebellion, and international relations are articulated in such a way that the voices of the subaltern resonate beyond their "closed communities."[59]

Latin American scholarship from the late 1960s through the 1980s turned to new models for understanding class struggles, the emergence of political economies, and grassroots rebellions, breaking with the developmentalist paradigms of the past.[60] What was most exciting about this work consisted of its acts of recovery: connecting the "voices of the vanquished," mainly peasants, Indians, and the poor, to larger issues of state formation and class consciousness.[61] Assuredly, regional studies provide up close, micro-analyses of communities that may otherwise remain unnoticed. If nested within a larger framework, such studies can also provide valuable connections between the local, regional, national, and international spheres in order to generalize about broad themes of medical practices, nationalism, and state-building. My particular focus on "diseased relations" is meant to articulate the relation between a regional analysis and the international history of disease and public health. My intent here is to explore the impact of disease epidemics and public health movements on local societies as a microcosm for understanding cross-cultural responses to global disease patterns.[62] Europe and the United States are still the best-represented countries when it comes to this hybrid of political sociology, medical history, and ethnography. In comparison, a relatively small amount of contemporary scholarship has so far addressed epidemic diseases in Africa, China, India, the Caribbean, and Latin America.[63]

While this book relies primarily on narratives and records that reflect the "civilized" viewpoint—even as civilization was defined by wildly varying "scientific" determinations of disease, treatment, and prevention—I try, as well, to read the subtexts within these texts, taking advantage of the mass of ethno-historical work that has been done on the Maya, as well as studies on medical anthropology, peasants, modernity, and nation-building. The classic treatment of public health history, between the 1920s and the 1970s, was written within the paradigm of a teleological determinism in which the environment and populations exist as problems to which scientists find solutions. The new environmental history sees these public health projects differently. My analysis of public health programs in Yucatán takes them to be elements in a unique space wherein the complexities of identity formation and nation-building merge with struggles to survive and combat disease. Studies linking the political culture of empire to public health and hygiene projects in postcolonial contexts such as the Philippines, Africa, Latin America, and Southeast Asia have already begun to explore the interconnectedness of colonial authority and postcolonial nation-building in the human condition.[64] Such work has taken its cue from Warwick Anderson's observation that the way a nation frames disease, the environment, and race are all part of the "same maneuver" in European colonial administrations.[65]

The following chapters analyze specific disease prevention campaigns not only in relation to their mechanism and goals, but to their larger cultural and political meanings. In effect, I am exploring the political unconscious of Yucatán's disease moments, which loom large in its nineteenth- and twentieth-century history.

CHAPTER TWO

THE POLITICS OF PREVENTION

The Maya, Smallpox, and Vaccination Campaigns

IN DECEMBER 1852, the director of vaccine propagation and conservation for the state of Yucatán, Dr. Manuel Campos, wrote a resignation letter to Governor Barbachano in which he voiced his frustration with what he saw as a highly inept state bureaucracy. The forty-one-year-old Campos wrote that he felt like a tired and much older man, stating, "I have fulfilled my duties and cannot possibly devote any more time to an endeavor that seems to elicit little or no support."[1] Throughout his term as director of vaccine propagation and distribution between 1846 and 1852, Campos had pleaded with medical students and colleagues to take positions as *subvacunadores* (sub-vaccinators), even though he could promise them little pay and most needed to fill positions in locations far from their presumably urban homes.[2] The salary for a sub-vaccinator was minimal, or in some cases, the job was accepted on a voluntary basis.[3] To supply them, he had had to beg the government for money to buy new equipment, which had to be shipped to Yucatán from elsewhere, and had worked without pause to send the vaccines anywhere they were needed—only to learn that in many cases they never arrived or were never used. The mournful tone of his letter clearly reveals a deep sense of hopelessness. Despite all the potential offered by the vaccination campaign, he had seen that promise wasted and needless suffering and death from smallpox come about as a result.[4]

A native of Campeche, Campos had witnessed continual preferential treatment in state vaccination campaigns toward the urban center of Mérida and its surrounding towns. As founder of Campeche's medical school in 1849,

Campos had always been a fierce advocate for the decentralization of education and culture from Mérida. An enthusiastic advocate and administrator of smallpox vaccine in the early years of his medical career, he noted that the number of epidemic deaths in his hometown seemed to be disproportionately greater than Mérida's. Thus, in his career as a physician and public health administrator, he sought to mitigate these inequities. Campos was one among those of the peninsula's policy makers and *políticos* who saw Méridanos as parasitic on the wealth and benefits brought to the entire peninsula by their port city of Campeche. Old regional rivalries resurfaced during smallpox epidemics as disparities in access and funds marked disparities in power and influence between the two urban centers.[5]

Campos eventually rebounded from his disillusionment with administrative duties, accepting an invitation three years later to teach general medicine and surgery at the University of Yucatán. He still took time to write in the press, advocating the benefits of disease prevention through vaccination campaigns.[6] Many of Campos's colleagues shared his dissatisfaction with the inefficiencies of Yucatán's smallpox prevention campaigns. Regional differences aside, why did medical doctors keep encountering so many obstacles to rational medical therapy in a countryside eminently threatened with epidemics? Why were their efforts to safeguard the most vulnerable members of their communities often repeatedly thwarted by lack of funding and miscommunication? Embedded within these vaccination programs lie clues that point to the strategic function of vaccination programs in the state's long-range program of civilizing the Maya and modernizing the region according to the European standards adopted by the creole elite.

In this chapter, I take the smallpox prevention program to be paradigmatic of the role public health campaigns played in the process of modern state-building in postcolonial Yucatán. Ultimately, physicians and statesmen did try to mitigate the vulnerability of the vast Maya population to a plague that had intermittently caused such tremendous death and cultural havoc down through the centuries of Spanish rule; yet the success of the anti-smallpox campaigns was impaired by three interrelated factors. First, long-seated regional tensions between the urban port of Campeche and the capital of Mérida supervened upon the implementation of vaccination campaigns throughout the peninsula, creating rivalries and forms of sabotage that ultimately strained the relationship between Yucatán and Mexico City as well. Second, the elite contempt for and misunderstanding of the Maya, especially in regard to their own culture's development of etiological precepts and therapeutic preferences, created a two-sided complex: on the one hand, the representatives of the government came to regard Maya practices as things to be crushed rather than as settings to be adapted to; and on the other side, the Maya increasingly came to regard the programs as aimed not so much at improving the health of the people as in taking away their rights. Third, Caste War violence severely depleted funding for the anti-smallpox campaigns and inhibited vaccine distribution and production during particularly critical disease moments.[7] When it came to representing the history of Yucatán and the cultural differences between indigenous and creole populations in the scholarly literature, these factors have often been understood ideologically through a crude contrast drawn between modernization and false folk belief. A better approach is to seek to understand Maya views about disease and vaccination in order to comprehensively understand all the dimensions of the disease eradication programs. From this point of view we can see how these programs functioned to enact the further spiritual conquest of the Maya.

Regional and National Tensions: Yucatán's Divided Path to Prevention

The narratives associated with nineteenth-century smallpox campaigns reveal that the old colonial church infrastructure that took care of the sick had crumpled, leaving a great deal of responsibility for anti-smallpox work to fall on the state as politicians and medical policy makers like Campos strove to insert a full-scale vaccination regime in a region where the Maya peasantry's painful memories of smallpox devastation coincided with memories of conquest, subjugation, and death. In the collective memory of the nineteenth-century Maya, smallpox was not just a present and future menace, but it marked the transformations brought about by the brutal conquest of the region by Francisco Montejo in the 1530s, which had been preceded by the devastating smallpox epidemic of 1520 that resulted in a death toll estimated at 500,000.[8]

The logistical obstacles involved in acquiring, propagating, and funding smallpox vaccination campaigns were, in part, derived from the fragile relationship between the periphery and the center. In the management of this relationship, the provision of national resources for public health services was inequitably applied. These problems were not hidden at the time and were attributed by the popular press to the Caste War. While the war may have eaten up funding, in reality funding was insufficient to begin with. That, combined with the difficulty in servicing a state that did not have a proper railroad service until the 1880s and did not link its internal railroad service to the national system until 1910, contributed to ineffectual vaccine distribution.[9]

Transportation proved a significant challenge even before rail services arrived in Yucatán. In 1846 only limited road service connected Mérida to the towns of Izamal, Tekax, Campeche, Sisal, Motul, Tecóh, Peto, Tizimín, Sotuta, Yaxcabá, and Valladolid. Several small towns remained a great distance from these throughways, and during the rainy season, many roads flooded into impassable mud pits. Not until 1881 did a rail system connect Mérida to Campeche. Port service offered no better solution to distribution problems since many carriers found the region's major ports of Campeche and Progreso difficult to access. The French geographer Élisée Reclus explained that the ocean at both Campeche and Progreso was shallow enough that steamboats had to anchor pretty far from the coastline, at least eight kilometers away at Campeche.[10] Undoubtedly, Yucatán's tenuous relations with Mexico City coupled with geographic isolation constituted a significant problem in acquiring vaccines from the capital. The marginalization of several small towns far from road and rail services within Yucatán further exacerbated the distribution of medical supplies and vaccines throughout the peninsula.[11] In fact, Yucatán's peculiar isolation contributed to its Caribbean orientation, underlying separatist movements and the forging of closer relations with Caribbean nations and the United States.

In fact, Yucatán's short-lived epochs of self-rule in the 1840s were not easily forgotten by Mexico City and thus marked the state for the administrative equivalent of punishment, insofar as Yucatán's needs were low on the list of national priorities. However, Yucatecans were not the only Mexicans fiercely holding on to a regional identity distinct from that of Mexico City. Mexico's northern states of Sonora, Durango, Chihuahua, and Baja California enjoy a long history of geographic, cultural, and political distinctiveness as *norteños* in contrast to their *chilango* counterparts in Mexico City.[12]

Distinctiveness also appears to have bred isolationist tendencies. For instance, throughout mid-nineteenth-century smallpox epidemics, requests for smallpox vaccine from all parts of the republic cluttered the national office of the Consejo de Salubridad (Health Council) in Mexico City.[13] Some territories were more persistent in their requests than others, particularly central states such as Puebla, Michoacán, Aguascalientes, Coahuila, and Veracruz. However, many of the peripheral states, such as Sonora, Chihuahua, Chiapas, and Yucatán, only appear to have made sporadic requests. Whether the lack of requests for vaccine in these peripheral regions points toward self-sufficiency, reliance on outside sources (such as the United States for assistance in providing smallpox vaccine), or Mexico City's punishment of these areas, this chasm between periphery and center played a central role in the development of Mexico's modern health-care system.[14]

Just as Mexico's northern frontier's separatist tendencies inflected its relationship to the center in terms of its elementary provision of state services, so, too, did strained Yucatecan–Mexico City relations hamper the distribution of vaccine to the region. Regionally, vaccine sites and public health assistance lay primarily in Yucatán's capital city of Mérida, thereby neglecting a significant portion of the peninsula's Maya and mestizo peasantry living in rural communities, fighting in the southeastern tropical rain forests, or laboring on haciendas.[15] For instance, in the southeastern port city of Bacalar, a notorious rebel stronghold during the Caste War, residents claimed they had been "sacrificed" in a "holocaust" perpetrated at the hands of their disgraced country. Residents complained they had no access to vaccines or medicines because rebel fighting isolated their communities. Bacalar residents blamed a mandatory, state-imposed five-peso transit fee for their inability to escape their "deplorable circumstances" to seek out medical care or to tend to sick family members in other districts.[16]

Rivalry between Campechanos and Yucatecos extended over many social, economic, and political issues, but underneath these issues the main point of contention was port access. Access to the principal ports on the peninsula was rooted in Spanish colonial administration. Yucatán primarily functioned as an agricultural region throughout the colonial period, while Campeche emerged as its port in the 1770s when, under reforms promulgated by reforming minister Jose de Gálvez, Campeche was given the privilege of being opened to trade with European merchants based in Veracruz.[17] This privileged position continued well after the colonial period.[18] Ultimately, overtures on behalf of Yucatecans to outsiders for vaccine and medical supplies refueled old rivalries between Campechano and Méridano elites. As early as the mid-sixteenth century, Méridanos sought to bypass Campeche's privileged position as Yucatán's premier port by investing in the development of a new port city—Sisal, a coastal community located directly north of Mérida.[19] In broad terms, Campechanos were mostly Liberal and federalist leaning, whereas Méridanos tended to gravitate toward centralism.[20] Meanwhile, Campechano and Méridano elites engaged in spirited polemics in their respective publications, each time strengthening the disdain between the two groups, drawing it to the forefront of regional culture.[21] In September 1857, Pablo García, a

Campeche native and a staunch supporter of regional secession, complained to Yucatán's military head, Manuel Cepeda Peraza, that Campechanos were tired of "disingenuous and false promises" from the Yucatecan state. García, declaring himself the leader of secessionist interests in Campeche, continued his rant against Yucatecos: "It is not our fault," he asserted, "that you have insulted us and trampled upon our rights, abused our gentleness and our temperance and placed our state in a weak and vulnerable prostrate position."[22]

By midcentury tensions between the two regions had severely complicated the logistics of importing and distributing vaccines. The animosity finally culminated in 1862 with national recognition of Campeche as an independent state with García as the new state's first governor. Although this produced a new formal political reality, on the ground, many local leaders and citizens found themselves still caught between the two rival capitals since Campeche still functioned as the major port of entry for the peninsula. Some public health officials were unsure about where to make appeals for more vaccine directly after the separation.[23] While the lines seemed to be clearly drawn for those who lived in the urban centers of Mérida and Campeche, confusion regarding the administration and supply of medical goods and services only served to further alienate rural communities on the Yucatán-Campeche border.

In response to vaccine shortages, local leaders barraged state and national public health administrators with requests for vaccine, supplies, and more medical personnel. Local leaders soon discovered that their requests would receive more timely responses if they were phrased in terms of contagion. For example, in April 1855 the prefect for the district of Tekax, Eumesindo Ruis, wrote a letter to Yucatán's governor to report that the commissary of Oxkutzcab Pueblo had no pus vaccine and no one to administer the fluid if and when any arrived.[24] Ruis begged the governor to "appoint an intelligent administrator of vaccine for this community so that at the very least we can curtail the progress of this awful epidemic, that in all probability will infect everyone in these towns and in this district."[25] Ruis's decision to play upon overriding fears concerning the spread of the disease proved effective with public health and city officials, who were being pressed by a mounting level of public hysteria focused on "the pox." The greater the death count, the more damaged the reputations of state public health officials and institutions. The prefect received a very prompt reply verifying the shipment of more vaccine to Oxkutzcab.

In Campeche's Hecelchakán district (northeast of Campeche), authorities were unable to acquire vaccine in 1850 and part of 1851. The information provided in the archives for vaccinations in Campeche covers only the months of July, August, September, and October of 1851 (see table 1).[26] The complete absence of vaccination records during the rest of year indicates either that there was not enough vaccine to go around, thus halting vaccination efforts, or that bookkeeping was faulty. However, what can be inferred from the available information is that children were not as likely to be vaccinated if they lived outside of Mérida. Similar to the situation in districts surrounding Mérida, Hecelchakán's population depended on Campeche, as its closest urban center, to supply it with fresh vaccines. Since Campeche suffered from a lack of organization and distribution of its vaccine, its satellite communities also did.

To compound the problem, roads connecting Campeche to many of the pueblos were in poor condition. In 1850 the rainy season was so severe that the roads were almost impassable, and the following year brought fever, crop rot, famine, and elevated levels of illness for all inhabitants.[27] Moreover, the administrator in charge of pus vaccine (the *vacunador*) for Hecelchakán complained vigorously that fewer and fewer children were appearing for their vaccinations, making it difficult to determine how much vaccine should be prepared or acquired. Vaccinators received a small annual salary of 100 to 150 pesos, while subvaccinators only received 80 pesos annually and were responsible for most of the work, including overseeing the distribution of the vaccine to all districts and the collection of trimester payments and records.[28]

Table 1: Vaccination Statistics for 1851

Partido/Locale	Children Vaccinated
Cacalchén	55
Campeche	853
Homun	80
Izamal	383
Mérida	2,750
Motul	1,384
Tekantó	87
Teya	60

Source: Compiled from Pérez Galaz, "Situación estadística de Yucatán," 424, 454, 456, 581, 593.

Vaccination campaigns in districts where vaccine was scarce virtually slowed to a crawl, so much so that by 1851 towns like Hecelchakán could neither acquire nor administer smallpox vaccine. Low turnout meant that left-over vaccines spoiled; in addition, funds would be cut to districts that reported low vaccination counts.[29]

As the result of disagreements between Yucatán and Mexico City, policy makers pursued alternative routes to acquiring vaccine, food staples, and assistance during smallpox epidemics. Although the Yucatán received shipments of vaccine from central Mexico's national public health branch, the Superior Health Council, correspondence between Yucatán, New Orleans, Havana, and British Honduras (Belize) suggests an ongoing effort by Yucatecans to supplement supplies by acquiring vaccine from neighboring governments.[30] These efforts helped shape diplomatic exchanges between Yucatán and the Caribbean nations throughout the period of the smallpox epidemics. In July of 1855, Mexico's secretary of state, Antonio Aguilar, responded to the Yucatecan governor's recent accusation that Mexico's central public health committee had been neglectful in covering expenses the state incurred while obtaining vaccine from Havana. Aguilar stressed that the governor's administration should pay in full for the vaccine from Havana. He instructed Yucatán's government secretary that legislation introduced in March of the previous year clearly stated that only during active outbreaks would funds be sent to cover the full cost of the vaccine. Clearly, Aguilar doubted the severity of Yucatán's smallpox epidemic when vials of vaccine were being requisitioned from Havana. Aguilar drew the attention of the governor's staff to a circular distributed on July 30, 1853, justifying the national government's right to limit funds for vaccine.[31]

Limited access to national ports further complicated the acquisition and distribution of smallpox vaccine, giving local politicians reasons to denounce discrimination against Yucatán. Yucatán still depended on the port of Veracruz for access to the world market, as it had since the formation of the Gálvez regulations. Restless Yucatecan merchants began to explore alternatives to this arrangement, while state officials filled the channel between themselves and Mexico City with multiple complaints.[32] In February 1855, Mérida's district prefect grumbled in a letter to the governor that ever since the shipping route between Veracruz, Havana, and the United States had been severed, obtaining vaccine had become nearly impossible. The prefect also stressed that the welfare of several newborns relied on their timely vaccination. Newborns were among the most vulnerable to the smallpox virus and thus were liable to become infected if viable vaccines were not available to forestall the spread of smallpox in the community. Such an occurrence, the prefect underscored, could not then be blamed on the vaccinators or administrators in charge of vaccine conservation. Even the disruptions of the Caste War were not as important in interrupting the flow of vaccines as the Mexican state's regulations concerning the legal trade in and delivery routes of the precious fluid: "The loss of all of the pus vaccine could be avoided if within the peninsula there was a way of bringing it in besides from Veracruz, Havana, the United States and of the British Empire . . . the more forces and diligence that are directed towards this branch, the more successful the results that can be reached, which are desirable for the benefit of humanity."[33]

Granted, Yucatán's two secessions from the Mexican republic in the 1840s may account for the central government's failure to heed this particular state's demands. But Yucatecans were more entrepreneurial than to count solely on the council and forged agreements with government consuls in New Orleans and Cuba to circumvent direct orders from the central Mexican republic.

Misunderstandings and Misconceptions: Maya, Creole, and Smallpox

As we come to understand the European-Maya encounter during smallpox episodes, I want to emphasize that European understandings of smallpox derived from radically different historical experiences than those of the Maya. For Europeans, encounters with smallpox began with variolation, which was first used by the Chinese and later adopted in the Middle East and Europe. Smallpox was a disease in which the causative agent eluded scientists, and European-trained scientists relied on empirical observation to eventually cure smallpox. In other words, the pride of science was that it explained the causes of physical events according to physical laws. This fundamental notion held by Europeans that illness and disease could be explained by way of rational scientific deduction is important, because what European colonizers and their followers in the Americas drew upon to control smallpox in New Spain rested on these basic scientific principles.

Throughout the late colonial period, Spanish colonial administrators in the *protomedicamento* (the colonial advisory committee on medical matters) utilized dangerous methods to prevent smallpox, such as arm-to-arm inoculation, involving direct subcutaneous transference of the pus from an infected individual's pustules to a healthy individual, and variolation, an "injection" into a healthy person of diluted forms of a disease.[34] Development of a non-human-derived vaccine to prevent smallpox began with Dr. Edward Jenner's cowpox tests in England during the early 1770s.[35] Dr. Jenner noticed that some of the women who worked at dairy farms seemed to be immune to smallpox, and those who did develop it experienced a milder form of the disease, and their recovery was far more likely. Intrigued, he investigated possible immunological links between the type of pox that appeared on the udders of cows and the human manifestation of a similar pustule. Once the pus was extracted from the cow, the fluid was inserted—by means of a lancet or puncture—into a healthy individual's skin, which provided immunity with less risk than for those who were immunized with pure smallpox vaccines via the arm-to-arm methods.

Jenner's conclusions were not altogether embraced by the medical community. He confronted adamant opposition, riddled with criticism for his reckless experimentation with human life.[36] Aside from the fact that inoculation with smallpox pus was terribly inconvenient and dangerous, newly immunized individuals were contagious for up to two weeks and had to be quarantined. More important though, Jenner's development of a non-human-derived vaccine did curtail the dangerous practice of arm-to-arm inoculation. Since arm-to-arm inoculation required an active outbreak of smallpox in order for the pustule or variole to be harvested for the viral fluid, it was of little use as a preventative. With Jenner's vaccination method, the public would not need to wait for an active outbreak of the disease to become immunized. By propagating cowpox in the udders of cattle, the entire vaccination process could be monitored and administered in the one location. Vaccination with cowpox eventually encouraged many nineteenth-century medical professionals to believe that smallpox was preventable.[37]

In contrast, many nineteenth-century Maya believed that independent and willful forces in nature caused diseases, including smallpox. For instance, in the late colonial books *Chilam Balam of Chumayel*, *Chilam Balam of Nah*, and *The Ritual of the Bacabs*,[38] diseases were associated with different types of winds or *ik*. These "personified evil winds" were seen as harbingers of disease and could, on occasion, assume the form of "little people, who performed petty mischief at night. Some of them acted of their own volition, while others may be induced to act by spirits or sorcerers."[39] Ralph E. Roys has contended that reference to the so-called *males de aire* did not appear until the late colonial period.[40] It is likely that, given the Spanish inability to totally acculturate the Maya, the nineteenth-century postindependence Maya believed in the same causes as their ancestors had and likewise visualized disease and illness in terms of semipersonified forces.[41]

The vacunador sent to a Maya village confronted a population with a long-developed understanding of smallpox. Within this environment, he advocated a therapy he could not fully explain. Nobody knew anything, really, about the immune system or germs in the early to mid-nineteenth century. However, what the vacunador did know was that when he scratched a person with a needle dipped into a lymph solution cultured with cowpox, that person developed a minor illness, perhaps with a few pustules, and then the infection passed. In the event of a smallpox outbreak, that person would not be infected. The vacunador then had to explain this curious process to Maya peasants and compel them to let him stick their children with his needles. Likely those who saw others scratched with the cowpox needles and then experience a skin eruption concluded that vaccination was risky. This method raised concerns among many potential subjects. Moreover, the vacunador attempted to carry out his obligations as a representative of state power who rarely understood the needs of Maya villages.

Therefore, the preventatives carried into small towns by vacunadores, and the reception these preventatives received in the countryside, came with political and moral meanings. The creole elite accepted vaccination into the community by adhering to norms expressed by experts—whether they understood them or not—concerning the spread of disease and prevention. The Maya understood vaccination as a possible preventative for a disease that killed and had killed their ancestors since Europeans arrived in the sixteenth century. The act of vaccination itself, the piercing of the body followed by the eruption of a mild case of the disease they wished to avoid, held no particular empirical power for the Maya. The vacunador was thus thrust into the midst of a moral clash. The vaccinator's position was truly an intermediary position, bearing similarities to a position once occupied, at one time or another in history, by the priest, the tax collector, the surveyor, the teacher, the commissar—all figures that represent either the state or the entitled institutions of the powerful.

What was perhaps most devastating to the morale of all those who suffered from smallpox, other than the obvious physical discomfort, was the absence of a healthy caretaker, whether this be a doctor, family member, or community healer. Often entire families and towns were stricken with the disease, leaving almost no one to tend to the sick during the critical phase of delirium. If the smallpox sufferer was not properly hydrated and fed during this period, death was almost certain. It was simply easier, and probably less frightening, for many Maya to stay home if they contracted the disease.

Not surprisingly, many residents of Yucatán probably found inoculation and vaccination—which involved the most intimate of contacts, the disturbance of the skin through pricking—frightening and thus avoided such preventative methods. The Maya likely chose to continue with their own medical practices, such as the ingestion of herbs and the repetition of prayers.

The Maya also integrated European notions of the body's humors into their therapeutic framework. Maintaining balance within the body required regulating the body's humors along a "hot" and "cold" spectrum. Humoral medicine is a largely medieval, Western system of conceptualizing the body. According to this theory, humors exist as four fluids secreted from the body and are responsible for a person's character and health. These fluids, blood, phlegm, and yellow and black bile, were classified as either hot or cold. An imbalance in the body's temperature meant illness. The illness and its proper therapeutic could then be identified by examination of bodily secretions.[42] Within this context, smallpox qualified as a "hot" ailment requiring "cold" treatments such as draping cold, soaked banana leaves across a victim's pustules and sores.[43] This treatment appeared in a home remedy book, *El libro del Judío ó medicina doméstica*, compiled in the late eighteenth century by an Italian physician, Dr. Ricardo Osado. Dr. Osado lived in Ticul and in Valladolid under his true name, Giovanni Francesco Mayoli, and dedicated his life to collecting botanical information. A local practitioner, Osado adapted his own medical knowledge to local indigenous traditions of healing and curing in order to construct a system of diagnostics and therapeutics best suited to the needs and outlooks of indigenous communities. Osado's work was not circulated before his death in May of 1770.[44]

After the publication of *Medicina doméstica*, the book was widely circulated and became a commonly consulted sourcebook for Maya communities with limited access to medical facilities and personnel. Dr. Osado's instructions for treating smallpox victims followed the hot-cold paradigm. Osado recommended the use of herbs and tonics known to be "cold"; if a high fever persisted, the patient should take two spoonfuls of "various leaves of *ajeno* [an aromatic and bitter adornment plant], *poleo* [a plant used to make mint tea], and a single *limón* fiber, *X cabalhau che* [*contra yerba* or literally "counter herb," because only the roots of this tree are used and are good for curing chilling in the stomach or body], and the heart of a sour orange, liberally sweetened with bee's honey."[45] According to Alice Le Plongeon, the wife of infamous French archaeologist Augustus Le Plongeon, Dr. Osado's book was "held in great esteem by the people there, as well as by many of the inhabitants on the mainland and so highly appreciated that those who possess copies, either in print or manuscript, can hardly be induced to let them go out of their hands."[46]

A close examination of the linguistic derivations and roots of Yucatec Maya words used to define smallpox during the nineteenth century can serve as a window into Maya disease etiology. Nineteenth-century Yucatec Mayan language included about half a dozen interrelated definitions for smallpox; most shared a common root in the word for fire, *k'ak*.[47] Singularly, *k'ak* was used as a general definition for smallpox with large and painful pustules on the body. *K'ak* may also have been used as a general referent for persistent fevers and eruptive types of illnesses. Additionally, built into many of the definitions of *viruelas* (smallpox) was a division between *viruelas blancas* (white smallpox) and *viruelas negras* (black smallpox).[48] For instance, (*ah*) *pom k'ak'* was a name for smallpox, but literally translated and separated, *pom k'ak'* or *viruelas gruesas* (thick or fat smallpox) meant an illness with a puslike substance (the root *pom* refers to copal incense but can also refer to animal fat or tallow).[49] *T'uch k'ak'* is considered viruelas blancas, or smallpox that did not consist of separated, squeezable (*tupido*) pustules (*granos*).[50] (*Ah*) *ek'pets'k'ak'il* denoted black confluent smallpox,[51] when the pustules ran together to form more serious ulcers.[52]

Because the outward physical manifestations of smallpox resembled those of other diseases like measles and scarlet fever with their rashes, high fevers, and delirium, it is not surprising that some terms in the Mayan language came to conflate all of these diseases.[53] The *h-men*, or healers, among the Maya of the nineteenth century possessed specific medical knowledge regarding several different types of blistering fevers. Differing only slightly in physical exhibition, the gradations of these dissimilarities are nonetheless important because they illustrate the existence of a complex network of therapeutics and etiology that was already in place when the Yucatán public health administrators launched their vaccine campaigns to combat successive waves of disease throughout the mid- to late nineteenth century. We should also consider whether the Maya of Yucatán were really "resistant" to statewide modernizing campaigns or whether the resistance was tactical and local and directed not at modernization as such, but at particular and perhaps collateral grievances that arose because of this or that program. Scholars have found this to be especially true in regard to rural education.[54] James C. Scott has shown the dominated do not necessarily resist directly, but obliquely, and often without thinking in terms of resistance.[55]

Similarly, my conclusions do not point toward definitive Maya resistance to vaccinations and vaccine legislation. Rather, the ambiguity of Maya responses to state vaccination campaigns points to evasion or a disinterest tightly bound up with a collective memory of the conquest and colonization, aggravated by the sociocultural fissures reopened by the Caste War. Ongoing animosity between Mayas and whites, as evidenced by a millenarian sect of Caste War rebels calling for the removal of all *dzul*es (foreigners) from Maya ancestral lands, cast suspicion on those Maya who engaged in smallpox prevention through vaccination in the village culture. If, however, there were a number of Maya who took a more benign view of smallpox vaccination, it was still the case that the real challenge to the legitimacy of state public health programs was posed by the self-sufficiency of alternative local Maya healing practices long situated within communities. The Maya did not have a division of social labor that strictly separated the health-care function from other functions in the community—rather, it was a symbolically potent vehicle of community identity.

The Limits of the State: Vaccine Propagation, Distribution, and Social Disruption

The smallpox vaccine arrived in Mexico from Spain in the early 1800s by way of an expedition sanctioned by the king. That expedition was under the command of his personal physician, Francisco Xavier de Balmis (1753–1819). Balmis's expedition attracted the attention of the progressive European medical establishment, including Jenner himself. It had not been long since Jenner published work that established cowpox pus as an inoculative agent for smallpox, thus rendering obsolete the previous method of variolation. Balmis took twenty-two orphans, from three to nine years old, and inoculated them with the cowpox vaccine. Setting sail on November 30, 1803, from La Coruña, Spain, Balmis had ensured noninterference with his mission by obtaining safe passage from all the belligerents in the Napoleonic wars who, at time, infested the ocean.[56] During the voyage, physicians used the arm-to-arm inoculation method to keep the vaccine fresh. This involved extracting pus from the pustules of one child to be spread on the scratched arm of another child. So, it went until they finally arrived in Caracas with vaccines ready for inland immunization.[57]

Balmis arrived in Sisal on July 10, 1804, and was promptly escorted by state authorities to Mérida. In Mérida, Balmis immediately organized a provisional vaccination council, along with councils in Campeche and Valladolid.[58] While in Mérida, Balmis trained local physicians in propagation, preservation, and application of the smallpox vaccine. During Balmis's residency in Yucatán, he learned that vaccination was well under way in some parts of the peninsula with stores of fresh vaccine that he had not approved. Balmis feared the product nonlegitimate and possibly dangerous or harmful for human application.[59] Subsequently, Balmis's "legitimate" vaccine was taken to Mexico City and looked after by just five physicians throughout the rest of the nineteenth century.[60] Unfortunately for Balmis, his public questioning of the stores of illegitimate vaccines raised doubts about the one he hoped to administer. When he arrived in Veracruz ten days after his Sisal sojourn on July 14, 1804, "a visible lack of enthusiasm for vaccination . . . further exacerbated Balmis's flagging morale."[61] Within this context, the continued use of dangerous and complicated procedures involving human propagation and extraction of lymph fluid via arm-to-arm inoculation continued, which threatened to undermine the distribution of Balmis's cowpox serum. As late as the 1890s the Superior Health Council of Mexico City rationalized arm-to-arm inoculation as necessary in order to propagate a "legitimate" smallpox preventative.[62] This double form of vaccination—bovine and human—continued well into the early twentieth century. By 1915 the use of animals, cows and pigs in particular, became standard for the development of vaccines. Not until 1919 did national legislation bring an end to the use of human vaccine propagation altogether—a full two decades after England outlawed similar practices.[63]

The heroic age of the vaccine was soon succeeded by the bureaucratic age of the vaccine, as the manufacture of the cowpox-infected lymph fluid became a technical matter. Understanding how to store lymph fluid after extraction evolved into one of the greatest obstacles public health officials faced.[64] Angela T. Thompson outlines three methods used to preserve vaccines in her study of smallpox epidemics in early eighteenth-century Guanajuato, Mexico:

> To understand why the Balmis expedition and subsequent vaccination programs required careful organization, the difficulties of preserving the vaccine must be appreciated. Unfortunately, cattle infected with cowpox were not available everywhere to provide matter to make the vaccine. Where infected cattle were not available, communities had to secure vaccine from elsewhere and preserve it by one of three methods. One was to vacuum-seal the vaccine. Another involved crystalizing or drying it, either in threads or between glass slides. These methods were unreliable, for they frequently failed to produce a live vaccine. A third method that preserved the vaccine

> alive, *brazo a brazo*, or arm to arm, was much more reliable but difficult to maintain. In the arm to arm method, the vaccine was administered to a child through a scratch on the arm. After about nine days, a pustule would develop sufficiently for matter to be extracted and rubbed into a scratch on another child's arm. The process would then be repeated with another child and so on, thus preserving the vaccine literally arm to arm. A drawback to this method was that it required a constant supply of individuals who were not already immune, for the vaccine would take only in people who had not previously been exposed to smallpox or cowpox.[65]

In April of 1855, the prefect of the district of Mérida, José Cadenas, wrote to the governor of Yucatán to request more vaccine. In his correspondence, the prefect requested funding for a trip that Dr. José M. Domínguez was planning to take to New Orleans in order to obtain "pure" vaccine. Domínguez planned to employ the Balmis method, traveling on a boat with six children who would be inoculated with smallpox, not cowpox, when they arrived in New Orleans. Domínguez chose the more dangerous method of inoculation using human subjects to cultivate the virus. The double culture of inoculation and vaccination was clearly in play. It facilitated a polarization both within the medical community and among residents as to which vaccine was more safe and effective. Cultivation of a vaccine propagated in an animal, not a human, was readily available, yet Domínguez doubted its efficacy. He chose instead to propagate the vaccine utilizing dangerous and controversial methods. On the return trip, the doctor and his assistants planned to capture the fluid from the pustules of the infected children to prepare vaccines in Mérida. Cadenas requested complete financial backing for the trip from the municipal treasury. In support of his proposal, Cadenas explained that the method Domínguez proposed was "almost completely secure, provided nothing [was] to go wrong."[66] He argued that the benefits realized from such a voyage would be extensive, providing the weakened immunities of Yucatecans with the defenses they desperately needed. Furthermore, the doctor reasoned that given the appearance of smallpox in New Orleans, and cholera in neighboring Mexican states, it would not be long before the peninsula was enveloped in a dual epidemic. Three days after Cadenas's request was drafted, the office of the governor approved funds for the trip.

Despite the appalling use of orphaned children as guinea pigs, and the potential loss of human life, not to mention the moral and religious implications, expeditions similar to Dr. Domínguez's of the 1850s continued between Yucatán and the more developed medical infrastructures of the United States and Europe well into the final decades of the nineteenth century.

Fears circulated that the cow-based vaccine could create bovine side effects, infect the bloodstream, and produce malformed offspring. In Campeche residents wondered "if someday we are going to find ourselves crying over this anguishing epidemic that has befallen us, discouraged by the vaccine that has altered our blood . . . that when [the epidemic] returns it rears a more monstrous and horrendous face."[67] By the late 1850s, problems associated with the distribution of the cow pus vaccine and its rather limited usage time provoked controversy concerning its effectiveness.[68] However, as the vaccine began to noticeably reduce the number of smallpox deaths in a few regions, demand for the vaccine grew. District leaders from all corners of the Mexican republic requisitioned additional shipments and begged for funding to propagate their own vaccine.[69]

In Mexico, the acquisition and propagation of cowpox vaccine depended upon national and state government funding, which went to local district leaders who distributed it to local cattle ranchers in order to set up cow pus manufacture. There were limitations placed on where, and how long, a rancher could raise livestock for the purpose of vaccination propagation and the notion of actually raising an animal to infect it naturally increased anxieties in farming communities. Often the license that proved a rancher's right to raise *ganado vacunado* (vaccine cattle) had to be resubmitted to state officials when the land changed ownership in order for the permission to be extended to the new owner.[70]

Inherent contradictions in land laws and regulations concerning the raising of ganado vacunado can been seen in the case of Manuel Correa, a resident of the district of Umán (located about thirty kilometers south of Mérida). Correa tried to obtain a license to raise ganado vacunado on lands that had already been granted such permission when their previous owner, Nicolas Pisté, had applied for it to raise vaccine cattle and other commercial-grade cattle in 1818. The chain of ownership to the finca went, then, from Pisté to a Mateo Dzul and then to Juan de la Cruz Gomes. Dzul, but not Gomes, had applied for permission to raise ganado vacunado on the land.

In September 1825, Gomes was granted the license to raise ganado vacunado by the newly independent government. However, when Gomes applied for the same right in 1852, judges in the first circuit denied his request because the now defunct República de Indios for the pueblo of Bolón had issued the original grant of permission. Furthermore, following the same reasoning, the judges ruled that Correa's claim to the lands, as indicated in the original 1818 petition, could not be legal. In sum, the court vacated the documents Correa produced. The license awarded in 1825 to raise ganado vacunado was only a "gift" from the government and could not be repeated.[71] The judges ruled Correa must also comply with laws established in 1827 and 1841. The 1827 and 1841 land laws permitted the occupation of fincas (small ranches) that had passed to new owners without informing members of the surrounding districts. Those lands that had passed through the hands of various *castellanos* (Spaniards) more than twice were not extended the same rights. The express permission of the surrounding owners of fincas had to be obtained in writing if the land in question was to be populated. Correa lacked such an agreement with the pueblo of Muna (in the district of Umán). Therefore, the judge's final ruling was that within thirty days, Correa was to be evicted from the site with all his cattle and horses, must close the well on the property, and could not return to the land for any reason. Additionally, Correa had to pay the costs incurred in responding to his request and the appropriate fines for his infraction.

Given the circumstances of land seizures and privatization of lands during the 1840s and 1850s, it is curious Correa even brought the matter of cattle licensing up in a court of law. Undoubtedly, Correa's interests would have been better served had he not pursued legal channels to secure his land title. Most Mexicans realized the law was often predatory, and many preferred to go around it. In fact, Correa's legal troubles were situated within the broad-reaching land reforms of the 1840s and 1850s. Demonstrating consecutive ownership of lands during this period proved nearly impossible, and many lost family lands to the government. Once seized, the lands were declared *terrenos baldíos* (vacated public lands) by the government. Beginning in 1842, Governor Miguel Barbachano offered terrenos baldíos to soldiers "in lieu of money." While rural peasants did experience a modicum of success in holding on to their lands through a system of *denuncias* (claims), the majority of these "public lands" were purchased by elites or transferred to soldiers along with other wealthy individuals whom the state could not afford to repay.[72]

The Correa case raises more questions than it answers regarding the state's pursuit of vaccine propagation and sanitized livestock. On the one hand, the government was always searching for vaccines as part of its public health agenda, even going so far as to scour New Orleans for them. But this case seems to imply that the regulations and taxes on legally raising and slaughtering ganado vacunado were so burdensome that the benefits of doing so seem minor or nonexistent. Ironically, the unfortunate circumstances that led to Correa's eviction were a result of his efforts to comply with state policy regarding the renewal of permission to raise ganado vacunado. Countless notarial (tax and land) documents for the Caste War period indicate that it was not unusual for the owner of a parcel of land to produce documents that proved rightful ownership predating independence, only to be denied those lands later, based on amendments to the national Constitution. Yet, if Correa had not called attention to himself by complying with national and state laws for raising ganado vacunado, he might have been able to continue raising cattle as others before him apparently did, without permission from the state.

After an initial period of profitability in raising ganado vacunado, the miniboom in vaccines peaked *before* the outbreak of the Caste War in 1847. Noticeably, regional land legislation and local efforts to raise ganado vacunado were not in sync, and they subsequently posed a number of insurmountable obstacles for those enterprising ranchers who tried to raise the animals. Part of the initial lure of raising ganado vacunado was the prospect of possible long-term revenues generated by the expected demand for vaccine and stimulated, cattle ranchers hoped, by the public health agenda of the state. State laws passed in 1846 and 1850 required all primary schools to help their students by acquiring trained professionals for vaccination.[73] By the 1860s, physicians began to recommended revaccination for smallpox in order to maintain uninterrupted immunity. Such a requirement sent a message to ranchers that vaccine would always be in demand. In effect, farmers could make money both raising ganado vacunado and on the meat and other byproducts that came from the slaughter of infected cows.

Many ranchers who raised a few head of ganado vacunado on their fincas likely sold them "off the books" to either community leaders in dire need of the vaccine or brokers who devised their own systems of distribution by way of Havana and through remote rebel territories in the southeast across the Río Hondo into British Honduras. At some point in the chain of purchase, however, a trained physician or vacunador had to intervene to extract the pus from the cattle, making it difficult for ranchers like Correa to continually evade the state's representatives in a process that was apparently very carefully regulated by both public health and civil officials. Perhaps Correa had made himself known to the state because compensation for a rancher's vaccine would not have been as high if he sold cattle to nonlicensed vacunadores. Interest in a rancher's ganado vacunado could have also come from local priests or foreigners. The possibility of an illegitimate market in *pus vacuno* is reasonable considering the inability of public health commissions to meet great regional demand created by shortages of the vaccine.

If this hypothetical black market in ganado vacunado in fact existed, we could reasonably infer ranchers might have created their own commercial networks for the product. Yucatán is no exception to the rule that smuggling is one of the mainstays of peripheral economies. Ultimately, contradictory and inflexible policies made the legitimate raising of ganado vacunado a risky venture, especially in the context of the fines and evictions that marked the period of heightened civil unrest. As a result of these perverse economic pressures, it became too difficult for local ranchers to develop vaccine resources in compliance with state policy.

In Mérida, public health officials were confronted with a particularly gruesome challenge to public hygiene with regard to the slaughter of vaccine cattle, which occurred just twenty-one hundred meters from the public Parque Central (Central Park). Despite legislation geared toward public sanitation passed during the 1830s cholera epidemic, the sanitary conditions surrounding the public slaughter of livestock in many cities and pueblos stood in stark contrast to the strict regulations the state imposed on the licensing and taxation of ganado vacunado. The conditions of the public *rastro* (slaughterhouse) in Mérida were quite unsanitary, and the minister in charge of local sanitation, Pascual Lizarraga, was often criticized for lacking a basic understanding of veterinary science, knowledge considered invaluable when determining how an animal should be slaughtered. Furthermore, inspections were often haphazard, and inspectors were often corrupt enough to be bribed to overlook infractions. Commonly, animals were butchered in the evening and the meat left hanging in the open air until the market opened the following morning. Such conditions lured unpenned animals (according to several residents of one of Mérida's suburbs) to the site of such carnage where the scenes of dogs and pigs pulling at the newly slaughtered flesh disturbed the passersby and the smells wafting through the neighborhood sickened the residents.

Regulations on the slaughter and sale of livestock, such as the 1849 law stipulating that no one could slaughter an animal intended for distribution and sale outside of the public rastro, were difficult to enforce.[74] For those who had to drive their cattle some distance to a rastro, selling livestock that had lost weight on the trail and paying for drovers in order to comply with existing legislation meant less profit. Slaughterhouse fees often were quite high; for cattle a payment of eight reals had to be made to the local *alcabala* (boss) before they were killed, in addition to the fee for portioning of meat and use of the facilities. Similarly, if the owner failed to produce the proper license for his operation, then he or she would be fined for the slaughter and the infraction and charged a fee for use of the rastro. Given such costs, one can imagine a scenario wherein the value of the cow or pig itself no longer surpassed the fees and fines applied at the time of slaughter. As an added incentive to ensure compliance, livestock "police" milled around the rastro collecting a standard 4 percent cut from each slaughter for themselves.[75]

The collective effect of the regulations was to change the traditional organization of livestock raising, making it more costly for small landholders. The shift to bigger landholders took place at a time when more plantation-style farms in general were starting to emerge in the peninsula. At the same time, the regulations created a new "vision" of what it meant to raise animals and own land, which was no longer defined by traditional, unwritten codes or the knowledge handed down from father to son. According to Rugeley, the 1840s also saw the enclosure of terrenos baldíos, "unfallow land," which concentrated agricultural capital into the hands of a few "nuevo riche."[76] In the 1850s Yucatecan statesman, lawyer, writer, and newspaperman Justo Sierra O'Reilly wrote in his *Consideraciones*, "The señores and the nobles were owners of immense cultivated territories with slaves. Under the same method [employed] today: the hatchet and the torch."[77] Public health concerns played an important role in the synchronization of these factors for the landowner. First, public health policy regarding the safety of animal and human interactions served as a justification to elevate standards for landowners who wanted to raise livestock. Second, public health policy provided a means through which the state and powerful elites could focus on the small landholder by establishing new ground rules in the name of public safety and regional stability. Combined, these factors made it more difficult for small landholders to raise livestock and compromised their ability to hold on to their property.

In the 1850s, a vision of public health began to emerge that tentatively set aside the liberal individualism premised on the individual's control over and responsibility for his or her own body as the basis of the social order, and instead subtly shifted the governance of collective habits to the public sphere, thus extending the reach of the state into private life. Suggesting that disease proliferation could flourish in uncontrolled public spaces, like rastros, cemeteries, boarding houses, taverns, markets, hospitals, schools, and bordellos, shifted the onus of blame from the individual and at the same time limited the individual's freedom of action by curbing the behavior of the collective public. This meant reshaping an unpredictable, fluid environment containing a menagerie of beasts, insects, plants, soil, humans, and (although this was not known at the time) disease pathogens.

The convergence of popular notions about disease origin became intertwined with emergent scientific theories and the chaos of everyday life to create "diseased moments." These "diseased moments" constituted a crucible containing a heightened sense of fear and worry about death, infection, and one's livelihood. The threat disease epidemics held over populations made it socially possible for statesmen to enact social legislation on a scale otherwise impossible outside of the confines of "diseased moments."

Matthew Restall contends that the smallpox epidemic of 1856 was the most devastating since first contact between the "Old" and "New" worlds in the sixteenth century.[78] In Yucatán the smallpox epidemic of 1856 devastated entire communities. During one of the most "powerful and disastrous" epidemics in history, communities struggled to vaccinate and revaccinate residents while in the midst of a concurrent cholera epidemic and the violence of the Caste War.[79]

In February 1855, on the eve of the 1856 smallpox outbreak, prefect José D. Villamil of Mérida wrote to Yucatán's governor stating he would be unable to provide smallpox vaccinations for his district.[80] Villamil blamed the ongoing revolt of the "barbarous" Maya for blocking vaccine supplies from reaching the interior. Furthermore, Villamil explained that rebel tactics of burning down entire villages made communication with eastern towns nearly impossible and subsequently attendance at vaccination appointments had dropped considerably.[81] "Those in charge of administration of the pus vaccine in this city [Mérida]," Villamil claimed, "complain that each time the number of children that appear for inoculation is less and less."[82]

The horrors of the 1856 smallpox epidemic enforced upon the minds of Yucatecan politicians the need for a ready, continuous flow of smallpox vaccines. The system of smallholders raising ganado vacunado had proved insufficient, and the transport of the vaccine from central Mexico along roads to Veracruz and then by boat to Campeche was too dependent on the federal government's whim and subject to too much loss to be the sole source of supply. The quest to locate regionally viable sources of vaccine and the need to transport the vaccine so that it neither spoiled nor was spilled encouraged the continuation of Balmis's dangerous methods of vaccine propagation and immunization using a chain of human carriers as hosts to carry the disease. The human subjects selected were those on the bottom of the social hierarchy: foundlings, African and indigenous slaves, and convicted felons (such as army deserters). During these "propagation journeys," the victims were given doses of live human lymph or cow pus vaccine subcutaneously with a lancet. As their infections progressed on the journey and the disease took hold of their bodies, their pustules were harvested and applied to the next victim in order to keep the vaccine alive until the ship reached its destination and the vaccine could be applied en masse. If, by chance, one of the victims died during the journey, it was considered a necessary sacrifice for the good of the many.[83]

Restructuring Vaccination: Sanitation and Disease Proliferation at the End of the Century

Between 1850 and 1900, changes in smallpox science improved vaccine efficacy and application. The period of time between vaccination and revaccination became more standard, and the development of microscopy in the 1830s facilitated the diagnosis and classification of diseases. In 1842 Italian pathologist Adelchi Negri created cow-to-cow chains for the transmission of cowpox, making the Negri method of vaccination propagation the more common method in Naples, and from there the practice spread throughout Europe.[84] The emergence of germ theory in the 1870s laid the groundwork for scientists Robert Koch and Louis Pasteur to discover the microorganism that caused smallpox (although this discovery had to wait until the twentieth century when the causative factors for contagious disease were isolated), so that by the late nineteenth century, Western medicine finally had a causative story about smallpox, in addition to an empirical preventive.[85] At the International Congress of Health in London in 1891, Dr. Sydney Monckton Copeman, FRS, presented his work on standardizing the use of glycerin as a preservative to keep the lymph moist. Glycerin preserved the potency of the lymph for a few months with virtually no contamination.[86] As improvements to smallpox vaccine propagation and preservation progressed, legislation throughout Europe and the Americas emerged to make smallpox vaccination compulsory. In 1853 Britain passed an obligatory smallpox vaccination law and Germany followed in 1874, Mexico in 1898, and Brazil in 1904.[87]

The passing of obligatory vaccination legislation often met with resistance, however. Many claimed that forcing vaccines on people, particularly on schoolchildren, constituted an "immoral . . . interference in the natural order of life, or an infringement upon personal autonomy."[88] Such measures not only frightened laypersons, but also seemed to cast serious doubt on the judgment of policy makers and modern medical science. During the last years of the nineteenth century, regional public health administrators in Mérida labored to propagate vaccine by utilizing unvaccinated children from surrounding districts.[89] Children were vaccinated with bovine- and human-procured lymph fluid, and once the children produced pustules, physicians extracted fluid from the pustules and transferred the fresh fluid to the next child in a chain of arm-to-arm vaccinations designed to keep the vaccine fresh. Using chains of children to keep strains of both human and bovine vaccine "alive" continued even after the introduction of Negri's glycerinated cow lymph. Even more astounding than the continued use of children to propagate and preserve vaccine was an apparent agreement among physicians that animal-procured lymph fluid was much safer than human-procured lymph fluid because human lymph vaccine could transfer syphilis to its recipient. In regard to the use of human lymph vaccine the Hahnemann Society in Madrid in 1867 noted, "Today, by good fortune, we are convinced that arm-to-arm vaccination can communicate syphilis."[90]

Despite the known faults with human lymph vaccine, many communities, particularly those located great distances from urban centers and professional medical assistance, chose to utilize the pustules from an active outbreak for inoculation in the absence of preserved bovine fluid or even "human-stored" bovine fluid. Such practices facilitated the creation of dual methods of smallpox prevention. In his report to the Second Pan-American Medical Conference, Dr. Govea of Tamaulipas, Mexico, conceded that "the superiority of animal vaccine over that of human, is now an undeniable point," but bovine-derived lymph did not store well and did not produce harvestable lesions in children. Furthermore, Dr. Govea pointed out the vaccine often lost potency while in transit. He advocated teaching residents a simple "operation" to harvest pustules. On-site harvesting was seen as a far more practical solution because residents could easily be trained to perform the procedure and would not have to wait in a crisis for medical assistance or vaccine to arrive.[91]

In fact, Yucatán's Consejo Superior de Salubridad (Superior Health Council) worked to establish a system of harvesting smallpox pustules by ordering communities to send unvaccinated children to Mérida to be exposed to smallpox and have their lesions harvested. On September 7, 1897, the Superior Health Council's Saturnino Cervera Guzmán asked the governor for assistance in propagation efforts:

> I have the honor to convey information from the Council which has . . . in light of the unification of our population to the Capital [Mérida]

> by railroad, decided that whenever there is a need for the fluid [vaccine], children who are not vaccinated should be sent to the Capital so that their pustules may be [later] utilized in the area of their residence, Izamal has found themselves in this situation, [and] I beg of you, if you think it fair, to order the jefe político of the above mentioned *partido* to remit four or six robust, unvaccinated children for the previously indicated objective.[92]

The day after Guzmán sent his letter to the Superior Health Council, the administration responded they would do everything in their power to ensure that the municipal authority of Izamal acquiesced in the propagation efforts. Regardless of regional efforts to propagate a human lymph vaccine for general use, it remains unclear whether Izamal's municipal leader complied with such a difficult request. In any case, the town was hit particularly hard by the smallpox epidemic in 1897. Those fortunate enough to have gained immunity to smallpox still experienced the dark pallor the epidemic spread over everyday life and especially any event involving a concentration of people. Most notable was the suspension of the annual Izamal fair by public health and state officials who declared "it would be dangerous for the public health."[93]

Some municipal leaders may have willingly sent select unvaccinated children from their districts as sacrificial lambs, if they received assurances that more vaccine would reach their communities in time to prevent an outbreak.[94] On September 29, 1897, the director of Yucatán's Superior Health Council, Saturnino Guzmán, received word from the jefe político of Motul regarding the appearance of one child in the community with "pustules ready to begin inco-bation [*sic*]"; therefore, the jefe político informed the council he would be sending "four robust, unvaccinated children to the capital so that later, when they are in Mérida, they may serve to propagate the vaccine in this [Motul] area."[95]

Despite the known risks and sacrifice accompanying requests for uninfected children to be used as propagation vessels for vaccine, many public health officials insisted that this was the only certain way to safeguard their supply of the precious fluid. Compliance also had to exist on the local level. It was in this vein that in December of 1897 the political leader of Motul wrote directly to the governor's office requesting medical assistance for smallpox patients. He stated that "already the number of those infected had reached four, and one seven-year-old boy, Esteban Chan, had died the previous day."[96] Although young Esteban's body was buried according to health codes and the

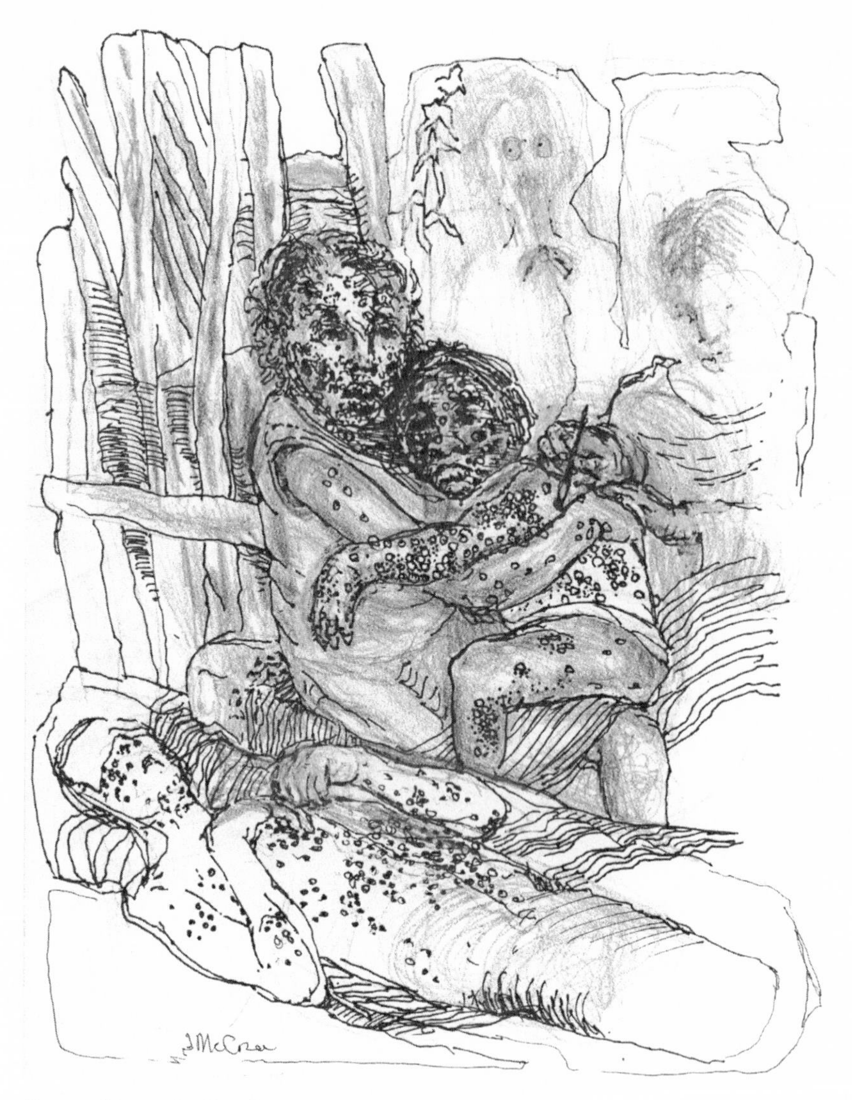

Figure 1: *Harvesting Smallpox Pustules* by Judith B. McCrea.

other victims were quarantined, the *jefatura* (town council) feared the disease would spread. Given the history of the rapid spread of the disease, local public health officials were understandably wary of their ability to contain it and begged their superiors for as many preventatives as possible.[97]

Municipal authorities were ultimately responsible for removing children from their homes and delivering them to the state capital. This task naturally provoked resistance, and there is every reason to think that many local leaders did not report cases of unvaccinated children to avoid these situations or perhaps simply ignored requests in the interest of self-preservation. Weighing the consequences carefully, some authorities must have pondered which was the worst-case scenario: making themselves targets of retaliation by wounded parties in the district or risking punishment from state officials in the form of limited funds and assistance.

In fact, secondary reactions—and deaths—related to bad or tainted vaccines compelled public health officials to consider sanctioning new propagation techniques and revaccination.[98] These efforts likely encouraged public health officials to revisit their measures of success in relation to smallpox prevention and containment. Clearly, more was at stake than simply vaccinating as many people as possible. Public health bureaus understood that a system was needed to monitor vaccine production and distribution. On-site supervision by medically trained personnel was desperately needed to replace the ad hoc vacunador system. The emergence of germ theory in the mid-1880s grounded disease prevention agendas in new ways, at last giving regional public health practitioners a sense that they could causatively map infection and thus scientifically eliminate disease and unsanitary environments.[99]

The popular creole belief that the Maya were too backward to fully implement vaccination as well as other modern disease prevention methods in their communities was reinforced by the emergent science of sanitation and hygiene. Sanitation science made clear connections between disease and filth. In his inaugural address to the Second Pan-American Medical Congress, held in Mexico City in November of 1896, congress president Dr. Domingo Orvañanos outlined the vital role of hygiene in overcoming disease: "What branch of Medicine can boast, as Hygiene can, that it prevents the development and propagation of disease, and that it procures the welfare of the populations and the lengthening of the average life?"[100] Public health officers now saw what might have been considered feed for animals or garbage to be recycled as filth and a site for the spread of disease. Within the context of public health and sanitation movements of the nineteenth century, we need to consider the term *filth* on a conceptual level. For instance, when discovered in stores of animal fodder or animal refuse used as fertilizer, "filth" evokes a certain moral vocabulary. "Filth" thus provided a new perspective through which sanitarians and medical professionals could view human habits and lifestyles. Rudi Colloredo-Mansfeld's work on race and hygiene in modern Ecuador, for example, argues that a preoccupation with racial and national hygiene, whether real or imagined, determines one's ability to fit into society; dirty bodies and clothes do not simply convey poverty but also speak to social, economic, and moral status.[101]

The new picture of the world of disease, with its flow of invisible germs carried by a host of pests, created the momentum for the initiation of controls over the human environment, such as a strict adherence to cleansing and fumigation routines. As the U.S. foreign consul in Progreso, Edward Thompson, noted in December 1900, most of the peninsula's unsanitary conditions could be found in Maya mud-and-thatch houses, so that even "under the most favorable of circumstances sanitary decrees are carried into effect among them with the greatest difficulty."[102] In fact, many foreigners regularly connected "filth" in the countryside to the Mayas' unhealthy living conditions. The continuance of the Caste War in the remote southeast of the peninsula also contributed to the image of the peninsula as a turbulent, poverty-stricken "Indian" backwater.[103]

While the entire peninsula often bore the burden of such an image, in truth by the 1890s only the southeastern portions of the peninsula remained consistently immersed in Caste War violence. Henequeneros in the northwestern zones called upon the federal government to help them secure the territories surrounding their profitable export haciendas. President Díaz declared the Yucatán beyond repair without the help of the republic. "I am convinced," Díaz explained, "that Yucatán cannot by itself, as it has not been able to do for more than half a century, recover, pacify, and maintain the southeastern region, much less colonize and develop it. . . . I believe firmly that only the Nation has the means to achieve such goals."[104] The regional divide between northwestern and southeastern Yucatán created the perception of zones where "pacified" Maya toiled on henequen plantations and "uncivilized" rebel Maya wandered the intemperate jungles of the southeast, and views of the indigenous people extended from this polarized view of "tamed" and "untamed" Maya. We should note, however, that despite Mérida's apparent transformation into a "civilized" modern city, by the 1880s the urban capital still did not have a sanitation code that allowed civil authorities to fine residents and businesses for throwing waste into the streets.[105]

Thompson's observations also illustrate the disjuncture between what medical professionals understood to be the truth about disease proliferation and what laypersons believed. Within the framework of an invisible threat, even the advent of germ theory did not preclude a reliance on older etiological tenets. For instance, zymotic theory contended that a disease could be passed via chemical or "animacular" infestation or invasion. An outbreak could be assisted by the existence of one or more factors such as festering waste (filth, soil, excrement) as well as the foul vapors that filth tended to produce, unfavorable climatic conditions, and a weakened personal constitution. Ultimately, these understandings of disease etiology gave rise to modern sanitation and hygiene movements. By the end of the century, a failure to comply with the "gospels" of modern "sanitary science" was seen by the new "converts" as the principal cause of illness.[106] If disease then ceased to proliferate, not only could modern sanitary science take credit for it, but also the political elite could take credit for good, well-informed leadership. Dr. Domingo Orvañanos's speech on sanitation to the American Public Health Association in 1908 spotlights Veracruz and Mérida as locales where the successful combination of hygiene and disease prevention led to a marked decrease in yellow fever. Dr. Orvañanos celebrated: "We owe these results to the energy, intelligence and labors of the President of the Supreme Board of Health of Mexico, Dr. Eduardo Liceaga, and to the President of the Republic, General Diaz."[107] Field doctors, who were sent into rural towns for on-site monitoring of vaccinations and quarantines, had been educated in programs that included sanitary sciences.[108] To rid the areas of smallpox once and for all, many doctors began to combine new doctrines of sanitary science, such as fumigating and sanitizing, with long-established methods such as quarantine.

As part of an overarching modernizing campaign to combat disease, the state began to send recent graduates from the regional medical school in Mérida to the countryside to provide prompt and safe quantities of vaccine for some of the more vulnerable sectors of the population. The move to send doctors into the countryside was likely due to the frustration many public health officials developed in implementing vaccination campaigns during the mid- to late nineteenth-century epidemics. Irritation, as well as political pressure, likely increased with repeated smallpox epidemics in the latter half of the century. In particular, epidemics in 1889, 1897, and 1899 inspired a reorganization of public health efforts throughout the peninsula. The state's failure to procure enough untainted vaccine for the entire population reached a nadir in 1880s Yucatán with the death of a local woman on board a ship used for a "propagation journey."[109]

In 1883 writer Fabian Carrillo Sauste published a commentary regarding the deplorable state of vaccination in the peninsula. According to Carrillo, the state director of vaccine had publicly declared that his personal efforts to obtain a good vaccine stock failed due to the total lack of volunteers and cooperation from all of the sectors of society. The director also observed that propagation of the vaccine via arm-to-arm methods only deepened public fear of the vaccine—"Personal force is useless and does not produce good results because of the lack of good turnout and cooperation from all sectors of society"—and thus, this method would no longer be used. He called for an immediate reorganization of the Public Health Authority's vaccination division as well as higher annual salaries for the director of vaccine and the subdirector; the subdirector would receive 240 pesos and the director, 600, a significant increase from the 150 pesos the director received in the 1850s.[110]

The sending of doctors into the field, in Yucatán as well as elsewhere in Mexico and Latin America, facilitated state-building goals aimed at purging the nation of any remaining influence of the Catholic Church.[111] The state's efforts to undermine the authority of the church in the rural countryside stemmed from an ongoing effort to gain more control over the most autonomous Maya communities where the church had built strong traditional ties. In diminishing the church's role, the political elite hoped to mobilize the pool of agricultural labor, thereby providing entrepreneurial landowners greater access to inexpensive wage labor. Drawing from the Reforma of 1856–57 and President Juárez's Leyes de Reforma, politicians and public health officials often sought to design policies specifically to displace the clergy's monopoly over such rites as marriages, births, and burials.[112]

State attempts to undermine church authority at midcentury can be seen in the restructuring of vaccine programs so that a town's vaccinator could no longer be an untrained priest, politician, or midwife.[113] By the late nineteenth century, only licensed medical doctors were allowed to monitor outbreaks and educate citizens in matters of quarantine, sanitation, and other aspects of disease prevention. The program did indeed succeed in providing some rural regions with personalized medical care, but at greater cost to the community, as public health officials and district politicians had to work together to locate the funds for the doctor's salary, housing, transportation, and equipment. Additional funds were needed for the purchase of smallpox vaccine and its safe transportation to disparate locales throughout the peninsula. Faculty at the medical school and public health officials were hard pressed to find young doctors to work in remote regions with little pay and for indefinite periods. Throughout the Porfirian period, the lack of personnel to administer the vaccine complicated the establishment of vaccination sites and times outside of Mérida.[114]

The war against smallpox in Yucatán, fought in the many villages scattered throughout the peninsula, can be traced through the correspondence of local leaders, subvaccinators, and field doctors.[115] The petitions from villages requesting supplies and funds vividly illustrate the everyday obstacles local leaders faced in their attempts to prevent smallpox in their communities, both from the powers above, with their rules and fines, and from the pressures below, as villagers demanded help with disease. Ultimately, local officials were bound by a legal framework that did not take into account such long-term obstacles as limited state funding, rebel activities, and a severe shortage of productive adult males (a demographic fact that began to show up by the 1880s).[116] In the 1890s, an increase in national funding to the regional medical school coincided with the reorganization of the Health Council, which in turn afforded public health officials the opportunity and manpower to send newly trained medical school graduates into the countryside to oversee vaccination and monitor active cases of smallpox.[117]

Among the correspondence one finds many allusions to the complaints of young medical school graduates and vaccinators about the conditions under which they were forced to work. Typically, the few trained doctors who did practice medicine in Yucatán did not want to work in the desolate henequen production zones or in dangerous rebel areas. Dr. Alfonso Peniche Rubio claimed it would be much easier to transfer smallpox victims to districts outside of war zones where they could be cared for properly given that these pueblos "never have physicians available, they are always out of medicine and supplies . . . and the disease simply multiplies in severity here."[118] Moreover, there was no prestige to be gained by working outside of Mérida; a doctor lived on reputation, and it rankled field doctors that anti-smallpox work entailed little or no recognition. They could well see, of course, that doctors who established their practices in Mérida were building their client bases. Reflecting the disparity in the state's attentiveness to the public health, Mérida doctors had a variety of resources and funds that simply were not available to those in rural districts.[119]

The correspondence of Anastasio Monsreal illustrates the plight of the field doctor. In August of 1897, Dr. Monsreal accepted a rural post, in the mostly Maya-populated town of Halachó, that many of his colleagues had declined.[120] He arrived to find a handful of persons suffering from smallpox.[121] Almost immediately afterward, and concurrent to his appointment to the district's Superior Health Council in Maxcanú, Monsreal began to send regular updates to the governor's office regarding the condition of the *virulentes* in Halachó. For several months, Monsreal's correspondence remained brief, relaying only the most recent deaths from smallpox and assuring his superiors he had control over the situation. But in December of the same year, the death of a fourteen-year-old girl took Monsreal by surprise, as he was unaware of the girl's condition. Monsreal blamed the girl's death on her father's "ignorance and the fact that he has an attitude of superiority and he took it upon himself to not consult a doctor."[122] He examined the girl's corpse and concluded she had died of severe hemorrhagic confluent smallpox.

Monsreal informed the Superior Health Council in Mérida that the victim's straw-thatched house was located just a few meters from the center of town. To make matters even more embarrassing, upon further investigation Monsreal found that the entire family was suffering from smallpox: José Higinio Flores was afflicted with confluent smallpox with complications in his lungs, and Monsreal gave him a generally bad prognosis; eleven-year-old Miguel Flores was in grave condition with hemorrhagic confluent smallpox; Josefa Almeida, fifty-year-old mother of Miguel and the deceased Pastora, was in the eruptive stage and diagnosed to be in fair condition with discrete smallpox; and finally, sixteen-year-old Juana Flores was in the final stages of the disease, or *período de descamación* (scab-forming period), and considered in fair condition. Shortly after Monsreal finished his examination of the remaining family members, he ordered armed guards to surround the house and promptly began routine fumigations of the structure and its surrounding area.[123]

After the discovery of these "hidden" cases of smallpox, we can trace the disintegration of the relationship between Monsreal and the citizens of Halachó in the correspondence to the council.[124] Monsreal was evidently put on edge. Suspicious of everyone, he believed that a local conspiracy to deliberately conceal smallpox victims was at work in Halachó and perhaps throughout the entire partido of Maxcanú. The fact that his reputation as a competent physician was at stake undoubtedly made interaction with the citizens of Halachó tenser. In a letter to the head of the Superior Health Council, the mayor of Halachó summarized the situation: "[We] insistently propose that the stated objectives of Monsreal have become ignoble and thus the atmosphere among the masses [has worsened], which it is believed will make the fulfillment of his job difficult." The mayor and other authorities from Halachó suggested that with "all due respect to Monsreal, the attitude that they spoke of will ultimately cause more concealment of smallpox cases."[125]

These circumstances did not improve, tainting the relationship between Halachó's citizens and Monsreal. The community probably lost trust in Monsreal after the death of the young Flores girl. For many local Maya, the appearance of a pox-infested corpse near the city square, while a certified doctor lived in town, cast fear and suspicion on the doctor and his abilities. Clearly, for many of Halachó's citizens, a smallpox victim's prospects did not seem any better under the care of Monsreal. It is reasonable to assume that some residents of Halachó who were infected with smallpox preferred to die at home, without armed guards surrounding their homes and without the intrusion of an outsider. Thus, Monsreal's actions actually promoted the very secrecy that he began to suspect everywhere.

The Flores family was not the first to have hidden an occurrence of smallpox from the town doctor. In Monsreal's correspondence to the Superior Health Council he speculated that many other clandestine cases likely existed. Undoubtedly irate that several cases of smallpox were intentionally hidden from him, Monsreal demanded that local officials question José Flores, the father of the family, about the reasons he had not sought Monsreal's assistance. Flores's only reply to this question was, "Perhaps it was fear."[126] After seeing the local officials at work, Monsreal made a direct plea to his superiors to help him with the delicate politics of the situation. The director of the Superior Health Council sided with Monsreal and advised him that they would have a word with the local leaders in Halachó on his behalf. Meanwhile Monsreal recommended Flores be given the harshest punishment possible for having concealed his family's situation from town officials. According to the correspondence, the governor's office agreed to remand Flores to the court for a sentence that would include lengthy jail time or a heavy fine or both. However, there is no indication in corresponding court files that Flores was ever fined or jailed for his "crime." The attention Monsreal drew to the Flores family did, however, serve to isolate the family from their own community. In the end, the records show that Monsreal accomplished little by making an example of the Flores family. He may have heightened the level of anxiety throughout Halachó, but there is no indication he created an atmosphere of compliance.[127]

It would be easy to portray Monsreal as a small town martinet. But that would not be the whole story. For we must remember that he was one of a handful of doctors who traveled to a remote disease site outside of Yucatán's urban areas specifically to investigate the area's epidemic potential and to treat those in need. Often these doctors were appointed at the last minute and subsequently integrated into an ad hoc local Superior Health Council. Paid very little (about thirty pesos a month on average), they arrived in their villages as the face of the public health initiative, replacing the untrained local leader or priest who previously had cared for the sick. We can assume that, very often, the leader or priest had earned the community's loyalty. Thus, a doctor like Monsreal often encountered a barrier of distrust and resentment from the beginning. This simply aggravated the miscommunications between the townsfolk and the medical establishment, which, even in the best of circumstances, bedeviled workers in the rapidly changing field of public health. It is easy to suppose that the use of force in the name of the community's "health" weakened the overall legitimacy of state medicine in the eyes of the citizens it was ostensibly helping (and surely Dr. Monsreal was not the only doctor to use his powers to fumigate and isolate to the full extent). For instance, in Mexico City public health inspectors blamed reductions in juvenile vaccinations on "mothers who hide their children for fear of losing them to extracted lymph. As a result we cannot compute the number of vaccinated against the number of those who should be vaccinated."[128]

In Halachó, Dr. Monsreal's suspicion that he was being lied to may have been exaggerated, but he certainly proved unable to convince the community that he was there to safeguard them. James C. Scott's notion of the public and hidden transcript is useful in understanding José Flores's motivations for hiding his own and his family's illness. Utilizing Scott's work, we can see that someone like José Flores, already undoubtedly heartbroken over the death of one child, made his decisions about whether to seek medical assistance or "hide" his family within a "restricted social circle." Like others who see themselves as subordinates, Flores exercised power over his own "restricted social circle" that included his family and home. José Flores and his family were then "afforded a partial refuge from the humiliations of domination, and it is from this circle that the audience (one might say 'the public') for the hidden transcript is drawn."[129] Flores's indirect resistance—the hiding of his family as they suffered from a highly communicable disease—also drew upon the image Flores knew the elite held of him, as a slow, ignorant, and uniformed peasant. Yucatán's public health council used their procedures to block Flores's plans, but ultimately Flores's resistance was made complete by way of his noncompliance.[130]

Given these face-to-face obstacles, the last thing field doctors like Dr. Monsreal needed was bureaucratic inefficiency. But the institutional support was a work in progress. The archives from the governor's office and the Superior Health Council contain numerous letters of resignation from vaccinators and doctors who were irritated and disillusioned in the 1850s, as the state began to stake its claim to its citizens' health.[131] Often positions were left vacant for several years until a replacement, if any, could be found.

In 1889 smallpox vaccination became compulsory for the entire population. To implement this program, doctors and health-care officials had to face down a profound animosity against legitimate state-supported medical practices. Trust was particularly eroded in the face of repeated smallpox epidemics.[132] In 1897 another smallpox epidemic exploded, resulting in dramatically high concentrations of mortality in rural zones. By the 1890s, regular collection of vaccination and smallpox mortality statistics showed that entire pueblos and haciendas remained untouched by the programs envisioned in the progressive legislation.[133] Legislation implemented almost forty years prior, mandating vaccination of children before their fourth birthday, had not been effectively adopted, to no one's surprise. In fact, 43 percent of the 127 who died of smallpox in Hunucmá were children under the age of ten.[134]

I would also note that the high mortality rate in 1897 may have provoked regional public health officials to turn more resources to the task of cultivating local reproduction of human smallpox vaccine. Children, most especially orphans, were still enrolled in the same arm-to-arm method used by Balmis in 1804, and the increased attention to vaccine supply paid off: by 1900, Hunucmá consistently produced enough vaccine from humans and cattle to meet local demand.[135] Typically, many local leaders scrambled to obtain enough pus vacuno (pus vaccine) to meet the demands of their districts well into the early years of the twentieth century.[136] As Mexico entered the twentieth century under the auspices of a Porfirian culture that proclaimed its modernity to the world, isolation and a lack of information continued to leave entire pockets of the Yucatecan population unvaccinated and vulnerable.

To be sure, public health administrators always faced the same obstacles to local compliance during smallpox vaccination campaigns. Initially, the renewed anti-smallpox program seemed to generate significant increases in the number of vaccinated persons in some regions, particularly after mandatory vaccination legislation passed.[137] For instance, during the first half of 1889 a census for Motul indicated that fewer than 4 percent of the population remained unvaccinated.[138] The highest concentration of those who remained unvaccinated lived either on church grounds or on haciendas.[139] However, the numbers for other districts seemed dreadfully low, indicating either blatant noncompliance or ignorance of the vaccination legislation. Similarly, according to records sent to the Superior Health Council in February 1889, 46 percent of the population in the small pueblo of Sitilpech remained unvaccinated.[140]

Many municipalities like Espita were nonetheless made well aware of the mandatory vaccination policy by the circulation of broadsides and serial publication announcements in the state publication *El Siglo XIX*. Prior to 1901, vaccination rates remained relatively low in Espita, and local and regional officials reasoned it was related to rumors that the vaccine was tainted or bad.[141] By 1901, the vaccine supply no longer appeared to be tainted, but despite marked improvements in the quality of lymph vaccine, fear of vaccination endured. In 1925 Yucatecan physician Dr. Alvaro Avila Escalante wrote in his *Historia de la medicina en Yucatán*, "Residents of pueblos maintain false ideas about liberty." Escalante argued that as a result these residents "descend into beliefs that they have the right to not be vaccinated, to hide the sick and to throw into the four winds their contagion."[142] Such logic helped to absolve public health officials for their own mistakes during smallpox epidemics while simultaneously condemning the Maya for their noncompliance.

Conclusion

The experience of Yucatán in the most successful disease prevention campaign of the nineteenth century against smallpox points to both a grudging progress as compared to the horrific epidemics of the sixteenth and seventeenth centuries and the problems caused by the peninsula's peripheral location vis-à-vis Mexico. On the one hand, it is symbolically important that Balmis, whose expedition to bring smallpox vaccine to Mexico is generally considered the beginning of the modern era of smallpox eradication in Mexico, disembarked first in Yucatán.[143] On the other hand, the lymph vaccine that Balmis brought ended up in Mexico City, administered and hoarded by the National Health Council. The supply of vaccines and their distribution and administration all depended on institutions of public health that were rocked by the events of the first half of the century: independence, Yucatán's regionalist aspirations, the war with the United States, and the beginning of the Caste War. Within the framework of the new technologies to combat smallpox epidemics, the epidemics unfolded as disease moments that revealed holes in institutions, biases in attitudes, and deep cultural conflicts.

The cycles of smallpox epidemics that swept through Yucatán in the mid- to late nineteenth century significantly altered the relationship between the state and the inhabitants as the state took on the role of the final arbiter in all health matters. Folded into the civilizing and modernizing campaigns, which were the guises under which the creole elite fought the tumultuous Caste War of 1847 through 1902, smallpox vaccination campaigns served to put a face on the government in remote villages and provided the foundation upon which modern secular health services were built in southeastern Mexico. The result of this outreach was the penetration of the organic structures of Maya culture and an attack on the elaborate techniques and theories of health care that the Maya had built up over the centuries since the *conquista*. These indigenous techniques failed to prevent the epidemics; the vaccination method, on the other hand, seemed, over time, to work. Suffering from the aftereffects of both disease and vaccination (if they submitted), the Maya were, in the end, further demoralized in a period during which their system of land tenure was under attack and the need for free, mobilized labor to work on sugar and henequen plantations was growing. Like the Flores family, indigenous communities maintained with the state tentative, if not strained, relationships made up of accommodations interspersed with covert rebellions. As public health initiatives were reorganized in the last decades of the century, the Porfirian mode of modernization finally caught up with Yucatán.

For Yucatán's policy makers and bureaucrats, the smallpox epidemics brought out numerous anxieties concerning the acquisition, propagation, transport, and preservation of the smallpox vaccine. Many local leaders like Señor Velasquez of Bolonchenticul and doctors like Anastasio Monsreal became frustrated with working under the double pressure of an inefficient bureaucracy and a surly and hostile rural population. It is also apparent that the elite's image of the "barbaric" Maya Indian superstitiously resisting civilization, whether by clinging to the church or to old beliefs, hindered the ability of leaders to understand some of the more tangible reasons as to why vaccination was not entirely successful throughout the peninsula. In fact, throughout the world nineteenth-century public health officials scrambled to propagate and distribute enough vaccine during devastating epidemics of the 1850s, 1870s, and 1880s through 1890s.

As remarkable as the gains of the public health agenda in some areas of Yucatán, like Mérida in 1900, was the lack of progress of organized vaccination campaigns in many other areas, where the landscape looked the same in 1900 as it did in 1847, at the inception of the Caste War. These gaps in public health were made manifest by the 1897 smallpox epidemic, where the same lack of resources that had bedeviled officials in past epidemics, and the reversion to old techniques of making vaccine in order to cover gaps in supply, showed structural weakness in the state's public health capacities. In the final analysis, an overtaxed and overburdened administrative framework in Yucatán could not effectively communicate the benefits of smallpox vaccination to rural communities and their leaders.

Vaccination campaigns were retooled to address gaps in distribution, and enforcement of the mandatory vaccination law implemented in 1898 was tightened. But strict public health policies facilitated a reliance on non-state-sanctioned medicinal practices that were more convenient and less invasive—such as consultations with *curanderos*, herbalists, and Catholic priests—or non-action. The Maya populations in rural areas may have chosen to avoid state public health campaigns by avoiding vaccination and hiding victims of smallpox, thus underscoring popularly held notions among statesmen that the indigenous population remained obstacles in Yucatán's modernizing process. Certainly the Catholic Church sought to hold on to whatever power they could, particularly during the initial Liberal attacks on religious privilege during the Reforma of the late 1840s and 1850s.

The cleavage between secular and religious realms of authority, between the church, the state, and the Maya, left a space open in the sociopolitical landscape in which each faction saw an opportunity for gain and a threat of loss. An exploration of the power struggles over sacred burial grounds and burial rites during the mid-nineteenth-century cholera epidemic underscores the overriding vigor with which elites vied for power over the traditionally sacred domain of the dead. That this battle was fought partly in terms of the health of the living introduced a distinctly secular and modern element into the struggle, as we will see in the next chapter. The struggle to determine how the dead were disposed of crossed all classes, involving the upper echelons of the church hierarchy and the lowliest of gravediggers; however, this foray into the business of death was ultimately connected to the status of the Maya—their rituals, meanings, and worldview—in the modern order that the creole elite sought to build in Yucatán.

CHAPTER THREE

ON SACRED GROUND

Cholera, Burial Rites, and Cemetery Management

EARLY ONE OCTOBER MORNING IN 1853, don Esteban Herrera walked slowly toward his local church in the town of Cacalchén. As he would later testify, Herrera, the village's *juez de paz* (magistrate), was tired and worn after having spent the night in consultation with the priest and laying out about fifteen bodies end to end on the patio of the small church. He was plagued with visions of the pinched and bloated carcasses, victims of an ongoing cholera epidemic. In the last few months, demand for burial plots had far exceeded the capacity of the church grounds. Consequently, the bodies lay exposed until he could decide what to do. Herrera felt that the only realistic option was to bury the bodies outside of the pueblo in what would be a new general cemetery. But this plan touched on anxieties concerning the disposition of the dead felt by the many citizens of Cacalchén, who had experienced the loss of friends and loved ones to the illness. Many felt helpless and unfairly punished. Furthermore, it was easy to perceive the hurried construction of the new cemetery as another interruption in daily life exacted by the disastrous cholera epidemic.[1] As Herrera approached the gated entrance to the church patio, he picked up a tree branch and began to work his way through the dozens of dogs and pigs.[2] Herrera was frustrated that the priest permitted the families of the deceased to leave the infected bodies out overnight. He thought it was unsanitary and barbaric to allow the air to become infested with disease-causing "miasmas," harmful or poisonous airborne menaces thought to emanate from noxious wastes, decaying bodies, and, in particular, diseased corpses such as the cholera victims. Herrera's ideas about disease prevention were common among

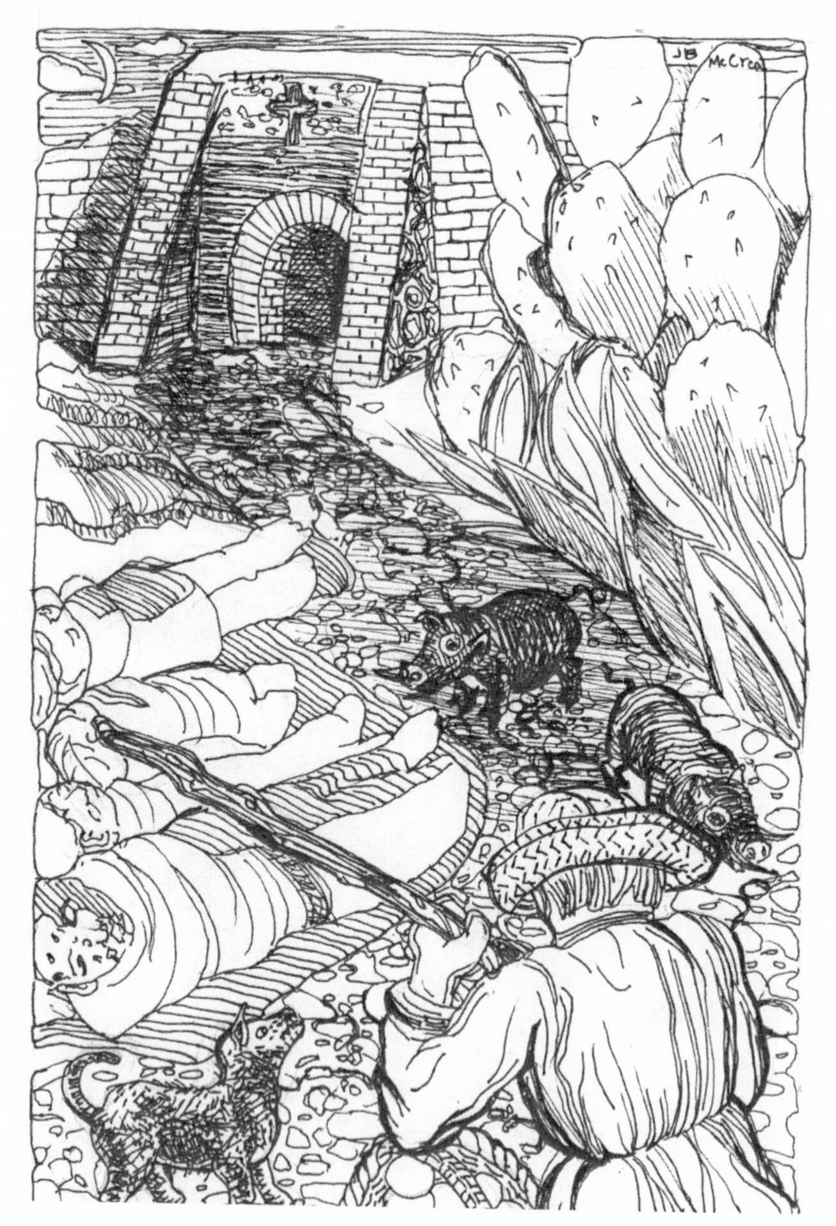

Figure 2: *Don Esteban Herrera and the Cacalchén Cemetery* by Judith B. McCrea.

laypersons and medical professionals of the time, who were dealing with a violent disease for which they had no ready-made theories. When cholera came to New York City in 1832, for example, a doctor there ascribed it to "a general distemperature of the air."[3]

Other issues plagued Herrera as well, like the reminder he received from the local priest about a Catholic canon that required a twenty-four-hour waiting period before burying the deceased. Then there were the residents, already aggravated and tense from the epidemic. Herrera knew that if he tampered with either Catholic or Maya burial traditions, especially overnight vigils and processions to the gravesite, he would face fierce protests. But if he was to obey the state public health laws, as was his civil duty, he would have to order immediate burials for disease victims. By the time Herrera had chased the animals out of the church grounds, a few laborers had arrived, and he ordered them to prepare the bodies for transport to the graveyard site outside of the pueblo. This provoked a number of complaints: one laborer asked Herrera how could he request such a thing, while another explained that the family of one little girl was still busy preparing her procession. The workers all grumbled that they had no time to work in their milpas (small agricultural subsistence plots); they wanted to know when promised grain supplements for their extra labor would arrive.[4] As we will see later, the way Herrera interpreted his job in this time of cholera brought down upon him the wrath of his formerly peaceful village. In this diseased moment, the structure of power was stripped of any disguise or ornament in the eyes of the townspeople, and the promise of power—the protection of the villager's life and limb—was considered to be broken. In this way, an epidemic was not only an event in natural history, but one in political history—a theme that will be developed in this chapter.

Herrera's problem was one shared by many local leaders in Mexico's southeastern states and the Yucatán Peninsula during the cholera epidemic of 1850–55. For religious and civil officials, this time of accelerated death presented a dramatic increase in workload, ultimately compromising community support networks as daily lives were thrown into the chaos of the epidemic. The struggle to locate suitable burial grounds and conduct a proper burial encompasses terrain wherein policy makers vied with clergy for authority over the sacred realm of death and the secular causes of disease. Coincidentally, the cholera epidemic erupted during a period in which Liberal reformers were seeking to curb the power and influence of the church after Mexico's independence from Spain was won in 1821. This supervenient set of political issues intensified the conflict over burial rituals and the management of cemeteries. In the political codes of the time, Liberalism in Mexico stood for secular nation formation and economic development by way of promoting Mexico's entrance into the global economy.[5] For the indigenous Maya, recently released from the subservience to the church enforced by the Spanish Crown, this age of Liberalism provided new opportunities. The Maya found they could publicly assert their right to manage their own rituals for healing the sick and mourning the dead without interference from the church. Negotiating for control over these rituals ultimately compromised the authority of state-sponsored public health campaigns. Consequently, the Maya were placed in the middle of a dispute between church and state over the sacred terrain of death.

As we saw in the previous chapter, the Maya and Yucatecans all confronted the catastrophe of smallpox epidemics. While the cause of smallpox remained unknown at the time, prevention presented certain dilemmas brought about by the dual use of inoculation and vaccination with human- and animal-derived serums. Yet the gap between cause and empirical evidence, plus continual waves of the disease, created an uncertain public health structure to contain smallpox until the very end of the century. With cholera, the disease moment had a different structure. Not only was the cause unknown until Robert Koch's discovery of *Vibrio comma* bacteria the 1880s, there was also no empirical tradition to rely upon. Instead, the medical establishment was divided worldwide between those who blamed cholera on distempered or "miasmatic" air and those who, following John Snow's research in London on the 1854 plague, blamed it on unclean water.

Further, some statesmen claimed that quarantines did no good, whereas others claimed cholera was contagious. Evidence connecting ships to the spread of cholera was especially damning to the former claim. For example, Dr. Augustin Pellarin's careful tracking of a cholera outbreak in 1865 on board the French ship *Sainte Marie* demonstrated the clear link between illness on board a ship and the appearance of illness at the port of entry. Landing at Pointe-à-Pitre, Guadeloupe, on October 20, 1865, the *Sainte Marie* had already lost one crewmember to an "undefined" illness before docking. The reaction of the regional officials figured into the dispute over quarantine as crewmembers disembarked directly after landing, returning to their homes and jobs. Within two weeks, the governor of Guadeloupe declared Pointe-à-Pitre and all island dependencies in quarantine. But it was too late. The disease spread quickly throughout the islands, killing just under twelve thousand people within six months.[6] Slowly, it became clear that the dejecta of the cholera victim spread the disease, inasmuch as it got on hands, into water, and into the systems of the victims, though the medical establishment was largely concerned with bad air up to the 1850s. The cholera pandemic of the 1850s was a "diseased moment" in which no faction in the struggle to contain cholera in Mexico was scientifically "right." Like almost no other disease of the nineteenth century, cholera illustrates the ways in which politics proceeds under cover of public health.

My examination of the 1850s cholera epidemic is divided into two levels of discussion. This chapter explores the struggle between the state and the church over control of major rites of passage in the lives of Yucatán citizens, which played out during the cholera pandemic that swept across the globe with fearsome rapidity. The next chapter explores the 1850s cholera epidemic in relation to the Caste War and the direct relationship of the state to Yucatecan pueblos.

In Mexico the pandemic intensified church-state struggles over the control of sacred domains. This study of graveyards and burial rites is situated within a broader understanding of Mexico's sociocultural, political, and economic history. The blurring and redrawing of the line between public and private spaces has provoked emotional and highly politicized debates over who should possesses authority, and to what degree, over birth, marriage, and death in many modernizing societies. Conflicts concerning interment customs were common in Britain as well as Mexico during the pandemics of cholera. Sheldon Watts has written of British reformers using the public health menace posed by the corpses of cholera victims to "smash" the moral worlds of the working class by banning wakes and the funerary ceremonies customary to the burial of loved ones.[7] The interment of the dead, particularly during disease epidemics, inserted powerful secular forces into the symbolic interactions that had formed the relationship between the household and the church or the gods. The historical roots of the conflicts over the regulation of cemeteries and the dead in Mexico may be found in the records of Spanish colonial administrators. As we shall see, postindependence narratives and quarrels recorded in newspapers and archival accounts show how claims concerning burial procedures and cemetery management restructured relationships between priest, parishioner, local magistrate, and citizen.[8]

This social theme becomes especially charged in an epidemic, when the sheer number of the dead and the fear of infection create stress and panic not only among the public, but among bureaucrats charged with controlling public order. In the 1850s, the popular recollection of the first cholera pandemic of the 1830s was still fresh. Having observed that cholera spread via shipping, physicians, public health workers, and police carefully watched the ports and tried to maintain control on the transference of goods and peoples when word about a second pandemic began to circulate in the United States and the Caribbean. Yet the disease could not be stopped from entering Mexico.[9] Cholera made its appearance just as Mexico was undergoing one of its chronic periods of acute political instability in the struggles between the Liberals and the Conservatives. The Conservative faction was in retreat under the onslaught of legislation introduced by reform-minded statesmen such as Miguel Lerdo de Tejada, the secretario de fomento (development), and Benito Juárez, the secretario de justicia (justice), and new laws were passed aimed at minimizing the privilege and power of the Catholic Church and military. The unlucky coincidence of the cholera pandemic of 1850–55 falling in a period when, in any case, the Mexican state was determined to take control of cemetery management and burials from the church was even more complicated in Yucatán, as Caste War violence threw into relief the contrast between tradition and the Liberal modernizers.

In Yucatán, the threefold intersection of the diseased moment of the cholera epidemic, the violence of the Caste War; and the governmental attempt to strip the church of its potent privilege as the ultimate organizer of burial policies and cemetery management helped transform the relationship between the state and its citizens during critical decades of postcolonial nation-building. Specifically, the way in which policy makers and clerics interpreted disease etiologies and concepts of contagion during midcentury epidemics informed their decisions regarding burial and death rites. The formation of new burial policies also underscored the sociopolitical agendas of Yucatecan statesmen who sought the triumph of "civilization" over the "barbarism" of the Maya in the Caste War. By identifying and demonizing rebels, statesmen delineated who would be included, marginalized, and privileged within the emergent nation-state.[10]

To understand how an outbreak of cholera could reinforce (and redefine) boundaries between those who were "civilized" and those who were "barbarians" in Yucatán, one need only consider its legacy as a disease bred in filth, unsanitary living quarters, and intemperate bodies. Drawing upon existing fears of the "other" or the "immigrant menace," cholera often reinforced existing divisions between elites, working poor, and rural peasants.[11] Cholera also killed at an alarmingly fast pace. Victims suffered from acute and rapid dehydration, explosive vomiting and diarrhea, and excruciating muscle cramps. In the final stages, the body is poisoned as renal failure sets in, flooding the body with toxins. Death could come after several hours or the malady could linger cruelly for days. After death, corpses were often bloated and took on a bluish hue that provided the disease with the name "blue-funk."

The first worldwide cholera pandemic in the 1830s originated in India where it was endemic, moved throughout Europe, and entered the Americas in 1832, traveling across the Atlantic to major port cities such as New York, New Orleans, Havana, and Veracruz. On the high plains of the American Midwest, Osage Indians lost about one-fourth of their population in 1834 due to "the cramps."[12] On July 30, 1832, thirty-nine people succumbed to cholera in New York City in one day. Many doctors simply stopped recording deaths. Dead bodies lay stacked in the streets awaiting burial, and coffin makers worked around the clock to meet demand.[13]

Cholera maintained a long history in the world's crowded urban centers where stagnate, contaminated water washed over food supplies and slid down the gullets of diners. Transferred through contaminated water supplies, cholera literally seeped into every fiber of daily life. In rural areas, where access to medical services remained scarce, cholera wiped out entire towns through shared sources of well and river water. Initial studies exploring the link between water and cholera began with British physician John Snow's study of waterborne bacteria in two London suburbs. Snow's work, published in 1856, concluded, "The population drinking dirty water accordingly appears to have suffered 3.5 times as much mortality [from cholera] as the population drinking 'other water.'"[14] In light of Snow's work on the origins of cholera, water sanitation became a primary concern for almost every region suffering from reoccurring bouts with cholera.[15] Snow's theories were confirmed in 1884 at the first international conference devoted to the cholera problem. At the conference, German bacteriologist Robert Koch presented his findings on the isolation of Vibrio comma, the bacterium that causes cholera. Cholera then became the first disease to be identified as water borne.[16]

Medical professionals throughout the world incorporated Snow's and Koch's scientific findings into existing etiological corpuses, often attributing the cause of infection to a combination of "bad air," "miasma," "bacilli," or "spores." For instance, in his address to the Tri-State Medical Society of Georgia, Alabama, and Tennessee on October 26, 1892, Dr. Joseph Holt noted that it is "never pleasant to risk immunity with sacrifice of considerable decency in having one's food swarming with bacilli and spores of cholera, or of yellow fever and small-pox in the air and over everything, killing pretty freely the unfortunate nonimmuned."[17] Dr. Holt combined old concepts of bad air "swarming" with the agents of diseases such as smallpox, yellow fever, and cholera with new notions that bacilli and spores in the air or on food caused illness. Ships in particular carried a reputation during cholera epidemics for harboring "bad air." Noting the need to protect mainland populations from tangible goods and peoples exposed to ship air, policy makers in port cities enforced strict quarantine and disinfection regulations for all incoming vessels during cholera outbreaks. In June of 1850, Yucatecan newspaper *Siglo XIX* ran an article by the French physician in residence in Campeche, Dr. Quin, about a small ship that left the neighboring state of Tabasco carrying two hundred men bound for Yucatán. Unconfirmed reports claimed that several of the crewmen and passengers died of cholera before reaching the port of Campeche. Dr. Quin advised, "If it is true, it will be fatal to offer help to those unfortunates on board, because the sanitary reality is severe, a justified position of observation should be taken from the peninsula, we cannot permit them to disembark, it is not possible to administer effective assistance, we cannot purify the air on board to a point of removing any doubt that miasmas continue to influence the healthy."[18]

While those in port communities understood the danger posed by incoming boats, cargo, and passengers to their health, for inland communities the connection between water and disease took a markedly different form. Yucatán's precarious water supply placed residents in a particularly vulnerable position in relation to cholera.[19] The peninsula's lack of internal tributaries or waterways complicated access to the fresh, clean water supplies that determined health and livelihood on a daily basis. Many rural communities relied on well water or water accumulated in natural sinkholes or cenotes for irrigation, cooking, and cleaning. If cholera bacilli infected one well or cenote, entire communities could fall ill within a matter of days. Without an alternative water source, cycle after cycle of disease persisted, depleting entire communities of nearly all residents and devastating the few who remained alive.

The immediate need of Yucatecan communities facing the casualties of the cholera epidemic in 1853 and in 1855 was to dispose of the multitudes of diseased corpses that accumulated so quickly and in such great numbers that they outran the capacity of traditional burial grounds.[20] The situation worsened with outbreaks of yellow fever in 1855 and smallpox in 1856.[21] Public health officials claimed that diseased corpses posed a public safety threat if they were not immediately and properly disposed of.[22] Drawing the dead into the realm of living law, public health officials crafted legislation specifically designed to avoid the spread of infection by mandating measures that would quarantine the dead and effectively neutralize any physical threat posed by diseased bodies, for instance, by forbidding wakes, traditional practices of washing the corpses, and so forth.[23] Such legislation posed serious challenges to Maya and Catholic rituals that included mourning for prolonged periods with the deceased prior to interment.

The principal actors in this important transitional moment—church officials, rural clerics, governors, legislators, public health administrators, doctors, local officials, and indigenous Maya—were all engaged with one another in a vast postcolonial struggle to extirpate (or preserve) vestiges of the nation's Spanish colonial past. Attempts to transfer power from Yucatán's Catholic Church to the Yucatecan state during the Reforma pulled the Maya peasantry into uncharted terrain, wherein religious loyalties and legislative compliance were not always compatible. Their relationships with local authorities, parish priests, and their communities were reconfigured as Liberal state officials widened their orbit of control over the ceremonies surrounding death and burial.

By situating local and regional struggles to cope with epidemic cholera in a larger matrix of tensions existing between Mexico's Catholic Church, Yucatán's nascent Liberal state, and medical opinion as reflected in public health policies, we can see Yucatecan politicians recognizing an opportunity to deal a blow to an already weakened Catholic Church with regard to the performance of funerary rites and the guardianship of burial grounds. Attempts by Liberal political elites to assert secular supremacy over the private lives of the suffering inhabitants during particularly harsh epidemics threw into question whose interests were truly being served. Yet the discourse of death was not unilaterally in the hands of the elite, nor was it simply a dialogue between the powers of the state and church. Rather, ordinary Yucatecans also invoked the language of health and public safety to promote their own goals, calling attention to the alleged negligence of state officials in protecting them from disease.

In October of 1855, a group of Maya villagers from Cacalchén,[24] referring to themselves as *los indígenas de este pueblo* (the indigenous of this town), filed a complaint with the superior tribunal justice of Yucatán against the pueblo's boss, don Esteban Herrera, for abuse of authority. According to residents, they, as citizens, had remained obedient to don Esteban Herrera for approximately five years and continued to show him respect when he was promoted from municipal justice of the peace to town commissary. The citizens of Cacalchén contended that they had remained silent and never raised their voices against their superior, "They were tranquil indígenas."[25] Yet they were finally forced to request Herrera's removal as magistrate because of his unfulfilled promises and the numerous abuses of his position. One section of the lengthy protest was devoted to Herrera's abuse of his position in demanding that residents work overtime and labor outside of their community boundaries. Allegedly,

Herrera took advantage of obligatory *fajina* labor agreements. The fajina in rural Yucatán often included work details in the *capilla* (small church) and community milpas. Commonly, surrounding the capilla grounds was a small area for grave plots.[26] The cholera epidemic of the 1850s unfortunately pressed against the limits of Cacalchén's capilla burial grounds. As a result, Herrera required his laborers to dig graves in a location outside of the pueblo. The villagers complained they were subjected to excessive and dangerous conditions and that cemetery work caused many residents to become ill.[27] The authors of the complaint also claimed the capilla priest was Herrera's accomplice in an effort to obtain free labor for the capilla and their private homes.

Herrera responded that there simply was no alternative but to require residents to dig graves outside of the pueblo because of the numerous deaths attributed to cholera. Cholera had claimed the lives of 933 people in the village, according to Herrera, in a matter of four months, from September to the end of December. Incredibly, the town's population had been halved.[28] Herrera's reply to the supreme justice drew attention to public health regulations that prohibited the burial of bodies within the patios and atriums of capillas. Herrera cited a legal article introduced in March of 1837 indicating that justices of the peace and commissaries were to "procure in each pueblo a conveniently situated cemetery."[29] Herrera admitted that several cholera victims were still "barbarically" buried in the capillas, but he was working to rectify the situation. It is possible that Herrera feared contagion if burials continued as they had in capilla atriums and near dwellings. We must try to imagine the suddenness of the epidemic and the inability of any of the participants to understand how contagion spread. It was invisible and fatal. Herrera was surely aware of the danger he himself faced. In his response, he claimed that he was only doing his job by deciding to locate burial grounds outside of pueblo limits for the well-being of all residents. According to Herrera, he acted with "humanity on behalf of the residents and the Indians of the pueblo."[30] Herrera also emphasized that most of the deceased were from the area, and thus he could see no reason that his request that the locals help bury their own should be considered abuse.

The subprefect of Motul district investigated the situation on January 16, 1855, and wrote to inform the justice of the peace of his findings. The subprefect's report exonerated Herrera and even praised him. He added it was natural that Herrera have some enemies, but people would always say bad things about Herrera because of his leadership position: "It is only natural, as in other epochs, that the workers hate their boss."[31] In the subprefect's cursory review of the Herrera case, Herrera decided to build a new cemetery outside of the pueblo because he had little recourse, inasmuch as the village of Cacalchén was suddenly inundated with an extraordinary number of corpses that could pose a danger to public health. The policy for these emergencies explicitly allowed the local commissary to use his discretion in such matters. Many Mexicans (following beliefs that were shared by European and American doctors) were convinced that cholera was transmitted by bad air. Thus, both popular and elite belief was that graveyards, located within town limits and filled to capacity with diseased corpses, might infect the air and sicken the entire community. In this context, Herrera's idea to build a cemetery outside of town was a seemingly reasonable alternative.

However, the subprefect ignored the laborers' claim that working in the graveyard caused more illness. In fact, many of the villagers must have wondered where Herrera's priorities lay. And whom was Herrera trying to protect during the cholera epidemic? If as many citizens in his district died of cholera as stated in Herrera's written defense, then his gathering of the labor pool posed a threat to the health of the village at least as great as the corpses piled in the church. Along similar lines, throughout the nineteenth century it was widely believed that contact with contaminated corpses was a risky endeavor. In Herrera's own filed responses, he never mentioned any measures taken either by himself or the capilla priest to fumigate the cemetery grounds or quarantine the diseased corpses. Yet, it is clear from Herrera's explanation of his actions that he was familiar with at least a few public health ordinances, which mandated such matters as the depth of graves, fumigations, and procedures for cleaning bodies.[32] Then why did Herrera not observe precautions in the new graveyard as stipulated by the public health policy of 1837, which he cited in his response? Municipal records also show that Motul district was assigned a public health council in May of 1850 and an agreement was formed in that same month to add more hospitals and quarantine stations in preparation for the cholera epidemic.[33]

Herrera was surely familiar with the common belief that cemetery work compromised workers' health, since nineteenth-century etiological doctrine held that airborne "miasmas" from decaying bodies infected the healthy. Surely, in a village suffering horrendous casualties in such a brief period of time, Cacalchén's residents had good reason to assume Herrera was needlessly placing them in danger. In addition, cemetery work was popularly disliked as degrading. Local work crews assigned to cemetery duties felt unjustly punished and complained vigorously when assigned to properties that included burial grounds.[34]

Cemetery work was also backbreaking labor. The limestone bed that the peninsula rests on made the task of chipping through the rock exceedingly difficult.[35] Furthermore, the seasonal late summer rains that usually preceded cholera epidemics brought an onset of tropical fevers that must have further complicated the burial of bodies. In fact, the rains, which would carry human waste runoff into the water supply, combined with the way in which the water supply was limited by the limestone subsurface was what made Yucatán villages so vulnerable to *Vibrio cholerae*. As testimony to the level of difficulty involved in burying bodies in Yucatán, cases were often reported of bodies buried in shallow group graves or in heaps aboveground—hidden only with a loose piling of rocks.[36] In instances of haste, rumors of live burials abounded, only serving to worsen the climate of fear so common during these outbreaks.[37]

The complaints of Cacalchén's indigenous residents reveal a gross and terrible failure of the institutions of governance. Herrera, the accused abuser, is an intermediary personage. Herrera was a village-level official who formed lateral alliances with other notables, like the priest, to handle a situation that was clearly a disaster. Investigation of the complaint against Herrera shows the indifference with which this information could be received despite the alarming circumstances bound within this "diseased moment." Half of the village of Cacalchén died in the space of four months. The discrepancy between the grounds for state interference and the success of that interference exposes the uneven nature of the relationship between resident and state. In this gap, one can infer a "hidden transcript" in which the people contrived their own explanation of these epidemics and of the state's indifference to the feelings of families.[38]

Late Colonial Hygiene Movements and Cemetery Sanitation

As I pointed out, state-church tensions over cemetery management and burial of the dead had already featured within postcolonial Mexican society. Undoubtedly, Spanish colonial traditions played a significant role in the creation of modern Mexican burial practices.[39] Strict procedures regarding corpse hygiene and burial locations were established in synch with waves of epidemic disease during the colonial period, in particular the major killers: smallpox, measles, and typhoid.[40] Local leaders consistently struggled to locate funds to build more cemeteries. Isolating those who died in epidemics required the combined efforts of priests and colonial magistrates, who had to compromise on reforming certain church traditions concerning burial. In particular, the tendency in the baroque period to bury the dead within the church or its immediate precincts was increasingly looked upon by medical authorities as a barbarous habit conducive to spreading disease. In accordance with King Carlos III's 1787 *cédula real*, colonial officials constructed cemeteries outside city limits. Unfortunately, in the case of late colonial Mexico, these objectives were never fully realized, and the church continued its practice of cramming entire families into crypts and mass grave pits within church grounds. The abundance of corpses was, of course, always acute during disease epidemics. Community members in the midst of epidemic episodes of smallpox, mysterious fevers, and other maladies feared the results of allowing the festering bodies of disease victims to be mixed with those who died of natural causes because family members would pay their respects to their dead loved ones and, presumably, be infected by the proximity of any actively contagious dead body. Yet space for the dead was at a premium, making such encounters hard to avoid.

Because of the limited amount of burial space in late colonial Mexico City, frequent exhumations were required in order to relocate corpses from crowded plots that were literally bursting through the soil.[41] As there was no consensus on how disease spread, it was reasonable to believe that any allegedly infectious bodies might contaminate the air, propagating further illness. Thus, one way of solving the problem was to effectively quarantine the infectious dead from the noninfectious dead, the latter of whom could be paid all the customary homage of traditional funeral rites and usages. However, as Western medicine turned more and more to lack of sanitation and hygiene as a cause of illness, any corpse became a potential multiplier of infection. Problems encountered in burying the dead led to an 1804 cédula real specifically prohibiting burials in *nichos*, under patios, and in church courtyards.[42] Despite these precautionary forms of legislation, and much to the disgust of colonial officials, many people's desire to have a family member or loved one buried under the gaze of saints within church grounds took precedence over royal decrees.[43]

Colonial officials also faced funding shortfalls in attempting to expand old graveyards and build new ones, since the Crown rarely made such funds available. The Crown's stinginess makes some sense: how could funds possibly be allocated to build or expand cemeteries when the empire was engulfed in debt? As Anne Staples so eloquently explains, "If they could not see to the needs of the living, it was more difficult to see to those of the dead."[44] The needs of the Crown were intricately bound up with the needs of colonial officials, whose subservience to the colonial order could be put at risk by either increased burial fees or a callous disregard for traditional funerary practices. William B. Taylor illustrates the clear connection between village insurrection and the raising of fees for burials, marriages, and baptisms during the late colonial period.[45]

The late colonial implementation of the Bourbon reforms was meant to tighten the grip of the Crown on its Latin American colonies. Restrictions on burial ceremonies and cemetery management emerged under the rubric of sanitation and hygiene doctrines. As early as the 1780s, Spanish ministers to New Spain were concerned about the practice of burying priests and wealthy elites under the floors of the church. In 1787 ministers in Veracruz, Mexico, ordered an end to such practices.[46] This initiative threatened to disrupt a long history of established pomp and circumstance accompanying funerals for the wealthy and the notables on church grounds. Furthermore, the placing of the dead as close as possible to saints and sacred shrines seemed to be a priority for many of Veracruz's elite and clergy, perhaps because of the belief that this ensured their placement in heaven.[47] Arrangement of the dead in close proximity to the altar reproduced the hierarchy of the living. D. A. Brading's work on Bourbon-era Mexico outlines a schedule of fees for burial and the regulations that allocated places for the dead and shows that only the Spanish received permission to be buried in the section of the church closest to the altar.[48]

Moreover, the reforms of the late colonial period, much like the ones set into motion by leaders of independent Mexico decades later, were justified firstly in terms of public health and secondly as a means to clamp down on what many officials perceived to be civil disorder in long and often drunken processions to gravesites and all-night vigils. In Yucatán, the attendees of these vigils were often Maya or mestizo, and they likely saw the suppression of traditional funerary rites as part of the dzules' (whites') endeavor to exert control over their communities by suppressing their cultural and religious practices.

Control of the Indian population here, as elsewhere, was subordinated in the years immediately following Mexico's independence to the politics of faction. What role would the Indians play in the formation of the new nation? How would they be integrated, if at all? After all, the church, and devotion to the Virgin of Guadalupe, encouraged many Indians and mestizos to fight in the wars for independence in the Bajío region in 1810.[49] But the church still held power after independence, and despite the Crown's seizure of all church property in New Spain in 1804, the church remained influential throughout New Spain during the final decades of rule under the Bourbons.[50] One of the first challenges the church faced after independence, after the Crown withdrew its patronage, was to address the needs of parishioners as citizens of the

Republic of Mexico, while keeping hold of privileges that the new state might have been tempted to take away. In the 1830s, state lawmakers began to see opportunities to assert their authority amid the overwhelming anxiety and hysteria that accompanied epidemics of smallpox and cholera. In response to the latter, lawmakers created emergency committees with the aim of firmly managing public order and minimizing hysteria. There had long been an intellectual rivalry between the Liberal elites and the church as the defender of the traditional order. These committees then became vehicles for Liberal-minded policy makers to wring power from the church by recommending a raft of legislation that would undermine the church's vast influence in the sphere of everyday life.

Mexican Liberal intellectuals, led by José María Luis Mora (1794–1850), began to lead anticlerical attacks in the 1830s with an assault against what Mora called "'the abuses of superstition' and upon 'the ambition and covetousness of the ministers of the altar.'"[51] In fact, Mora specifically criticized the church's monopoly on mortuary rituals and control of cemeteries in his indictment.[52] This transformation from the colonial forms of rule, which left many of the life passage rituals of ordinary people—most notably births and deaths—in the hands of the church, to independent systems of governance was not fully realized in some regions, particularly in the northern and southern periphery, until the Liberal victory that concluded the Liberal-Conservative wars in midcentury.

To forge the image of the Mexican republic in the minds of its citizens or create, in Benedict Anderson's phrase, an "imagined community," Liberal ideologues sought to set aside any mediator between the state and the individual. Laws such as Juárez and Lerdo laws, passed in November 1855 and June 1856, respectively, sought to displace the power of the church, limit its role in policy making, and reduce its privileges.[53] The Ley Lerdo did not single out the church—as many of the ultra-Liberals would have preferred—and also limited state ownership of public buildings such as schools, jails, and meeting halls. But the implementation of the Ley Lerdo did result in the mass auctioning of church lands and buildings, which subsequently passed into the hands of a few wealthy families.

The Liberal vision of Mexico should properly have swept away old forms. However, in public health, this was not the case. Instead, public health committees, legislation, and sanitation brigades of mid-nineteenth-century Mexico were grafted upon older institutions, such as the caste system and the protomedicamento (the colonial advisory committee on medical matters); the lines drawn between the colonial and postcolonial institutionalization of public health were rather messy.[54] As testimony to this murkiness, one need only examine the uneven regional implementation of the national Liberal legislation, crafted in the 1850s, that targeted church privileges and holdings. Yet neither the Ley Lerdo nor the Ley Juárez diminished the influence of church authorities on the regional level, particularly during moments of crisis associated with epidemics and warfare. Meanwhile, the federal state was too weak to speed up long-term change or enforce public health and sanitation legislation, busy as it was trying to ward off repeated threats to Mexico's national sovereignty, dealing with escalating international debt, and suppressing persistent rebellion throughout the countryside.[55]

One of the triumphs of the Liberals was to strip the church of its special privileges or *fueros* (including church courts and tithes). The very structure of the church's fees was subject to state mandates that forced a reduction in fees for such services as the last rites. Additionally, all cemeteries under church administration were placed under the control of state public health and hygiene divisions in 1856 and 1857. In many cases, fees for burials were terminated altogether.[56] However, every male taxpayer, including Indian *vecinos* (residents), was subject to an increased head tax, which included a percentage to be distributed to the church.[57] Church influence in state matters, such as the appointment of local *jefes* (regional bosses), was also questioned. In the Liberal vision of the Mexican republic, the breakup of church lands would result in the emergence of independent smallholders; the abolition of the church's power over marriages, baptisms, and last rites would create a more secular, progressive citizenry; and the state takeover of the recording of deaths and the handling of corpses would allow modern health-care policy to be implemented by the civil officials who took over these duties.

A key component in the state's attempt to weaken the church was the elimination of church fees for services. Sacramental fees were so high throughout the republic that, it was claimed, "in most cases it was the hacendado who paid the actual fees and then charged them to their peón's accounts. Marriage fees were so high that many couples did not marry."[58] A weakened church presented many advantages to the Liberals. For one thing, Liberal leaders hoped to encourage immigration, often from Protestant countries. For another, as historian Jan Bazant contends, "many liberals expected that if the land passed from the 'dead hand' of the church into the 'living hand' of capitalist-oriented landowners a significant economic boom and increasing stability would ensue."[59] Clearly, anticlericalism was ascendant in 1850s Mexico.

Ultimately, the Liberals' program did not produce the results they envisioned. The secularization of cemeteries robbed the church of power, but it also lifted the burden of expensive obligations to maintain cemetery grounds and oversee new construction,[60] which, since the sixteenth century, had constituted a sizable financial burden for local parishes.[61]

Yucatán's Major Political and Economic Turning Points, 1850–1900: Liberalism and Liberal Reforms

The reforms of Mexico's Liberal period, between the 1840s and 1860s, significantly reconfigured both Indian-state and church-state relations in Yucatán. However, the manner in which these relations were altered differed from central Mexico in that the majority of the population was still strongly loyal to the church, which operated as the surest anchor of colonialism. The success of Liberal reforms in Yucatán was hampered by the fact that the strong role the Catholic Church played in rural Maya communities made the church a necessary ally in early Caste War negotiations with rebels. Many of the rural parish priests in Yucatán were versed in Maya customs, and some even spoke Yucatec Maya, making their role as negotiators invaluable.

Because many priests like José Canuto Vela maintained strong relationships with Maya communities, the state desired to use their tacit knowledge and negotiating skills to prevent the spread of violence and insurrection during the early phases of the Caste War.[62] José Canuto Vela was commissioned by Yucatecan bishop José María Guerra to head a mission of priests to interview the rebels and draft a peace pact. Vela spoke Maya, a skill other powerful clergymen like Bishop Crescencio Carrillo y Ancona, archbishop of Yucatán from 1887 to 1897, did not overlook as instrumental in reaching the sentiments of the rebel Maya. Also well known for his skills as an orator, Vela delivered sermons in Spanish and Maya throughout the peninsula, particularly in rebel strongholds like Chan Santa Cruz in southeastern Yucatán.[63] Vela's relationship with parishioners illustrates vital linkages between indigenous communities.

Relationships between the state, Maya rebels, and the church shifted to address the circumstances brought about by the Caste War. While church officials maintained authority in many realms of Yucatecan society throughout the Reforma, ultimately Reforma legislation of the 1850s replaced church influence with state power.

By the terms of the Ley Lerdo, the state exercised control over burial rites by requiring death certificates to be endorsed by state employees. Additionally, strict regulations were implemented to quarantine any corpse considered dangerous to public health, making it that much harder for the family members and priests to perform vigils and the rites customarily given to the dead at the gravesite (for instance, the display of the body in the casket, etc.). Hence, by entering the private realm through public health campaigns and policy that made the state the intermediary in some of a family's most charged and intimate moments, the state forged for itself new tools for social control. *Social control* implies control over disorderly conduct, but the symbolic power acquired by the state in creating a collective imaginary of citizens was important. For instance, one of the weapons Liberalism used against the church was the inclusion of article 15 in the 1857 Constitution allowing for freedom of religion. The passing of the legislation in December 1860 articulating *libertad de consciencia* (freedom of conscience) allowed the state to take religion out of the educational curriculum. Libertad de consciencia helped bolster the state's efforts to enforce religious tolerance.[64]

Liberalism in Mexico was also in itself a key doctrine of nation formation and economic development.[65] Historian Annick Lempérière sees Mexico's reform laws, particularly Ley Lerdo, as a vehicle for the creation of "neutral spaces, ones liberated from religious connotations and identifications, at the disposition of state authorities, who could then utilize these spaces for the exclusive presentation of symbols and ceremonies that stressed national and republican identity."[66] On the regional level, state public health and hygiene departments absorbed these neutral spaces. Yet it would be a mistake to read this history in a totalizing manner that reduces the citizen to a passive bystander. As the state attempted to seize symbolic power over the disposition of the dead from the church, the neutral spaces that emerged were used as well by other parties. For instance, in Yucatán, the indigenous Maya seized the opportunity to assert the necessity of their own rituals for healing the sick and mourning the dead—rituals that ultimately came into conflict with the authority of the state and its public health campaigns.[67]

In their attempts to assert authority and prove their scientific knowledge in regard to disease epidemics, civil officials and the leaders of national public health committees utilized the print media to emphasize the importance of disease prevention and containment to a constituency of educated Mexicans. The print media ran serials about tonics and measures to ward off cholera during the first epidemic of the 1830s, broadcasting a clear message to every citizen: obey the public health policies in place and take personal responsibility for preventing the proliferation of disease in your own neighborhood and family to save the nation; above all, avoid superstitious practices.[68] For example, the Campeche newspaper, *El Fénix*, published a series of medical case studies, conducted by the "famous El Dr. Foy," that demonstrated the importance of personal sanitation and temperance in remaining healthy and disease free. The editor's introduction to the "Dr. Foy" serial stated that the doctor's advice on disease prevention was intended to awaken the public and avert "sleeping in the arms of a vain confidence."[69] Dr. Foy's advice about cleanliness and hygiene was probably read with great interest by the small group of educated Yucatecan elites among whom newspapers circulated. However, it probably found few readers among the rural, monolingual, and mostly illiterate Maya. In this way, the expansion of the media sphere among the urban elites increased the isolation of nonurban Maya communities, since the ebb and flow of mainstream disease prevention information no longer came through the church. As Maya isolation grew, so, too, did the elite notion that the Maya were either ignorant of or resistant to modern Western medicine.

Liberal policy makers thought restricting the role church officials played in community matters was a necessary means to legitimate state public health policies. Unless the role of the church could be minimized in community welfare and the ties between citizens and their parish loosened, reasoned Yucatecan statesmen, the peninsula would never emerge from the "backward" traditions of colonial rule. However, making the church dependent on the state for its maintenance and improvement funds irrevocably crippled many rural parishes, a situation that, while it ultimately undermined the power of the church and strengthened the role of the state, often left communities without an advocate to intervene against powerful exploiters.[70]

An additional blow to the church's ability to assert its traditional authority in many rural pueblos can be partially attributed to a lack of recruits to fill vacant posts left by elderly clerics. These vacancies were noted in 1853–55 when the second cholera pandemic entered Yucatán. Many older priests fell victim to epidemic diseases and "tropical" fevers during the second pandemic.[71] The decline in the peninsula's priest population left many pueblos without the services of priests to perform last sacraments, confessions, and burials.[72]

Nonetheless, scholars have argued that the church continued to play a critical role in Yucatán during a time when liberal reformers throughout the republic launched offensives against church power.[73] To some degree, the Catholic Church in Yucatán was spared the worst excesses of this anticlericalism; the Caste War perhaps best explains why. Church officials played a critical role as intermediaries between the state military and Maya rebels. Perhaps unknowingly, rural priests provided statesmen with an "in-field" monitoring system of the Maya masses, which was utilized by a struggling state militia in their attempts to contain the rebellion.

The Social Politics of Cemetery Construction

Disputes regarding where and how a person could be buried, especially during disease epidemics, surfaced as a pivotal issue in the struggle for legitimacy between the state and church. Yucatán lawmakers appealed for cemetery construction, or extensions of existing grounds, with increasing urgency during the 1840s and 1850s due to the extraordinary death toll from disease and violence. Local leaders found a way to acquire facile popularity by requesting additional burial grounds, since this need was sorely felt by afflicted families. Thus, the graveyard became a sort of monument to their own political careers while at the same time providing citizens with their own personal physical landmark, one that embodied valued notions of ancestry and *patria* (fatherland).

In an appeal to the governor of Yucatán in April of 1841, the vice-counsel of Great Britain, who resided in Villa del Carmen, a small island off the eastern coast of the peninsula in the modern-day state of Quintana Roo, requested an extension to the existing city cemetery in order to accommodate non-Catholic foreigners. The request was denied on the basis of the fact that additional cemetery space for non-Catholic foreigners could not take priority when space was so clearly needed for Catholic nationals.[74] Although most all of Mexico's cemeteries were supervised by city public health organizations by the 1840s, religious affiliation still seemed to matter a great deal in determining a family's burial rights. Clearly, state burial legislation, still in its infancy, was liable to quite malleable interpretations on the part of local office holders. The ruling by the state public health commissioner regarding the Villa del Carmen graveyard illustrates the ever-present tug of tradition on political decisions that were, supposedly, meant to elevate the political and secular over the religious.[75]

A decade later, the request for the graveyard was finally granted, and a cemetery was built on the edge of town facing the ocean. The approval for cemetery construction was granted with the strict proviso that only non-Catholic foreigners were to be interred in the graveyard. Thus, the old colonial social world was still preserved among the dead. Later on, the cemetery was moved to the margins of the city to make way for the growing population of Villa del Carmen. The cemetery also remained under the control of its respective foreign consuls. The citizens of Carmen were particularly proud of the "foreign" cemetery. They felt that the construction of the foreign cemetery set a good example of religious tolerance for non-Catholics and that their recognition of other "cults" in the current epoch was commendable considering "how reminiscent it [was] of the colonial period when any religious intransigence was prohibited throughout the Republic."[76] The Carmen cemetery marked a pivotal point for public health policy concerning cemetery construction in the peninsula. Separation from "living space" became a key feature of how cemeteries were organized and laid out during disease epidemics. Anxieties over the reproduction of pestilence contributed to legislation regarding when and where diseased corpses could be buried.[77]

Fear of contagion was also linked to those who traveled between ports where diseases were rumored to lurk, which was rational with regard to cholera. Newspapers and doctors plotted the first reports of cholera throughout Latin America against the arrival of ships and could often find the exact ship that brought contaminated cargo and people infected with cholera to a given landing. U.S. consul Henry Perrine's experience with the 1833 outbreak of cholera in Campeche is relevant. Perrine carefully tracked the ship that departed Tampico with sick aboard, evaded quarantine after docking in Campeche, and subsequently spread the disease throughout the port city and inland. Perrine explained after the ship "eluded" quarantine that "prevailing winds" helped spread the disease "towards all points of the compass, and of course to the Eastward, in the very teeth of the trade wind. . . . Some plantations to which no person has been admitted, have escaped the desolation of others around them, as we learn by persons who have left these still healthy positions."[78]

In general, the populace targeted foreigners, migrant workers, and military personnel as carriers of contagion. Therefore, a public health policy that required the quarantine of foreign victims of the disease both before and after death, based on risk factors and not religious orientation, would have made sound etiological sense. Instead, what we see reflected in the burial pattern in the Carmen cemetery is that public health officials did not determine the place of burial according to contagion, and this in a port city with a high immigrant population, but were influenced by a number of social factors, including the social status of those who requested cemetery construction and their relationship to civil administrators. Foreign-controlled cemeteries would also be difficult to tax. Moreover, authorities did not always regard the relinquishment of land for cemeteries as mutually beneficial to both the government and the immigrant community since it cost the state land that could have been developed toward ends that were more profitable.

In many cases, the conditions under which new cemeteries were constructed required that the official responsible obtain clearance in advance from the public health council. For many rural priests this requirement seemed unnecessarily intrusive, especially when the cemetery was intended exclusively for members of the church hierarchy. The extra steps that priests had to endure in order to obtain permission to move, extend, or build a new church cemetery must have seemed animated not by a regard for the public health so much as a disregard for the church.

To step outside of Yucatán, examples of conflicts about cemeteries abound in the archives for other sections of the country. A good example of the way these things went is an exchange that was initiated on November 26, 1852, by the priest for Santa Cruz y Soledad in Mexico City, José Antonio Fostanéll. The priest wrote the following note to the Federal District government: "Construction has begun on a small *panteón* in the interior holdings of this parish, ultimately all nichos [tiny spaces] will be well constructed, and ventilated according to all of the Salubridad's requisites for cadavers."[79] He then went on to explain that the bodies of many priests, buried in 1806, were exhumed and awaiting reinterment into better-ventilated areas. Fostanéll also added that he would personally supervise all the necessary public health precautions during the relocation.[80] By beginning work on a new panteón without first obtaining permission from state public health officials, Fostanéll could be seen as undermining their authority. For Forstanéll, the desperate need to relocate the bodies of the priests preempted the state's health codes, in effect placing the needs of the church above the laws of the state.

When the Federal District's public health commission responded by approving the panteón, they also took the opportunity to remind Fostanéll that it was inappropriate to begin construction without the necessary approval; however, as the bodies had already been exhumed, the commission granted the authority to proceed. They reiterated the benefits of burial regulations implemented in 1841, policies of which priests of Fostanéll's standing were well aware. Finally, the commissioner José Manuel Reyes emphasized that the inhabitants of Mexico enjoyed "great advantages that were not observed in the past" thanks to forward-thinking policy makers and their judicious public health policies.[81]

What is interesting about the Fostanéll-Reyes exchange is that Fostanéll initiated it after he had already begun construction on the new cemetery.

Perhaps someone passed by the site and warned the priest that he was in violation of civil code. The tone of Fostanéll's communiqué is drenched with indignation, as if compliance with civil policy was an obstruction to his lofty goals. From Reyes's perspective, Fostanéll's presumption that permission was merely a formality was unacceptable. Thus, Reyes's response brims with official verbiage—such as verbatim quotes of policy articles—to support Reyes's equally lofty goal of promoting the welfare of humanity. Ostensibly for Fostanéll's sake, Reyes paints a portrait of the importance of civic duty by outlining the great advantages that public health policies provided Mexico's citizens. Did Reyes expect the further circulation of his reply? We might ask why else would Reyes make such a fuss about a relatively routine permit in order to elucidate the value of civil policy. Surely, underneath the official business, Reyes was also reminding Fostanéll who was in charge in the new postcolonial order.

Ultimately, Fostanéll was not fined or charged with any misconduct, although he had undoubtedly placed the commission in an awkward position when he informed them that exhumations had begun; stalling the completion of the cemetery would have led to more trouble than it was worth, what with recently exhumed bodies awaiting reburial and, presumably, presenting some public health threat. Fostanéll's seeming resistance to cemetery codes also demonstrated to civil authorities that he believed himself above their reproach. However, Reyes's reprimand was intended to remind Fostanéll that appropriate procedures for cemetery construction had to be obeyed even by the church. Fostanéll's disregard for policy could arguably be considered a mishap or an oversight. What is interesting for the historian in this small episode of interaction between the two officials is that the language in which it was conducted mirrors the shifts in the sociopolitical orientation of Mexican society at large. It was a language edging toward contempt and violence, as though positioning the two players, Reyes and Fostanéll, in two different cultures and countries.

Maya Concepts of Death and Burial Rites

For classical Maya culture, the image of decay and disease surrounding the corpse so common in European representations of death had a much different meaning, as death held the possibility of reincarnation into new life forms (animal, mineral, or vegetable). It is possible that this belief survived to some extent among nineteenth-century Maya, making graveyards, for them, sacred locations where life either continued or was in transition. Yet here we hit upon a blank in our knowledge. Conclusions concerning nineteenth-century belief systems of the Yucatec Maya are suspect at best, given the biases through which our information about the Maya—from officials, travelers, and the military—are filtered. However, some speculation based on knowledge of ancient and contemporary Maya funerary rites can shed light on why the Maya resisted civil legislation that prohibited extended worship at the gravesite and required almost immediate burials of disease victims.[82] Many nineteenth-century Maya may have held on to a view of the afterlife that included reincarnation, as dictated in the origin myth of the Popol Vuh. They may have worshipped according to a syncretic combination of folk belief and Christianity. We know that one syncretic belief—that of the talking cross—played a central role for the Maya rebels in the Caste War. In any case, such beliefs would dictate that the deceased's family needed to remain close to the gravesite and to pray for the victim until his or her soul finished its journey. Therefore, nineteenth-century Maya likely did not view the graveyard, even at the peak of an epidemic, as a "cesspool" of infection, as did most educated creoles. It was common practice to mourn the dead for "a considerable time, in silence during the day and with loud wailing by night."[83] Fasting and abstinence were also part of the grieving process. Thus, the Maya view that their people's burial places should be in close proximity to their homes would have stood in stark opposition to state authorities' desire to isolate cemeteries outside of urban centers and to halt the practice of burying the dead under church patios.

The need to have a funeral ceremony for the deceased and to have the body buried close to home was also an important marker of status for the bereaved person in a Maya community. More was at stake for those who grieved than the individual right to continue with their nightly rituals at gravesites and burials under the patios of church floors; social standing as well was keenly articulated in mortuary rites. The more in attendance at a funeral, the more revered the deceased became after death. During both the colonial and national periods, funerary presentation and gravesite mourning were intimately intertwined with visual declarations of status. Anthropologist Aubrey Cannon contends, "Mortuary patterns are in a class with fashions in dress, luxuries and etiquette."[84] In Maya communities, public displays of grief and homage to the dead served as visual testimony to the deceased's life. The Maya custom of visiting the place of the dead one year after their passing is still in effect today. On the day of the visitation, the whole family, friends, and neighbors gather at the gravesite to pray for the "salvation of the soul of the deceased."[85] Special dishes (breads and tamales) are made, and typically a rice drink (*horchata*) is placed on the grave along with flowers and candles. Linkages between contemporary and nineteenth-century funerary practices facilitate an understanding of the ritual continuities that survived from the colonial era to the present day. The burial site has always been an important focal point for directing grief, prayer, and homage to the dead. Certainly, then as now, the location of the place of burial held a symbolic and social importance toward which public health officials and the creole elite were blind or dismissive. Moreover, nineteenth-century public health recommendations dictating the removal of diseased corpses from local cemeteries and a speedy burial violated Maya funeral rites on a very personal and intimate level. For instance, many Maya believed that if the body of the deceased were not properly bathed, cloaked, and pointed in one of the four cardinal directions,[86] their soul would not reach its proper destination.[87]

Conflicts of Custom: Burial Rituals and Public Health Policy

Thus it was that the burial place of the dead became a focal point in the matrix of struggles that defined all sides in Yucatán in the nineteenth century. While these struggles emerged over everyday occurrences of death, in times of crisis, such as an epidemic, the clashes became more overt, and the semi-covert strategies used by the church and the Maya to get around state directives came to the surface. State and national public health policy concerning the burial of corpses during disease epidemics aggravated already strained relations between the church and state over cemetery management.[88] Since Maya burial traditions had become syncretized with Catholic rites during the colonial period, the implementation of new public health policies radically disrupted these sacred rituals. In addition, under cover of the scientific fight against disease, political dynamics frequently governed policy, rather than it being a rational response to a particular disease epidemic. An examination of the inconsistencies in public health policy as it functioned within these disease moments reveals the disconnection between the rural indigenous Maya, local politicians, and national leaders, who were struggling for power over the community rather than for the protection of community members.

In Mexico City, lawmakers and elites manipulated, contested, and at times ignored official policies concerning the burial of cholera victims. Well into the cholera epidemic of the 1850s, the director of the Superior Health Council in Mexico City received several reports from state and local officials concerned with the upkeep of local graveyards. Many priests, local politicians, and police wrote to confirm that they were trying to uphold legislation that required cholera victims to be buried separately and in open spaces.[89] However, many of these letters also complained of the insurmountable challenges their writers faced in acquiring enough burial plots for *coléricos* (cholera victims). In essence, those engaged in the task of managing burials and handling diseased bodies attempted to communicate to the council that new burial legislation did not take into account the unique conditions of each cemetery, nor the near collapse of the system in the event of epidemic deaths. To the contrary, burial legislation actually impeded the ability of local officials to bury bodies in a timely and sanitary manner.

The need of families to grieve according to their customs created another layer of difficulties for those entrusted with the enforcement of burial legislation. Suddenly, family visits to the cemeteries had to be coordinated with civil officials and cemetery management: only a limited number of persons could congregate in the graveyard at one time—and never at nightfall.

If proper protocol was not followed, then complaints had to be filed, producing endless paperwork, fines had to be collected, and banishments enforced. For example, in a suburb of Mexico City, in the Panteón del Campo Florida, a government official named Noriega, after hearing several residents complain about the manner in which cholera victims were buried in the Florida cemetery, sent the councilman from the Eighth Quarter, S. Ramon Duarte, to visit the cemetery in order to "discover whether the dispositions of the Council were being upheld."[90] In a letter to the secretary of the council, Noriega wrote that Duarte had found that the bodies of coléricos were sometimes being buried in the same hole or ditches where rubbish was thrown—clearly a violation of council ordinances. Councilman Duarte spoke to the ecclesiastic in charge of the graveyard and recommended immediate compliance with council regulations. Duarte also explained exactly what those requirements were, so that a "complete and full understanding could be reached."[91] The council responded to Noriega's correspondence on January 23 and agreed that the cemetery at Campo Florida should comply, but without scheduling any further inspections. Given the massive number of corpses to be disposed of, it is likely that the violation of council regulations for coléricos at the Florida graveyard was not an exceptional occurrence. Although many local officials took legislation dictating where and when coléricos could be buried seriously, it is evident that sanitation violations at local pantheons and cemeteries must have eluded an understaffed and underfunded public health bureaucracy quite often during the chaos of epidemics. We also see evidence for this conclusion in the relatively light punishments the council administered when infractions were confirmed at local cemeteries. Consequently, we may ask to what extent cemetery maintenance figured as an important preventative against cholera infection in the minds of policy makers. The ordinary citizens of, for instance, Panteón del Campo Florida might have felt that the discrepancy between the rule and the enforcement showed either corruption or disarray in the government. We know, at least, that they were not at all satisfied.

The inconsistencies in burial policies throughout the republic motivated some Yucatecan lawmakers to consult sources outside of their nation's boundaries for advice. In May of 1850, Mérida's *El Siglo XIX: Boletín Oficial del Gobierno de Yucatán* published a series of articles from Havana's *Diario de la Marina*. One of the essays declared that burial of all corpses should not begin before a sixteen-hour waiting period had passed. In case of death by disease, the victim should be burned and all measures to ensure a thorough burning implemented for the well-being of the municipality. With the passing of new burial legislation, all interments in Havana required the presence of at least two officials to oversee the entire process.[92] Furthermore, no bodies should be buried in tiny nichos, or nooks, or in private patios. Additionally, no private burials were allowed, due to several reports of live burial.[93]

Yet Yucatán did not, like Cuba, adopt a homogeneous burial protocol. Different regions had different waiting periods, and there were no uniform burial policies in place to deal with the midcentury epidemics. In the Mérida-Sisal district of Yucatán, for instance, burial regulations only required a two-hour waiting period. Why the large differential in burial times? What was the reasoning behind burial policies? Furthermore, what were the factors that determined whether one waited two or sixteen hours before burial? To some degree, the variations in burial policies corresponded to the different schools of medical and scientific thought concerning disease prevention. While some public health and medical professionals remained firmly devoted to the benefits of quarantine, others were already beginning to notice that by the peak of an epidemic, quarantine seemed useless. By midcentury sanitation experts were proposing a solution to the disease's spread based on cleanliness, which meant street cleanings and public fumigations.[94] However, it is also reasonable to assume that local public health officials, when confronted with a variety of options, simply chose a system that best suited their district's access to graveyard labor, land, and medical supervisors. In fact, laypersons came to understand the practical connection between filthy drinking water and illness before the dissemination of Dr. Snow's findings in the mid-1850s connecting the two. José Miguel Ortiz, the justice of the peace for the small coastal town of Seybaplaya, located south of the port of Campeche, wrote to the district jefe político in August of 1853 to complain about the poor state of sanitation in his town. Ortiz accused the residents of allowing "water to stand and collect deadly venoms compromising public health."[95] Historian Nelson Reed also claims that Caste War rebels intentionally poisoned drinking wells with the clothes of cholera victims in an attempt to cripple state military advances against their strongholds in southeastern Yucatán, which points to a folkloric belief that water communicated cholera.[96]

The availability of labor could very well have been a key reason as to why Mérida's mandatory pre-interment waiting period was significantly less than Havana's. The labor pool for cemetery work was predominately derived from the Maya peasantry and subsequently had been weakened and compromised by the Caste War.[97] In the execution of Havana's burial legislation, an official had to oversee the entire burial or cremation process, but it would be impossible to fulfill such requirements during the height of an epidemic, when a shortage of labor of all kinds was extreme. Moreover, the pre-interment waiting period of two hours in Mérida would have given rise to hasty burials and backlogged interments, clearly exemplified by the Cacalchén case. In an effort to expedite burials during the cholera epidemic of the 1850s, the prefect of the Mérida-Sisal region decided to do away with official supervisions of burials. Hence, how proper pre-interment times were decided, and who made the official decisions, became the point of an obscure grassroots struggle between priests complying with the religious canon, including mandating an all-night vigil for the victim, and local officials applying the civil ordinances requiring almost immediate burial.

Specifically, a Yucatecan civil mandate passed in 1854 called for victims of contagious diseases to be buried no more than two hours after death to prevent the proliferation of "miasmas" into community air, in accordance with established medical opinion that blamed cholera on bad air. Whatever the doctors said, however, this particular dictum infringed on Catholic and Maya burial rites. In June of 1854, Mérida's governor, Rómulo Díaz de la Vega, wrote a memo to the superior political governor of the Department of Yucatán noting that the municipal commissary, don Estebán Campos, had ordered all victims to be buried within two hours after death.[98] Campos was concerned about the recent deaths of several victims of *vómito prieto* (yellow fever) in the Yucatecan port town of Sisal and thus ordered rapid burials to prevent the spread of the disease. However, compliance with the commissary's order was impossible because a certain Gómez, who held the only key to the cemetery, would not open the gate because he abided by church canons, which prohibited the interment of a body until twenty-four hours after death.[99] To further complicate matters, no medical doctor was allowed to examine the deceased because of Campos's concern regarding contagion from the corpses. With attention paid to every detail, the gatekeeper also insisted on seeing a medical doctor's report. Enormously frustrated, Governor Díaz de la Vega respectfully requested that authorities order don Campos to not impede future burials and to "avoid all manner of differences with ecclesiastic authorities."[100]

In the case of don Campos and Governor Díaz de la Vega, the church's struggle to maintain control over at least the most coveted elements of burial was more than symbolically important. The Díaz de la Vega–Campos interchange highlights the very essence of church-state struggles in the private sphere, with mounting state demands being met by various forms of resistance by the clergy. The interference with Catholic rituals was as much a political as a health matter, intended to undermine clerical authority in everyday affairs. Moreover, it is clear that the struggle for legitimacy between church and state often superseded the desires of residents who were quite directly affected by inconsistencies in burial and cemetery management. The citizens often seemed sidelined in these struggles, and one must read between the lines of official documents and newspapers to get a sense of how ordinary people improvised in the face of epidemic disaster. The struggle between Campos and Governor Díaz de la Vega continued throughout the 1850s and 1860s.[101] Whenever possible, Campos seized the opportunity to send workmen to the church burial grounds for routine fumigations, and he ordered exhumations for the purpose of relocation. Díaz de la Vega continued to write letters of protest fraught with a deep contempt for public health officials and their seemingly blatant disregard for sacred rituals. Díaz de la Vega always emphasized how much more complicated his job as a caretaker in the community was made by the ignorant policies of the public health department.[102] More importantly, Díaz de la Vega was angered by the usurpation of his local power, yet it is easy to imagine that Campos envisioned himself as the enlightened messenger of an informed doctrine for disease prevention.

By 1857, with the learning experience of two cholera pandemics behind them, policy makers devised a new set of public health policies for use in the capital. Juan J. Baz, governor of the District of Mexico City, revamped district laws regarding the use of cemeteries during epidemics. One important regulation required medical doctors to issue certificates of death (which would certainly take longer than the two hours Mérida's Campos envisioned between death and interment); in addition, all autopsies, embalmments, and mummifications were now to be performed under the supervision of the proper authorities.[103] Furthermore, cemeteries were to be divided into six parts: four sections for those who died of common illnesses, a fifth section designated solely for cholera victims, and a sixth for victims of other contagious epidemics. Additionally, exhumations, for whatever purpose, were strictly forbidden in the case of cholera victims. Due to the dramatic increase in deaths during the 1850s cholera epidemic, public health experts felt it was necessary to implement precautions within cemeteries to prevent the proliferation of disease throughout neighboring communities. The work of Snow and others in England, pointing to impurities in the water supply, had still not been absorbed in Mexico. Instead, medical authorities advised the maintenance of sanitary conditions in cemeteries that required more labor for routine fumigations and scourings. In the public's eyes, steps had to be taken to prevent the seepage of "miasmas" from the grave into their homes. These steps included disinfecting entire cemeteries with sulfuric dust, cleansing the victims of cholera (before and after death) with harsh bichloride of mercury (a highly poisonous compound used as an antiseptic), and burning all items in the victim's vicinity.[104]

While the new order for graveyards mandated the physical quarantining of diseased corpses, separate sections for children and the ecclesiastical orders were allowed to remain. The president of the republic himself, Ignacio Comonfort, ordered that archbishops and bishops be buried exclusively in the cemeteries of their convents and other privileged places.[105] Animals (for instance, dogs) were not to be allowed in the cemeteries, and customary dances and celebrations were no longer permitted for the death of children. Also, there were to be no burials in temples, chapels, sanctuaries, or other enclosed locations. Clearly, the separation of church and state in the Republic of Mexico was intended to extend to every level of social activity, in essence creating a new species of republican dead. Yet for Yucatecans, what might have seemed a tolerable imposition by the state in normal times may have been much less tolerable during moments of moral crisis. The ban on processions and all-night vigils for the dead were particularly difficult to follow. But perhaps the most devastating result of such legislation was the permanent separation of a deceased family member from family burial plots if they had the misfortune to die of an epidemic disease.[106]

But the church was not only experiencing trouble maintaining its traditional rites and ceremonies due to state laws; it had financial woes as well. In many ways, the costs associated with numerous burials crippled the church's ability to recover operating funds to maintain parishes and grounds. For example, the pueblos of Pomuch and Poc-Boc,[107] auxiliaries of the Hecelchacán parish, suffered severe reductions in their populations during the summer of 1855 due to successive waves of cholera and smallpox. In a quarterly report to the Department of Yucatán, the *cura* of Hecelchacán, Eugenio A. Ortíz, recorded only six contributors in Pomuch and five in Poc-Boc. Writing on behalf of his parishioners, Ortíz explained that the inhabitants of both pueblos felt that the required fees for the performance of baptisms, assignations, and marriages were prejudicial and unfair because of the high number of burials that both pueblos were obliged to finance.

During the most devastating epidemics, timely access to burial grounds and transportation of bodies required careful organization and labor that was often impossible to effectively coordinate. Again, U.S. consul Henry Perrine's account of the 1833 cholera outbreak in Campeche vividly illustrates how the sheer magnitude of dead bodies overwhelmed communities:

> Very soon, coffins ceased to be made, and graves to be dug. An armed force alone, could compel assistance for the dying or the dead of the hospitals. Propositions to burn the bodies, were substituted by shallow excavations in the sand of the sea shore, as a less laborious measure. The corpses of the most respectable persons were slung in net hammocks to a pole, and carried by two men, to some separate hole which they scraped among the bushes. The mass of dead bodies were piled up in loads like logs, and carted to the common ditch on the shore, where they were laid in rows an covered with a few shovelsfull of sand.[108]

In neighboring British Honduras, competent burial policies were also marred by inconsistent policies and a lack of manpower to facilitate proper management of mass graves during cholera, yellow fever, and smallpox epidemics. In 1852 the head of the Public Health Board, Dr. John Young, inspected a hospital in the capital and commented on the despicable conditions of the facility, which included damp areas stacked with cholera-ridden corpses.[109] Unable to transport the bodies promptly to burial locations, Dr. Young feared that patients in recovery could become ill simply by remaining in the hospital. Although the Public Health Board of British Honduras required immediate burial of all victims of contagious diseases, labor shortages in some districts prevented these measures from being realized.[110]

The labor problem was temporarily resolved shortly after Dr. Young's inspection with the recruitment of prisoners to handle corpse collection and interment. However, while this eliminated a need for labor, the possibility for further infection troubled many members of the board. Their concerns were medically sound. Throughout the cholera epidemic of the 1850s, many prisoners on graveyard duty reported feeling ill.[111] Although their illnesses were generally attributed to contact with corpses, contaminated soil, and dangerous miasmas, today we know that cholera was most likely to have been contracted when the prisoners were exposed to contaminated drinking water and the generally unsanitary conditions of prison living quarters. Much as the villagers of Cacalchén believed their lives to be endangered by coerced cemetery work, prisoners on corpse and burial duty at the gaol (jail) in British Honduras complained that their punishment exceeded their crimes.

Public health committees and policies were established with the intention of diminishing the disorder during chaotic moments, but in reality the conflict between public policy and custom did not encourage compliance. Moreover, the church and the parish priest could not be removed from their positions as central players in the burial proceedings of most Mexicans throughout the midcentury epidemics without creating the danger of a total breakdown of social order. The state simply was not strong enough or rich enough to replace them. Recognizing the continued presence of the church in such affairs, the state resorted to a series of stricter burial policies and enforcement tactics in the name of medical science, even as medical science became notoriously divided over the question of the cause and prevention of cholera. By 1859, Mexican law required that all burials, including those of the church hierarchy, be subject to review by judges and registrars. The law also dictated that more of the dead be buried in new graveyards outside of general municipal cemeteries located near residential structures. As a result, many citizens who wished to comply with both civil law and church canon were faced with payments to the city and the church for burials. The legislation of 1859 required clerics to appeal to their state governments for special permission to bury high-ranking church officials in their own parishes or haciendas. As this regulation came into force, a number of complaints were lodged against state governments regarding the exorbitant fees imposed to inter church officials on private grounds.[112]

Further burial legislation, aimed at resolving the church-state conflict, was passed in January of 1861. Benito Juárez issued a decree that synthesized the Liberal attempt at secularization by creating a consistent national code for processes. Future intervention in interments, on behalf of the secular and regular clergy, would no longer be tolerated. In addition, the decree stated that every burial had to be preceded by notification to the proper civil representatives, and likewise, all inhumations, in any location, would be subject to immediate inspection by appropriate authorities.[113]

Inspections by civil authorities required the payment of fees. Similar to colonial regulations regarding burial fees, the fee schedule depended on the social status of the deceased and the desired location for burial. Officially, burial sites based on caste no longer existed after Spanish colonial rule; in practice, many rituals of the colonial era continued with pauper graveyards located outside of town limits and burial within church grounds remaining a privilege only for those who could afford the high fees.[114] As a direct result of the burial legislation of 1859 and 1861, complaints regarding special privileges and high fees flooded state officials. Members of Mexico's elite were often enraged by the rule that they could no longer bury their loved ones within the church grounds, in family mausoleums, on family properties, and within the church itself, all because of restrictions linking issues of sanitation to an overabundance of corpses in small enclosures. As a result, if room was found in such sacred zones, the fee could be quite high. For example, in 1863 the civil registrar charged Pedro Macial Guerra sixty pesos for a permit to bury his late uncle, the bishop D. José M. Guerra, within the grounds of the Hacienda Cucul outside of Mérida.

Guerra wrote a lengthy letter to the governor explaining that the cost for a regular burial was five pesos and that the exorbitant charge was grossly unjust. Well versed in the rhetoric of law, Guerra cited several articles from legislation passed between 1859 and 1863, which he believed supported his argument about excessive fees and prejudicial treatment. Guerra wrote, "You could legally charge me seven, eight or nine pesos and stay within compliance of the law, but certainly not an augmentation of a quota at double let alone sixty pesos."[115] Almost immediately after the letter was dispatched, Judge Ancona, on the first circuit court, reduced the fee to thirty pesos, adding that such an amendment was more than fair since Guerra had requested a burial outside of the general city cemetery. Moreover, Judge Ancona explained that the quota on burial space was not applied arbitrarily and that the civil judge of the state capital was well aware of the laws cited in Guerra's correspondence.

The two appeals filed by Cura Eugenio A. Ortíz and Guerra, respectively, concerning mandatory state fees for burials demonstrate challenges to power on two distinct levels. Cura Ortíz drafted his as a collective plea from the citizens of the rural pueblos of Pomuch and Poc-Boc, which were, he wrote, overwhelmed by disease epidemics and simply could not afford to pay church and state fees together because of the hardships brought on by illness, crop loss, and warfare. The question for the state bureaucrat, and for the historian, concerns Ortíz's sincerity: was he really concerned about his parishioners' compliance with civil regulations and fees? Or was he perhaps aggravated by his own reliance on a rather inconsistent system of civil distribution of church funds, funds that the citizens seemed unable to pay? Clearly, Ortíz utilized the collective hardships of his parishioners as the basis for his complaint against the state's encroachment on his professional life and the financial stability of his parish. On the other hand, who else was keeping a modicum of order in Ortíz's parish?

In the case of Guerra, the circumstances certainly seem less dire. Nonetheless, the fee imposed is clearly punitive. Why would such a high fee have been applied? Was there a prejudice involved, perhaps a local grudge against the Guerra family? But equally possible may have been the state's attempt to collect fees from wealthy citizens in the absence of successful head-tax collection and a treasury depleted by the expenses of the ongoing Caste War. What is particularly salient in the language of both complaints is an underlying sense of injustice about having to pay fees during moments of painful personal loss. Underneath the public ire about burial fees, of course, is the question of what the state was good for, as its public health policies were proving insufficient to prevent epidemics. For some, it may have seemed as though the state had begun to operate as their once distant empire had—with little regard for the interests of those they ruled and taxed.

In many ways the leadership of postindependence Mexico was so deeply marred by rivalry between the church and the state that indigenous residents found themselves without even the nominal resources for appeal they had under colonial rule. The vexed politics of burial was one level at which such struggles were carried on. Did the mounting fees and restrictions encourage passive resistance by the inhabitants of Yucatán? Given an alienated church hierarchy and an understaffed government bureaucracy, many may have arranged private burials in locations of their choosing, thereby completely bypassing the authority of both the church and the state. In an effort to preserve burial traditions, family traditions may have become a more realistic and economical option. Although tracing gravesites outside of pueblo and city cemeteries would be a difficult task and rely almost completely on hearsay, there is some indication that many burials were never recorded and gravesites were left unmarked throughout the Caste War.[116]

The migration of many Yucatecans during the bloody Caste War undoubtedly displaced citizens from their homeland and their ancestral burial grounds. Where, then, were bodies laid to rest? In the case of many Yucatecan soldiers, death notifications were routinely sent to the family and the body buried wherever convenient, and often without distinctive grave markings. A report published in the Yucatecan periodical *El Regenerador* detailed the progress of Commander Manuel Cepeda Peraza's troops in their fight against los bárbaros in eastern pockets of the peninsula. The article explained that cholera hit the encampments around Temax hard and that most of the victims of the disease were buried "in transit," usually directly after their passing.[117] The wartime conditions of constant flight, mandatory military service, and migratory labor imposed on the indigenous population muddled notions of territorial loyalty and significantly altered local demographics. Furthermore, the erosion of a stable home life only made the process of locating and burying a family member more complicated. In the face of the collective grief of a stunned populace, loyalty to the customs of the church and to the laws of the emerging nation-state divided allegiances and created tensions on local, regional, and national levels, which were expressed in new discourses about science, medicine, and order. The irony is that the science and medicine were completely faulty. For those who wished to stay true to their religious beliefs and customs, particularly during moments of profound grief, the meaning of patria assumed a new face in light of church-state power struggles.

Conclusion

For nineteenth-century public health officials, acquiring control over cemeteries and burial processes increased the state's power over sacred territory and private spheres. In the eyes of church officials and parish priests, their expertise in cemetery and burial management rested on centuries of experience. With their very identity at stake, it seemed only logical to the church's hierarchy that they continue to watch over such sacred ground even as the nation fiercely secularized education, health care, and properties, effectively bankrupting the church by the 1860s. Ultimately, the appropriation of burial grounds by the state posed a serious threat to church power and leadership at the local, state, and national levels. Paradoxically, though, the state's dependence on urban-centered treatments, medicines, and hospitals actually strengthened people's reliance on smaller autonomous systems reminiscent of colonial enterprises. In rural pueblos, the limited access to medicines, medical clinics, and fees required by physicians perpetuated a dependency on the church and indigenous healers. Despite the creation of anticlerical civil policies, the parish priest remained a vital provider and facilitator for many rural communities throughout the nineteenth century. The tacit alliances formed between magistrates like Herrera and priests like the one in Cacalchén were often the only structure left to meet the onslaught of panic attendant upon sudden and devastating epidemics. Additionally, a productive exchange between Yucatecan communities and Caribbean regions was fostered during disease epidemics. In many ways, this informal Caribbean nexus allowed Yucatecans to circumvent dependence on the Mexican state for emergency supplies.

At a pivotal moment in the nation's formation, following the Liberal-Conservative wars of the 1840s and 1850s, the development of cemetery maintenance policies and burial procedures visibly embodied, on the village level, church-state struggles for authority over the intimate domain of death. Specifically, civil authorities utilized public health policies to limit traditional church participation in the major life passages of the Mexican family and advance the positivist civilizing campaign congruent with elite visions of the modern nation-state. To legitimate state power, statesmen subsequently merged their agenda to end the Caste War and civilize the region with disease prevention programs spearheaded by the medical community. In the process, public health policies and recommendations emerged to prevent the spread of contagion through improper handling of the dead, personal hygiene, and waste removal. In the next chapter and second level of this discussion, I focus on public health initiatives to curb cholera in the 1850s, which were concurrent with the most violent phase of the Caste War.

CHAPTER FOUR

CHOLERA AND THE CASTE WAR

Civilizing Campaigns and Disease Prevention

IN 1849 THE GOVERNOR OF YUCATÁN, Miguel Barbachano, started writing a column in *El Siglo XIX*. Barbachano had been governor since 1843—a fateful period for Yucatán that saw the overthrow of Santa Anna, the Mexican-American war, and the brutal commencement of the Caste War. Barbachano had long been the head of one of the two major factions in the creole governing class, the other being an old rival, Santiago Méndez, whose base was in Campeche. The idea of writing a column may have been a savvy political maneuver to garner sympathy and support for his administration during this difficult era of war and disease, yet one is struck by the note of arrogance in Barbachano's commentary on the war, disease, hunger, orphans, widows, and poverty. Barbachano complained, "Obstructions met me at every step. . . . I am not asking much, only that we acquire the means to put an end to the eye sores of hunger, nudity, public begging, and prostitution [*hijas sin hogar doméstico*] all of which are an embarrassment to the pueblos and to my administration."[1] About the Caste War he remarked, "How is it possible that all of this evil has been paid out to the children and the adults, the elderly and the sick, the maidens and the pregnant, when the truly guilty are those malicious who enter with hostility to commit crimes and introduce such anguish. . . . How is it possible that all of this misery falls on the poor?"[2] Barbachano's remarks point to the elite perception that Yucatán's problems were a matter of protecting the helpless. By bringing aggressors who harmed the innocent to justice, Barbachano simultaneously civilized the peninsula. Civilization, as Barbachano's list indicates, is firstly a matter of putting on a respectable appearance.

Barbachano himself had been educated in Spain, a fact that nineteenth-century Yucatecan historians such as Gustavo Martínez Alomía liked to emphasize, and was an "intelligent youth, of distinguished manners, [who had] been educated in Europe" and had acquired a sense of how things "looked" to the European.[3] Thus, his concerns underscore a desire to remove the embarrassing "eyesores" of humanity from public sites, as though these eyesores were the problems in themselves. Such convictions aligned perfectly with the nineteenth-century agenda of civilizing non-Western peoples, which followed from the early modern desire to Christianize non-Western people, and turned it into a secular program for the more thorough assimilation of the indigenous into a capitalist labor market. The marginalization of "barbaric" or "savage" customs, or the physical extermination of the indigenous "other," then laid the groundwork for modernization and economic transformation.[4] Furthermore, while the rhetoric of improvement might well have gained the loyalty of the elite, the working class, poor, and indigenous were well aware that behind public health projects meant to be for the benefit of all lurked a set of gains for the wealthier and the more powerful. Public health projects then invested elites with control over their workforces and security in their private domains.

We saw in the last chapter how Mexico's Liberal order, taking state power, fought against the colonial legacy of the church over the symbolically important power to control the rituals surrounding the dead, including those determining their final resting place. Public health officials worked with state bureaucrats and local lawmakers to impose a new order in the midst of the disorder of epidemics, with mixed results. Because cholera was both new and devastating, the challenge to the church monopoly over the last rites, which was a challenge to the church's power to sanction and intervene in the major life passages of the citizen, was coordinate with the campaign to prevent the spread of the disease. The historic paradox here is that during the first and second waves of the cholera pandemic, the medical establishment was mostly wrong in its ideas about what caused the disease and how to treat it. Neither the científicos nor the clerics knew enough about cholera to understand the dangers of *Vibrio cholerae*'s waterborne spread, or how human dejecta acted as a vector.

Even so, the state embraced the licensed medical community as the sole experts on health, and the state designed policies aimed at protecting the public from disease while simultaneously advancing the civilizing mission as a justification for ending the Caste War by any means possible and taming the rebellious Maya. Justifying its policies in terms of modern medical science, the state probed ever more systematically into ordinary, private domains, from brothels and taverns to private residences, churches, and (as we have seen) graveyards. However, this alliance with medicine was not simply an act of the state, but an act, as well, of the medical establishment, which began to see disease in terms of community and environment. Materially, medical personnel hoped to gain higher salaries, funding for specialists, and improved facilities, as well as power. Everything, then, depended on the state's capacity to assert order, which, in the Yucatán context, meant bringing to an end the Caste War as the first step in modernizing the pueblos.

This chapter examines the historical conjunction of the most violent stage of the Caste War, which fell between 1847 and 1852, and the beginning of the second cholera pandemic of the 1850s. Together, the state and the medical community authored the concepts and agenda of a campaign for "civilization" that would give modern medical science the sole authority to define and act on health issues. The formation of this power complex occurred against an utterly desolate background due to the devastation wrought by epidemic cholera and the Caste War, opening the door for contestation along two critical fronts.

First, there was the conflict between the state's governing elite and the people. As a consequence of the Caste War and disease, many Yucatecans found themselves stripped of their communities, land, and family wages. Very early in the Caste War, as both sides committed atrocities, Yucatecans lost confidence in the state's ability or even desire to curb violence. They saw little benefit in obeying a state that could guarantee them neither security nor property. During the Caste War and the cholera epidemic, many small rural communities ended up practically disenfranchised as a result of the uneven application of land laws and changes in the laws regarding final will and testament certifications. Often public health policy took no account of long-practiced daily routines, family traditions, and rituals, simply banning them. Health guidelines as the state public health committees formulated them had one overriding goal: to sanitize and civilize the body politic.

Second, the medical community was not close to a consensus in the 1850s on disease prevention and therapeutic methods in regard to cholera. The main theory, before Snow's demonstration in London, was that "bad air" caused the disease, and the main therapies, such as bleeding, often made things worse for the patient by further dehydrating him or her. In Yucatán, the difference between medical factions was interfused into the conflict between urban elites in Mérida and the port city of Campeche. The 1840s and 1850s witnessed acute squabbling between Yucatecan and Campechano elites over access to the peninsula's main port of Campeche, the distribution of funds, and persistent secessionist sentiment. This spilled over into the questions of funding public health initiatives and what these initiatives should be. The sheer volume of publications in the form of serial medical advice columns in periodicals and the circulation of medical pamphlets serve as testimony to the primacy of health and war in Yucatecan society at midcentury. Evident in these publications is the common ground shared between state's civilizing campaigns and its goal of safeguarding the health of the populace.

The rivalry between Campeche and Mérida thwarted the implementation of more pervasive disease prevention programs throughout the peninsula, whatever these might be. Among medical professionals, uncertainty over the origins of cholera pulled doctors into opposing camps over the issue of contagion. The medical community also quarreled endlessly among themselves about quarantine, which had a different meaning for a port city like Campeche than it did for Mérida. Such infighting was indicative of a medical community teetering on the brink of collapse, just as the infighting between statesmen in Campeche and Mérida reflected a divided and weakened state unable to quell violence.

The Caste War and the Nature of Cholera

The Caste War literally mobilized disease and death throughout southeastern Mexico. There were even accusations that some army detachments did this intentionally, as in the story told about Chan Santa Cruz. The Maya had dug a well there and soaked clothes from cholera victims in it. Then, when the state's soldiers invaded the village, they drank the well water and were struck with illness.[5] However, the real threat that roving bands of rebels and regional armies posed was less intentional. They left behind wastes, brought diseased people into regions without disease, and disrupted the traditional infrastructural systems in the pueblos. Caste War rebels and the state military lived in unsanitary conditions themselves, making disease prevention near impossible. Cramped sleeping and bathing facilities and a lack of access to potable water compromised food preparation and placed these seminomadic soldiers and rebels at a higher risk of death from cholera and a host of other gastrointestinal maladies while simultaneously transforming them into agents of disease proliferation among civilian populations.[6]

Many rebels crossed the Río Hondo to seek safe haven in British Honduras and unconsciously brought with them disease.[7] As a result of the Caste War and rampant disease proliferation, relations between Yucatán and British

Honduras (and, by implication, Britain) deteriorated. Moreover, leaders in British Honduras feared that the constant traffic of bodies and goods across the still unsettled border between the two nations would ultimately compromise the health of those communities living along the border. Thus, the government of British Honduras took up the weapon of the quarantine and applied it energetically in the ports and along the shared border with Mexico.[8]

From Mérida's point of view, Yucatán's Caste War may have been merely another civil breach; however, it was, in fact, "the largest and most successful peasant rebellion in Latin American history" and one of the most important, having a profound effect at the grassroots level on the white-mestizo interaction throughout Mexico.[9] Enrique Montalvo Ortega argues that both the Caste War and the Mexican Revolution of 1910 demonstrate "the capacity to confront and transform the prevailing oppressive conditions, and in both cases there can be seen a strong spirit of rebellion against such conditions and those who created them."[10]

The Yucatecan press of the 1850s placed blame for violence, pestilence, and barbarity squarely on the shoulders of "vengeful" Maya. Public opinion among the creole elite was laced with loaded descriptions of the Maya as "barbarians" who impeded economic growth by burning down productive export haciendas, stealing cattle, and living in squalor and filth with their animals. News periodicals and medical circulars criticized the rural poor for their "ignorance" and "passivity," portraying them as members of society who either would not or could not comply with sanitation regulations.[11]

In this way, the war froze into place a preexisting prejudice among the white elites that the Maya were obstacles to modernization and economic prosperity. Yucatecan newspapers wailed that the state was fighting against hunger, disease, and war all at the same time: "Hunger, disease, and war are plagues sent from the sky to try our patience or punish our evil deeds, there is not much difference in how we proceed against these elements or in their origin, and in the end we value the same men as instruments: of good, of justice and indestructible laws."[12] A history of Yucatán's cholera epidemic that treated it purely as a matter of health would distort its social meanings, which were enmeshed with those of the Caste War and the struggle between factions to control the state.[13]

The Caste War was a civil war fought mostly in the areas surrounding the colonial capital of Valladolid, located in the southeast of the peninsula.[14] But defining the Caste War as a war of ethnic revivalism or a battle between whites and nonwhites is thoroughly myopic, especially as Maya fought on both sides.

The literature on Mexico's nineteenth-century millenarian movements has focused attention on the deep mistrust, and sometimes hatred, for modernity that often shaped such rebel groups.[15] Focused as it was on the conduct of the war, the Yucatecan and national government was completely unprepared for the cholera outbreak in 1853. They could not fully respond to the need for assistance throughout Yucatán. This long war, although stifled within a few years in the north, lasted fifty years in the south of the peninsula, and during that time Yucatán suffered a catalog of disasters worthy of the book of Revelations: famine, crop rot, locust invasions, and other natural disasters, besides, of course, constant epidemics. The loss of life directly attributable to the Caste War through disease, battle, or starvation is estimated at over 24 percent of the peninsula's entire population.[16]

The prosperity that Yucatán's liberal elite hoped would come about through the loosening of economic regulations and the concentration of land wealth was enormously threatened by a war that encouraged resistance in the cheap rural workforce on which that prosperity was supposed to be built. In scope and kind, Yucatán's civil war was unlike any other indigenous revolt that took place in other parts of Mexico during the nineteenth century.[17] Some creole intellectuals did recognize that the factors behind the Maya insurgency were more complex than simply barbarism and consisted of such things as loss of land, famine, and even disenchantment related to the unfulfilled promises from the wars for independence of 1810 through 1821. At the beginning, however, outsiders and some elite Yucatecans believed that the Caste War rebels intended to rid the peninsula of all "whites."[18] Yucatecan authors Justo Sierra O'Reilly, Serapio Baqueiro, Juan Francisco Molina Solís, and Eligio Ancona all commented on the abuses endured by the Maya over the centuries.[19] Molina Solís and Ancona both explained that fissures within the ruling classes only complicated relationships between the Maya and whites even more as the Maya were treated to inconsistent policies and behavior by the "white" institutions and that perhaps this led to their eventual distrust of all outsiders. This distrust was particularly acute in the 1840s when the Maya were recruited by elite factions and armed to fight in the Liberal-Conservative struggles of the 1830s and 1840s. In the end, elite promises to the Maya were never delivered.[20]

Such disenfranchisement may have inclined some Maya to join in Caste War violence as cruzob rebels in the southeast or declare themselves neutral in the conflict—pacíficos—while others sought refuge on the British side of the Río Hondo and remained there well after the termination of the Caste

War in 1902. The government undertook a strategy of forced relocations during the initial phase of the Caste War, as panicked hacendados sold captured rebels into slavery on Cuban sugar plantations between 1848 and 1861.[21] The war campaigns deftly protected large landowners by removing rebels who burned fields and threatened to impede commerce; meanwhile, health campaigns were administered as metaphoric spin-offs of the military campaigns, protecting the body from illness as though it were an investment. For many rural communities and hacendados alike, accessing medical professionals and supplies meant absenting oneself from the household at a crucial time in order to travel great distances for assistance. The circulation of medical pamphlets designed to assist rural populations with home-based treatments addressed these concerns in part—for the literate members of society—but for those who could not read Spanish, few options were available.[22]

In a pamphlet published in September of 1853 entitled "Curative Methods to Combat Cholera, without the Use of a Physician or Pharmacy," Dr. Ignacio Vado Lugo, a bright young physician from Granada, Nicaragua, laid out simple steps for persons living far from professional medical assistance to care for cholera victims. Emphasizing the "primacy of hygiene," Vado suggested that once an individual contracted cholera, the "body of the patient, their clothes and their home, and all other things they have touched be cleaned." Those without access to fresh, clean water for sterilization could use a combination of "cold olive or almond oil."[23] Governor Miguel Barbachano appointed Dr. Vado to oversee and advise the Superior Health Council, which was reorganized in 1850 under national and state decrees. Dr. Vado ran the Mérida-based junta and taught at the medical school in Mérida that he helped found in 1832.[24] According to Dr. Vado, cholera was not necessarily contagious if one familiarized oneself with the disease and remained fearless.[25] Dr. Vado's contention that fear and panic served as catalysts for contracting cholera did not, however, eliminate the need for hygiene, sterilization, and quarantine.[26]

Panic in the face of a cholera outbreak characterized by its sudden onset and astonishingly quick course overtook small rural towns, fomenting a palpable sense of despair that some members of the medical community tried to address. Communal disarray was etched in the memories of those who survived the 1853 cholera epidemic. In a biographical note on Juan Pío Pérez in the introduction to Pío Pérez's *Diccionario de la lengua maya* (1866), Dr. Fabian Suaste connected disease and the Caste War as "a sudden double assault." He wrote, "At the time cholera morbus was brought into Mérida, advancing with so much speed and mortality, it seized the spirit of all, possessing [them] with depression and stupor resulting in a violent civil war."[27] At the national level, public health officials who saw cholera as contagious felt that the communication of the disease could be stymied. Others were convinced that cholera's vehemence was determined by the constitution of the person, whether healthy or degenerate, and for the latter, the disease would prove fatal. However, when responding to the outbreaks of the disease, the officials representing the state often found it difficult to convince the suffering population that local public health administrators had the situation under control. This claim contrasted strongly with what the people could see happening around them as neighbors, friends, and relatives were suddenly and swiftly killed by cholera and the survivors were afflicted with hunger and all the evil effects of infrastructural neglect.[28]

I cannot overemphasize how the unknown etiology of cholera, its rapid assault on the body, and its physical manifestations, such as severe diarrhea and dehydration, panicked witnesses. Cholera was different than other diseases; even after the death of the victim, the body might be subject to muscular spasms. As one nineteenth-century doctor wrote, "A very notable phenomenon is the occurrence of muscular contractions after death. It may be excited mechanically or may occur spontaneously. A case is related (Eichhorst) in which three hours after death the fibres of the biceps were observed to move tremulously, and then the entire muscle contracted, causing flexion of the forearm. Even the fingers performed movements like those made in piano-playing."[29]

Nineteenth-century doctors, describing the effects of cholera, fall into a language that is more reminiscent of the gothic novel than the objectivity of the scientific treatise. The disease was called blue cholera as well as Asiatic cholera and cholera morbus, on account of the distinctively blue hue of the skin of the face and fingers brought on by profound dehydration. One Indian doctor, Dwarka Nath Ray, described

> violent pain in the abdomen, with great anxiety; pain about the navel; purging, with extreme coldness of the extremities; the stools are slimy, green, mucous, black like dirty water, sometimes very offensive; urine scanty, sometimes a profuse discharge, turbid; retention of urine, threatening to uremia; voice weak, hollow, hoarse, or loss of voice; respiration short, and difficulty of breathing; pulse accelerated, quick and small, rapid, very frequently irregular, thread-like and often quite imperceptible at the wrists; external coldness, with cold, clammy sweat; cramps in the calves; twitching of the muscles;

exhaustion from the slightest exertion; the fingers and the toes are shriveled, the nails and the lips are blue; great emaciation.[30]

Sequestering convalescing loved ones and stacking the dead in cemeteries to await burial outlined the parameters of daily life for many Yucatecans during the epidemic. The fear of being infected was increased by the fact that

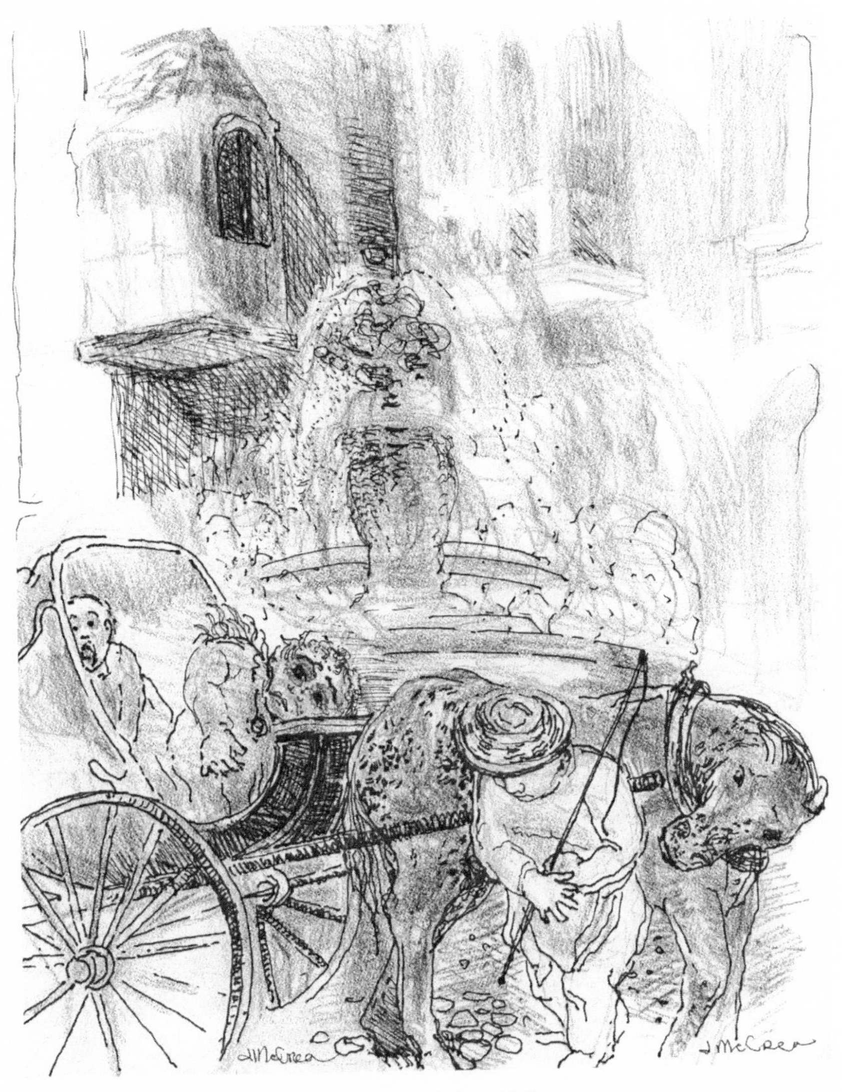

Figure 3: *El Cólera en el Paseo Montejo* by Judith B. McCrea.

authorities could only guess at the way in which the disease was communicated. However, local, regional, and national officials also saw the opportunity to reform public and private behavior. The chaos and despair endured by residents during the cholera outbreak of the 1850s was a strong impetus to reform or, as it was seen by public officials at the time, to advance civilizing and modernizing agendas while also combating disease. Beyond ground-level containment efforts, an examination of epidemic management in Yucatán reveals key information about how Yucatecans negotiated their relationship with the emerging nation-state. Regional state-building agendas brought cholera epidemics and public health policy together under a mantle of preventing widespread suffering, disorder, and confusion, but from the point of view of the citizens, the epidemic exposed the city and state governments' alarming negligence and incapacity. Citizens lodged numerous complaints not only about what was not being done, but also, on the grassroots level, about what was being done that ran counter to their own practices and beliefs.[31]

What was done to prevent the spread of the disease fell in the province of regulatory commissions throughout the peninsula. They curtailed the selling of fresh meats, fruits, and vegetables at community markets and cooperated with health practitioners who encouraged patients to boil water, avoid alcohol and spicy foods, and in general temper their activities. While seemingly oriented toward the preservation of health alone, these policies and recommendations also placed restrictions on freedom of association, which made governance of the public space easier. In regulating the venues and types of allowable association, statesmen laid the foundation upon which a clean, sanitary, modern infrastructure could be constructed.

During a town council meeting held on September 17, 1853, the alcalde (mayor) of Mérida, Juan Pío Pérez, best known today as a Maya linguist and the author of the *Diccionario de la lengua maya*, addressed the jefe político for Valladolid's district and asked what, if any, preventative measures he would be taking to stop the proliferation of cholera.[32] In the opinion of Pío Pérez, certain measures needed to be adopted in order to prepare "this city [Mérida] for the [disease's] violent attack on humanity." Vigilance should be exercised over drinking, especially on the part of the "worst sort"; the markets should be kept clean; and the Superior Health Council's programs should take precedence over other branches of government.[33] The following day the Superior Health Council reported that given the number of cholera cases in Valladolid, they were reinvoking the emergency-only articles for disease prevention passed in 1850. In particular, Article 8 was to remain in effect, which called for the establishment of four public *lazarettos* in the barrios (neighborhoods) of San Sebastian, San Cristóbal, La Mejorada, and Santiago,[34] almost doubling the existing number of lazarettos in Mérida.[35]

As the epidemic decimated the priesthood, which was already suffering from shortages due to the problematic relationship between the church and the state, there was a curtailing of masses and other religious ceremonies. The influence of the church was particularly strong in Peto where in 1849 the priest José Canuto Vela convinced rebel Maya to lay down their arms.[36] To some, it must have seemed as though the very fabric of life had come unraveled. Local leaders of parishes wrote to their regional bishops to request priests, but they also appealed to the governor for help and explained the extreme circumstances that blanketed their communities due to crushing disease and war.

In the town of Peto, the cura (priest) stated that all the pueblos he visited in his parish needed spiritual assistance.[37] Situated in the southeastern region of the peninsula near rebel strongholds, Peto was struck particularly hard by Caste War violence in the 1840s and 1850s. Peto's devastation included physical destruction to buildings, fields, and ranches, but the town also lost many of its leaders, educators, and intellectuals as they sought safe haven in Mérida and Campeche.

The lack of assistance in Peto during the 1850 cholera epidemics is not surprising.[38] Priests pointed out that they performed a civil service by diligently recording the number of deaths from cholera (as best as they could with no medical background for diagnosis).[39] However, priests were likely kept busy by other duties, such as the sharp increase in the administration of last rites and burials. Peto's priest emphasized in a letter to his superiors that "truly the deaths from cholera in the area has completely destroyed [the town] and also the war of the indios has taken its toll, forcing a few families to flee."[40] After the implementation of Liberal reforms in 1857, the limited resources of the church and its newly narrowed scope of control compromised its ability to effectively care for all parishioners, especially inasmuch as the church was having problems recruiting new priests. Since priests were also exposed to cholera victims, it is not surprising that weekly announcements throughout the 1850s reported the ill health or death of local priests.[41]

Thus, in order to implement public health legislation, the state had to employ its own workforce, which, of course, required more funding. Public health officials implemented state-of-emergency measures that subjected citizens to higher fines and jail time for violations. Yucatán's citizens suddenly found themselves confronted with a barrage of emergency-measure legislation dealing with the disposal of their personal garbage, access to water, places they could and could not consume liquor, and restrictions on where they could slaughter animals—the latter being particularly intrusive to rural smallholders. Prohibition of the sale of liquor, raw meats, and fruits likely stemmed from the influence of Paris's anticontagionist medical school, which held that cholera could not be communicated person to person. These doctors believed that infection was linked to a combination of external factors such as diet, personal temperament, cleanliness, and household sanitation. Across the globe, government bureaucracies became much more intrusive in the affected or threatened communities, subjecting households to routine inspections, and while the reasoning for such inspections was to protect the public from the proliferation of disease, the intrusions likely were not welcomed.[42]

Some of the many grievances that must have been felt with the state's seemingly inefficient public health agenda can be seen in the complaints lodged with Governor Miguel Barbachano's administration from March 1848 to August 1853. By the time Barbachano assumed the governorship of Yucatán in March of 1848, the state was well into the throes of an economic disaster. The bankrupt government regretfully announced that they would not be able to offer financial assistance to those who had suffered during the war. A *bando* (decree) issued by Governor Barbachano explained that that there simply was not enough money in the state treasury to support all the widows, orphans, and disabled soldiers.[43]

The federalist-leaning Barbachano constantly pleaded with the national government for more funds, medicine, and trained professionals. He pointed out that gaps in economic coverage for the peninsula's most vulnerable and isolated populations exposed the state to charges of inefficiency, negligence, and corruption. When Governor Barbachano began publishing his column in *El Siglo XIX*, he was motivated, in part, by the desire to spin his policies and cast blame on the indigenous rebels for the state's shortcomings. Barbachano's official correspondence from the summer of 1849 outlined the desperation of many Yucatecan elites and smallholders as the war against los bárbaros seemed to slip out of the grip of the government. Barbachano pointed to the poor quality of the federal troops sent to help fight the barbarous *sublevados* at the expense of the Yucatecan treasury. The soldiers were frequently sick; the Maya rebels outnumbered them almost two to one; the soldiers were poorly paid; and their physical well-being was undermined by food shortages.[44] Although Barbachano did not know it, he was describing an almost perfect target for *Vibrio cholerae*.

Widows and orphans of soldiers received little or no compensation for the death or disability of a veteran, a fact that contributed to the breakdown of family life. Often, wounded infantrymen went without any pay while suffering from wounds that made it impossible to work to support themselves and their families. As Barbachano wrote, "They ask for bread and there is none to give them." The list of those who needed assistance, in the governor's opinion, was virtually endless: widows, orphans, daughters, and mothers of the dead. According to Governor Barbachano, all had given of themselves in the glorious battle to promote civilization over barbarism and were then forced to suffer needlessly. The battle to conquer barbarism, Barbachano claimed, united the peninsula with the nation as the Mexican republic itself struggled to quell indigenous uprisings throughout the country's margins.[45] Barbachano implored his followers, his readers, to take up arms to assist their communities and to be charitable because he could no longer continue to confront the begging masses without some hope that the future would bring compensation for them.[46]

A clear consequence of war and disease, poverty and starvation left many of the region's poor and homeless with few alternatives other than scavenging off of the hacendados. "Stealing and begging for pieces of meat, bread, and corn," they were, in the words of the governor, "condemned to a life of indigence."[47] The governor pointed out that the rations for the infantrymen of four pounds of meat were not enough, nor were three bales of corn per week per family. The government could not be expected to solve such problems without aid. Yet, Barbachano threatened, if the government was not able to tap more money to spend, the troops would become demoralized, malnourished, and incapacitated. More wounded and dead soldiers, he pointed out, only meant more estranged and abandoned women left to loiter the streets.[48]

Barbachano's letters are not merely self-exculpatory, but testify to the attitudes of the governing elites on the eve of the outbreak of the cholera epidemic. The social breakdown that came as a consequence of the Caste War prefigured the breakdown caused by uncontrolled disease. The initial challenges of the Caste War were infrastructural and social. For state administrators piecing together legitimate claims to land, pensions, and inheritances, the destruction of municipal offices broke essential chains of title. The women on the street, often turning to prostitution, challenged the police. Public order was further challenged by out of work veterans. The ripple effects of the general breakdown in bureaucratic order can be seen during the Caste War and afterward as gaps in documentation, which prompted considerable confusion over the legal guardianship of minors. If orphans of the Caste War period could not provide certificates proving a "blood" relationship with a living family member, they were often remanded into state custody.

These effects were not contained in a short time period, either, but persisted for decades. An interesting case in the archives, which occurred in 1882, makes this clear. In that year, family members contested the guardianship of fourteen-year-old minor María Soledad Chable.[49] After the death of her father, her only living parent, all that existed of María's official records was a copy of her baptism record given to her deceased grandparents. The priest who oversaw María's baptism in the parish of Peto, Pedro Badillo, had the original baptism document translated from Maya into Spanish to assist María with her guardianship case. Since María was a minor when her father died, and she had no living grandparents, the question of guardianship remained open until her maternal uncle, Pablo May, claimed he had an agreement with María's mother to take the child. Pablo testified that María's mother on her deathbed made him swear to take care of her daughter should anything happen to her husband after her death.[50]

However, María's uncle and his sister Agipata, who were born before the early phases of the Caste War, lacked all documents legally linking them to María as a blood family member, due to the destruction of civil records. Accordingly, custody of María Chable was placed in the hands of C. Francisco Galera, the state official in charge of orphanages.[51] In October 1882, María was sixteen years old, which legally made her old enough to name her own guardian. She had an appeal drafted for her (she herself was illiterate) asking the judge at Tekax to release her from state custody. María had already run away once from the orphanage where Galera placed her. María, of course, wanted to be with her uncle, Pablo May, and he affixed to the appeal the testimonies of several community elders who attested to the fact that Pablo May was María's blood relative. After four years of appeals and litigation, the judge finally liberated María.[52]

Maria was, in a way, a late casualty of the war. Younger orphans, a product first of the war, and then of the cholera epidemic, posed a severe social problem. If a child was lucky enough not to contract cholera, or survived its ravages, his or her parents were often not so fortunate.[53] Thus, unless the child had other surviving relatives, they became wards of a state so strapped for funds for medical supplies and hospital beds that the orphans necessarily suffered. The justices of the peace of several Yucatecan districts attempted to assign children to any living relative who would have them or who could afford to care for them. As an alternative for children who had no one, arrangements could be made to have the child serve as unpaid labor, and in some cases, the church served as a safe haven. In the Tekantó parish the local cura established an orphanage where children could benefit from an education and regular meals.[54] However, there were likely just as many cases of children like María who ran and joined the throngs that Governor Barbachano referred to as "eye-sores."[55] By the end of the Caste War in 1902, the state treasury was completely empty, and a loan of 300,000 pesos had been made to "sustain the war effort" from Mexico's National Bank.[56]

In addition to these disasters, a severe crop shortage and famine between 1849 and 1850 depleted subsistence crops and in general worsened conditions in the region. The damage caused by the loss of subsistence grains, especially corn, was extremely detrimental to the overall health of the population—particularly the Maya, who relied on corn as a dietary staple. In an effort to prevent widespread famine, local jefes políticos made numerous appeals to state and national governments to lift import taxes on grains.[57] To compensate for a dramatic loss of labor in the agricultural sector, Yucatán's governor ordered *hidalgos* (peasants drafted to do army logistical work) to harvest all neglected milpas.[58]

Cholera and the Political Reconstitution of Yucatán

The Caste War violence, especially between 1847 and 1852, curtailed the state's ability to effectively govern the populace and supply people with necessities such as food, shelter, and medical supplies and services, forcing the state and the elites to fall back upon supplies from Havana, Belize, New Orleans, and Mexico City. In this way, the complex of humanitarian disasters was actually a driver that propelled Yucatán out of its isolation and made an orientation to the rest of the world, particularly the Caribbean, a necessity.[59]

State public health officials often turned to nearby Caribbean nations to supplement depleted resources, exchange information about the path of disease, and discuss preventative measures. The relationship between Yucatán and its neighbors across the Gulf of Mexico helped create an informal, trans-Caribbean network of assistance, and this relationship extended beyond polite exchanges of information and supplies. During the initial phase of the Caste War, Yucatán's hacendados brokered the sale of captured Maya rebels to the owners of Cuban sugar plantations. The carefully crafted exchange allowed Yucatecan elites to rid the peninsula of the constant threat rebel Maya armies posed to their personal fortunes and provided a much-needed workforce for Cuban sugar plantations between 1848 and 1861.[60] Thus Yucatán articulated its own form of autonomy during moments of crisis. By allying themselves more with their Caribbean neighbors than their own nation, Yucatán's government officials fostered their own set of rules and parameters for confronting disease and warfare better suited to the demography of Yucatán than the hegemonic programs and campaigns imposed from a distant national government.[61]

If Yucatán as a state became less autarkic because of the conditions produced by the Caste War and the cholera epidemic, the tightening of the chain of dependence was also felt internally, between the countryside and the towns and between the smaller towns and the larger ones. Many small pueblos were totally devastated during the cholera epidemics, which made them so dependent on larger towns that sometimes the smaller communities utterly dissolved and were annexed to larger and often distant municipalities. The former autonomy of rural areas was, in this way, crushed. Such territorial shifts also affected community identity. Eventually, the smaller communities ceased to exist, and a growing sense of loss emerged as communities faded away. Over time, the disintegration of communities and families became commonplace.

The case of the pueblo of Sucilá in the southeastern portion of the peninsula could easily stand for numerous others. In October 1854, the citizens of Sucilá wrote to their district prefect in Valladolid, complaining about their annexation to the *curato* of Kikil, in the neighboring partido of Tizimín. Apparently, this annexation had doubled the work of the partido's judge. The judge was already overwhelmed with work due to the recent surge in cholera deaths and the resulting paperwork of certifying the last wills and testaments of so many residents, and the petitioners complained that he had not certified the testaments of many who had died, thus leaving their family assets, especially land, intestate. According to the inhabitants of Sucilá, there had been no provision for new jueces de paz (justices of the peace) by the partido even after its boundaries had been expanded, and the caseloads accordingly increased, the previous year. The citizens of Sucilá were all the more irritated by the fact that officials had to depend on the municipality of Espita for administrative needs rather than the district capital, as they had in the past. Additionally, the populations of the neighboring pueblos Lóche and Río Lagartos had to compete with Panabá, Kikil, and Sucilá for access to the same judge who was located in Espita. After the jurisdictional reorganization had been completed, it became ever more difficult to obtain the services of a judge when one was absolutely needed. The complainants lamented, "Because of the recent trauma caused by cholera morbus many people have died without leaving a simple final testimony. All of this because the judge in Espita exercises prejudice against us." Apparently the judge in Espita still seemed to think that Sucilá fell outside his official jurisdiction, which was not true. If the inhabitants of Sucilá were lucky enough to convince a judge to come to their town, he always arrived late and charged exorbitant fees to compensate for the distance he had to travel.[62]

Sucilá suffered badly from the Caste War in 1847 and 1848, when Caste War rebels pillaged its church and treasury. According to one account, the rebels left nothing behind, even taking the coveted chalice and service for Communion from the local church.[63] As the petition shows, the villagers of Sucilá had seen better days. Like many others in the peninsula, the survivors had to decide whether they wanted to remain in the village at all. Aside from the need for judges to oversee an abundance of civil and criminal cases, what was particularly distressing for Sucilá's citizens was that they also needed judges in private residences to hear final testimonies of those dying from cholera. Since cholera victims could perish in a matter of forty-eight hours, there was little time left to put affairs into order, nor were there any special decrees that would allow the dying to choose, in front of witnesses, a representative who would have time later to deal with the legal issues involved in the disposition of the usually small landholdings. Sucilá's citizens explained that it was impossible, under such circumstances, to bring a dying patient to a district judge to hear their final wishes. Instead, many had to account for the final desires of loved ones verbally and then travel to a court in Mérida.[64] By the time these tasks were completed, the deceased's benefactor may have lost his or her inheritance, and sometimes it fell into the hands of the public collection house.

Sucilá's citizens believed that the dying had the right to keep final testimonies private. However, they reasoned, if they absolutely had to comply with the law requiring an authorized judge to oversee such declarations, then it was only fair that they have equal access to such services. The villagers were particularly resentful that the recent annexations increased the suffering of cholera-stricken families by adding new and bothersome legal complications. Finally, they ended their petition with the statement that they had suffered "consistent prejudices and administrative obstructions," which were almost too much, "compounding our troubles . . . we simply want to be left in peace."[65]

The Sucilá petition was signed by several residents, endorsed by the prefect of Valladolid, and afterward forwarded to the subprefect of Yucatán. On November 4, 1854, the governor of Yucatán, General Díaz de la Vega, Barbachano's successor, responded by granting the citizens of Panabá and Sucilá additional justices of the peace. The need for these new justices was plain; thus, he directed the prefect of Valladolid to fill the positions immediately and monitor the situation more closely in the future.[66] According to the original petition, several small villages such as Kikil had remained dependent on *cabeceras* or curatos to manage their administrative needs. However, recent circumstances had made it impossible for communities to demonstrate ownership of family properties if a justice of the peace could not be located.

Between 1846 and 1862, the number of pueblos in Yucatán dropped by thirty from 191 to 161. The number of haciendas also decreased from 1,265 to 1,049, and ranchos and *sitios* (small farms) dropped from 1,673 to 856.[67] The Sucilá case is a good example of how precipitously the community populations dropped during this period, with Sucilá's pueblos, haciendas, and ranchos decreasing from 1846 to 1862 by at least one quarter. Even Sucilá villagers could see that the annexation of a smaller curato to Sucilá territory disadvantaged the annexed rural communities. But such was the nature of the social disorganization caused by war and disease, which opened up opportunities for some, just as it ultimately opened up the opportunity for the creole elite, who were entrenched in positions of power within the state, to advance a civilizing agenda by putting systems in place to control epidemic cholera. The residents of Sucilá found that the concentration of legally distinct districts advantaged them by improving their access to public services. In this way, a seemingly subservient group could begin to have its own stake in the civilizing agenda pushed by the state.

The number of families who lost titles to ancestral lands due to the disruptions of the cholera epidemic and Caste War violence is unknown, since the violence made it virtually impossible for officials to track population movement.[68] Judging from earlier cycles of disease and rural depopulation, there are enough clues to suggest that loss of communal land was quite extensive. For instance, the Gómez family of Umán sold their finca, San José Tizimín, to Manuel Correa in August 1850.[69] Although Umán was not involved in precursory activities leading to the eruption of the Caste War, the town had been the scene of a famous incident in 1847 when the cacique, Francisco Uc, was arrested and charged with conspiracy, although in fact he had committed no other crime than that of being Indian.[70]

By 1850, the village was theoretically pacified. The sellers of the finca, Bernardo Gómez and his mother, Maria Ignacia, sold eighteen *mecates* for one hundred pesos to Correa. However, the vendors of the property did not have a title to the land because Maria's father, Bernardo's grandfather, Juan de la Cruz Gómez, died during the first wave of cholera in 1833. Gómez left no official will or documentation regarding inheritance of his land after his death. The suddenness of Gómez's death also meant that no one knew the location of the property title. When caciques like Uc were purged or the state government annulled their positions, it created large gaps in the traditional mechanism for keeping track of chains of titles. In the Gómez case, the owners called upon the local judge to draft a "transfer of property document" including signatures of several of Bernardo's neighbors, testifying that Bernardo and his mother were the legal owners of the land parcel.[71] It is evident from the records of this particular property sale that the absence of a title presented a surmountable, yet expensive, obstacle for the family. Yet one wonders what the legal consequences would have been if the Gómez family had been involved in a property dispute and had been forced to prove their ownership of the land under different circumstances? Would they have been evicted, or would the testimony of their neighbors have sufficed? If the Gómez family had gone to court, they likely would have lost their family lands. The state would have seized the lands and then possibly offered the family an opportunity to repurchase under a new mortgage agreement. Unless the Gómez family's standing in the community provided for their exception from the law, the oral testimony from neighbors and relatives, upon which they relied for confirmation of land ownership, would have proven to be insufficient.

Many families likely were unable to pay the required fee for a judge's services if their loved ones rapidly perished from disease—especially if the loved one was the main household earner. After all, the expenses of death were themselves quite burdensome even without the further expense of applying for and receiving proper documentation. Having lost most of their family to war and disease, many Yucatecans had little recourse but to relocate. The threat and devastation of disease literally pushed residents into remote pockets of the peninsula in their desperate attempt to flee the oppressive conditions of the Caste War, starvation, and disease. In effect, the war produced a "decivilizing" process that made its victims all the more vulnerable to the label of "barbarian" as the northern part of the Yucatán was pacified in the mid-fifties.

The Medical Community, the State, and the Cholera Quandary

"Cholera is not necessarily contagious, if fear can be overcome," stated Dr. Ignacio Vado in his 1853 medical pamphlet.[72] Dr. Vado postulated that disease sought out those predisposed to fear and attacked them more readily than others. This, he explained, secured the health of doctors who understood disease and illness better than most—that is, doctors and nurses and other medical professionals were "guarded" from disease because they did not fear it. According to Dr. Vado, those female nurses who wore appropriate uniforms rarely contracted the illness, despite their close contact with vomit, excrement, and sweat, and this should serve as an example to the public to show that education and a pious life ensure—almost always—protection from disease.[73]

Dr. Vado's notions were part of the lively medical discourse over cholera that pitted the contagionists against the noncontagionists. But this battle was waged largely over the heads of nineteenth-century laypersons, who viewed cholera according to their knowledge and experience of this and other diseases. The model of a contagious disease was smallpox, and for many, comparison between cholera and smallpox seemed self-evident. A compromise between older theories of contagion and burgeoning noncontagionist thought saw the evolution of contingent contagionists, who believed that cholera, while not inherently contagious, could become contagious provided the right combination of environmental conditions.[74] As John Snow, the London doctor who first postulated the connection between contaminated water and cholera, noted, the issue of whether cholera was contagious or not involved politics:

> The question of *contagion* in various diseases has often been discussed with a degree of acrimony that is unusual in medical or other scientific inquiries. The cause of the warmth of feeling that has been displayed has in most cases probably been unknown to its discussants. It is the great *Pecuniary Interests* involved in the question, on account of its connection with *quarantine* . . . if the doctrine of the communication of the disease must involve quarantine . . . it will always be very unpopular and . . . however conclusive the proofs may be . . . its advocacy [will be] extremely unpleasant to the medical man.[75]

Snow's hypothesis that cholera was water borne was, however, not completely accepted by the medical community for some years after he formulated it, partly because his proof was novel by the medical standards of the day: it was partly dependent on a statistical analysis of the outbreak of cholera in London neighborhoods correlated with their sources of water. What was known about cholera did not actually reach the public until long after the second pandemic passed. Snow concluded from his investigation that "the population drinking dirty water accordingly appears to have suffered 3.5 times as much mortality [from cholera] as the population drinking 'other water.'"[76] In light of Snow's and Koch's work on cholera etiology and prevention, water sanitation became a primary concern for almost every region that had suffered from reoccurring bouts with cholera.[77]

The international conference on cholera in 1866 still endorsed the old "bad air" hypothesis but combined it with a theory of assisting causes including "emanations from soil impregnated with organic matters, especially Cholera dejections, the sewers, privies and contaminated waters."[78] Within these guidelines, a filthy urban center, a neighborhood next to a cemetery filled with coléricos, or an especially unclean home could meet with harsh climatic conditions such as infernal heat and humidity to spur a contagious choleric outbreak if the disease had been introduced into the area already. But there were many variations on these notions of disease etiology. In the case of Vado's recommendations for preventing cholera, fear was the catalyst that, when combined with other factors, predisposed individuals to contract the disease.[79]

Throughout both of Mexico's cholera epidemics of the 1830s and 1850s, physicians, pharmacists, and laypersons advanced various treatments for the disease in numerous bandos and *informes* (reports). These popularized treatments and doctrines of healthfulness claimed to offer the public an alternative to institutionalized health care. Between the 1830s and 1850s, the Mexican medical establishment referenced the European and North American medical communities as writing the most informed small treatises on disease prevention and treatment.[80] Informes, typically including prevention tactics, home treatments, and burial precautions, ran almost weekly in several Yucatecan periodicals. Instructions for coping with cholera were also circulated and sold as instructive pamphlets to the public.[81]

Reflecting the creole elite's sense of Mexico's backwardness, they often privileged advice from foreign medical communities over that of local doctors and public health administrators. The case histories of notable Paris physician Quin ran as a serial in regional Yucatecan newspapers throughout both the 1833 and 1853 cholera epidemics.[82] But only a privileged few possessed the means to adopt the expensive preventatives recommended by Dr. Quin. In *El Siglo XIX*, Dr. Quin advocated the daily consumption of premium brandy and body rubs with rare oils. One can imagine that those who could afford such luxuries must have felt profoundly betrayed if they still contracted cholera.

Drinking brandy instead of water might accidentally have been good advice in that some fluids entered the deprived body. But in general, the cures recommended at this period, like the consumption of brandy, could actually dehydrate the patient more. Most therapeutic measures prescribed for cholera were as likely to worsen the patient's condition as to better it. Instead of rehydration, therapeutics promoted dehydration in the mistaken belief that the patient had to expel the cholera "poison." Even in 1831, Irish physician Dr. William Brooke O'Shaughnessy found success in saving cholera victims with intravenous injections "to restore [the blood's] deficient saline matters."[83] The patient was placed in a precarious position while the medical community bickered over the effectiveness of rehydration or dehydration for the treatment of cholera. While physicians wrestled with whether or not a cholera patient was infectious and should be quarantined, or whether hydrating a patient or depriving them of fluids cured cholera, physicians actually presented a health menace to their patients.[84]

Pamphlets from the first cholera epidemic in the 1830s were reprinted verbatim, without mention of new information. A certain Dr. Canú of Mérida penned a pamphlet describing several effective cholera treatments. Canú's treatments for cholera focused on directing illness away from the body with high-friction alcohol rubs. Canú stressed the importance of scrupulous personal hygiene and sensible dietary habits, clothing that allowed for ventilation, and breathing clean air. He explained that at the first appearance of cholera symptoms, one should purge the disease from the body by inducing vomiting with a combination of mustard, salt, and water.[85] If the stomach stabilized, then he prescribed a regimen of *aguardiente* (sugarcane liquor), more water, and thirty drops of opium.[86]

Dr. Canú's pamphlet was sold at the bargain price of one and a half reals—the inexpensive price was intended to allow the poor access to his "curious cures" and promote home health care for those unable to reach professional assistance. The editor of Canú's recipes for health, Joaquín Castillo Peraza, contended that anyone could administer Canú's therapeutics because, unlike Quin's recommendations, the instructions were clear and the ingredients simple.[87]

More often than not, though, these home remedies came with a whole host of bizarre side effects. Treatments that called for induced vomiting and the use of opiates often made matters worse. Physicians found "evacuation" methods to be "the vogue application of choice for combating cholera." Treatment required the patient to ingest "profound amounts of olive oil and warm water . . . until vomiting and evacuation occur[red]."[88] Commonly, such emetic-based treatments left patients profoundly dehydrated and even more vulnerable to death. Opium, used in compounds like laudanum, was also commonly used for the treatment of cholera for its anesthetic benefits.[89] The negative consequences of using opium-based tinctures like laudanum, such as addiction, overdose, and lethargy, paled in comparison to the benefits opium brought a patient as a general pick-me-up and painkiller. Tonic recipes included mixtures of calcified chalk, magnesium, fennel, and liquid opium. If the mixture did not cause vomiting when the patient drank it, then it often brought on a severe bout of constipation.[90]

Other pamphlets like Dr. Canú's were also in wide circulation. They were printed for different audiences at different social levels—for instance, by regional presses—and circulated as serials promoting home remedies during epidemics, encouraging residents to cope with illness at home.[91] These recommendations for home cures demarcate class divisions. Wealthy residents adopted therapeutics requiring importation of fine brandies, which suited their vision of the emerging nation—a nation with commercial ties to Europe. The least expensive regimen for treatment of cholera called for the use of aguardiente, a locally produced liquor, and these pamphlets clearly spoke to the poorer classes, though rural households of largely nonliterate peasants probably lived outside the range of these ultimately pernicious suggestions. The pamphlets' very existence points to the disjuncture between medical elites and the condition of the poor.

The search for home-based treatment options fostered a growing interest in therapeutics such as homeopathy and hydrotherapy by the mid-nineteenth century.[92] Interest in homeopathy and hydrotherapy represented a growing discontent with the results of state-licensed medicine but also underscored an elite vision of the nation-state where the diseased poor stayed at home for treatment using oils and tonics recommended by medical experts. *El Siglo XIX* ran serials focused on cholera cures; in one, Dr. Hanemann explained how homeopathy could prove effective in treating cholera if remedies were cared for properly. For instance, "copper containers from India," he argued, if not treated properly could change the color of liquid remedies to "a deep blue tint." Clearly, the practice of self-medicating with imported tonics presented patients and caregivers with even more precarious situations.[93] The therapeutic approaches that sought to achieve a practical quarantine by keeping patients at home not only accomplished the task of keeping people from infecting each other, but also relieved stress on the limited number of physicians. Many who contracted cholera also chose to stay at home instead of going to a hospital to "sleep in the same bed where there was a dead person" or "eat the same food given to other sick patients." The terror of contracting cholera in the hospital was also reinforced by hospital staff. One Mexican physician commented that in his hospital, "four die to save two."[94] While poor people's refusal to enter a hospital when ill certainly freed up valuable resources, fear of the hospital also undermined the state's ability to control the movement of the population. From a public health standpoint, without a system in place to account for all infected residents, there was no reliable way to determine mortality, proliferation, or even the usefulness of home remedies.

In light of the medical establishment's advice that worsened the disease and increased its mortality, it is perhaps not surprising that a slight predilection developed during the second cholera epidemic for alternative medicines. A few publications boldly endorsed Maya medicinal cures.[95] Such a trend reflected the willingness of the elite to adopt aspects of Maya culture they found the most appealing and useful, while simultaneously rejecting those elements they found abhorrent. The Mexican state ultimately focused on the promotion of ancient Maya culture and civilization, and the government capitalized on the international attention garnered by archaeologists like John L. Stephens and Augustus Le Plongeon to identify Mexico as the site of unique and glorious ancient civilizations.[96] Concurrent to the state's incorporation of the ancient Maya into national discourse, the civilizing campaigns aimed at "barbarous" Maya condemned the descendents of the ancient Maya to the margins. But the Maya did the same with Western medicine, choosing to employ only those elements that made the most sense within their worldview. Maya curatives were printed in the Yucatecan newspaper *La Redacción* as part of a series of methods a Dr. Vásquez used in combination with hydrotherapy.[97] Heralded for curing many cholera victims, Dr. Vásquez's methods were enthusiastically adopted.[98]

Although such practices remained outside of the spectrum of state-sponsored medical practices, the existence of these alternative cures illustrates the confusion that reigned within the medical community, which seemed impervious to its almost complete lack of prophylactic success with traditional emetics and the use of bleedings. For the rural poor, disease treatment combined different healing tactics. According to regional nineteenth-century historian Apolinar García y García, Maya shamans treated the diarrheas and vomiting associated with cholera and yellow fever with a combination of bitter *pozole* (a fermented corn beverage), boiled lemonade, and cooked *xkantumbú* (an indigenous herb).[99] They did not generally employ Western methods of purgatives.[100] The development of alternative methods such as those practiced by homeopaths offered Yucatecans a variety of choices; it also increased the number of treatments available to Maya healers. Thus it would be a mistake to think of "folk medicine" as remaining in a stasis while scientific medicine progressed. Indeed, scientific medicine proved amazingly slow at understanding the failure of its treatment program, as can be seen by the criticisms leveled at those, like doctors William B. O'Shaughnessy and Thomas Latta, who recognized early on the importance of replacing the liquids and salts being lost by the cholera patient.[101] Yet to some in the educated class, the use of local curanderos, *yerberos*, and midwives as medical authorities once again confirmed the barbarism of the indigenes.

The palliative benefits of homeopathy, combined with the use of indigenous plants and herbs, as well as consultations with Maya healers, eventually did coalesce into an informal, syncretic system of medicine by the early twentieth century.[102] And not until the first decade of the twentieth century did the Western medical establishment begin to understand the need for rehydration in the treatment of cholera. Although given the knowledge of the cause of cholera by Koch, the medical establishment did not understand how to use this knowledge to prevent the disease. Rather, it was used to justify the collective preventive measures that enforced the separation of sewage from drinking water and the filtration of the latter.

Bandos and circulars containing recommendations from the national Superior Health Council for cholera prevention were distributed throughout Mexico. For example, in the summer of 1853, when cholera was at its peak in Yucatán, Mexico City's Superior Health Council sent a circular to several regions in the republic. Of all the territories that received the cholera circular, Mérida was the second to the last to confirm receipt of the document, behind only the northern state of Sonora, thus confirming the peninsula's continued state of relative isolation from the rest of the republic.[103]

There were other problems with the communication of information as well. Commonly translated from French, Italian, or German into Spanish, medical advice pamphlets often could not be read by the peninsula's Maya-speaking and illiterate segments.[104] If they were read, dispensaries for the medicines they mentioned were hard to find. In fact, according to an 1862 census, only six new *boticas* were established in the entire peninsula during the 1850s, all of which were located in Mérida.[105] The standard opium-based medicines, and those containing mustard, sulfur, and laudanum, were thus often quite difficult to acquire and keep fresh.[106] The Yucatecan public health organizations and medical professionals seemed to have no consciousness of the constituency they were addressing and felt no compunction to instruct the population on more practical measures, instead of endorsing such expensive curatives.

In the 1850s, the successful treatment of a patient who already had cholera was always in doubt. What was less doubtful was the medical establishment's growing conviction that cholera could be prevented by taking sanitary measures on both an individual level (involving personal hygiene, dietary choices, and access to clean water) and a collective level (including disposing of sewage safely). Scientists examined the environment for clues about the proliferation of disease and looked to dietary habits, sanitary practices, personal hygiene, and regional climate. However, beginning in the second half of the nineteenth century, the old disciplinary boundaries between medicine and a host of other disciplines, like chemistry and biology, fell, along with old notions of humoral medicine. Bernard and Pasteur in France, with their knowledge of chemistry, and figures like Koch in Germany, who combined biology and chemistry, were leaders in the new understanding of disease etiology. The teachings of medical science started to change accordingly. Doctors, scientists, engineers, and military men (given the kinds of diseases that proliferated in armies) cooperated to form a new order of medical discourse, leading to a new professionalization of medical and health sciences beginning in Europe and the Americas.

By the late 1850s trials with sand filtration, "water systems," "dry earth systems," and chemical methods were already under way in most urban centers to sanitize and separate sewage and drinking water even though the origins of a cholera epidemic were difficult to track at midcentury. Although some emphasis had been placed on regulating water supplies and particular attention paid to ports of entry in Mexico during the first half of the nineteenth century, even after Koch discovered that *Vibrio cholerae* caused cholera, he was opposed by certain influential physicians who insisted instead that cholera-infected ground caused the disease. In fact, Koch's discovery of the means by which cholera was communicated did not lead to a cure. The route by which the injection of saline solutions was gradually adopted was not affected by Koch's discovery and did not follow from it. The paradox of the medical history of cholera is that, as Peter Baldwin puts it, "epidemiological knowledge and prophylactic practice proceeded in large measure independent of each other."[107]

It was not until the 1880s that physicians in Mexico incorporated Snow's 1849 fieldwork into an overarching etiological narrative connecting cholera to water, though British medical journals such as the *Lancet* and the New York–based *Scientific American* had introduced Dr. Snow's work to Mexican physicians in the late 1840s and 1850s.[108] Despite the anticontagionist school, the enforcement of quarantines continued at the discretion of local bosses and port captains whenever cholera was reported throughout the nineteenth century. Given people's awareness that cholera moved between different areas by boat, when cholera was reported in one part of the world, ports worldwide were put on alert. Thus, the second pandemic could be tracked from Egypt to Europe to America simply by drawing lines along shipping routes between various ports. Well aware of this, Mexican authorities tried to stop the disease's spread by quarantining ships from infected ports.

In December 1855, the president of the Superior Health Council of the Puerto de Campeche informed the governor of Yucatán about the crimes committed by one Manuel Gastanaga in charge of the ship *Guerrero II.*[109] Apparently, Lieutenant Gastanaga violated quarantine regulations while docked in Campeche. The president of the Superior Health Council, Simón Campos, claimed Gastanga's ship had just returned from Havana, Cuba, where cholera had broken out. Sanitation regulations required the ship be subject to a mandatory four-day quarantine and inspection, meaning no crew members or any cargo were to leave the ship until the council gave its approval.[110] However, as Lieutenant Gastanaga explained to Campos, the ship was exempt from quarantine regulations due to a written waiver from the *gobernador comandante general del estado de Yucatán* in the port of Lerma, located directly south of the port of Campeche.[111]

The lieutenant took great satisfaction in disregarding the authority of the Superior Health Council, and with the waiver in his hand, he proceeded to drink and carouse defiantly throughout the city of Lerma with other military officers. All the while Gastanaga mocked the rules that, according to him, summarily subjected ships and crew members to the caprice of local port authorities. Unbeknownst to Lieutenant Gastanaga, Campos had sent a spy to watch over the officer. After discussion with other members of the Superior Health Council, Campos informed the governor of the violation and recommended that Gastanaga be punished severely. Records do not indicate whether or not Gastanaga was punished at all. In fact, the matter appears to close with Campos's correspondence to the council.

Ships coming from dangerous ports were routinely quarantined and subjected to inspections from public health officials. During periods of epidemic, foreign vessels were prevented from docking altogether at Yucatán's ports. But the policies regarding quarantine and inspections for foreign ships were inconsistent enough to send mixed messages to the public: should they fear the entrance of diseases through foreign shipping vessels or not? Was the source of cholera within their communities? Did cholera erupt spontaneously, or was it triggered by outside forces such as a change in climate? Struggling with such unknowns made the business of developing and enforcing public health policy all the more difficult for state officials.

By the 1850s health officials could look back on precedents set during the 1833 cholera epidemic. At that time, a quarantine was declared on all ships arriving in Mexico from ports with reported incidents of cholera. The ships were fumigated, underwent onboard inspection, and all crewmembers were isolated for a period of time. By the time the trauma of the initial cholera pandemic of the 1830s subsided, medical professionals had become sharply divided over whether cholera was contagious and what exactly contagion meant in this context. The prevailing contagionist doctrines followed the model of smallpox, which is communicated by direct contact. But the contagionists were significantly challenged when applying this model to the pattern of cholera, for it seemed not to be transmitted only through human contact. Since cholera did not follow the rigid contagion parameters of smallpox, many doctors concluded that cholera was probably not contagious.[112] Public health officials and medical scientists reasoned that cholera was different from smallpox and clearly did not pass from person to person by direct contact; thus, it was not contagious.[113] At the same time, they knew the disease spread from one part of the globe to another, and they were aware that the spread of the disease often corresponded to shipping. How, after all, could an Asian disease affect the Mexican population except by some human agent? Yet cholera's completely unpredictable path and its reputation for sporadic resurgence did not suggest the kind of person-to-person transmission that had been proven conclusively with smallpox. Instead, cholera seemed to be linked, like yellow fever and malaria, to atmospheric or climatic conditions, typically emerging during the hot and humid summer months and after heavy rainfall and flooding. Public health officials could even time their campaigns to target the dangerous cholera months.

Throughout the second cholera episode of the 1850s, both Mexican and British officials (in British Honduras) chafed at mandatory quarantine regulations, goaded by businessmen who depended on open ports for export trade profits.[114] In an effort to underscore the uselessness of quarantine, the Yucatecan creole press printed articles downplaying the severity of the second cholera epidemic. The newspapers *El Siglo XIX* (Mérida) and *El Fénix* (Campeche) printed a report from the Public Health Committee of Tabasco explaining that the current epidemic did not appear to be as virulent as its 1833 predecessor: "It is certain that the Asiatic traveler of today is not present nor does it have as many of the horrible characteristics that the unfortunate and memorable 1833 epidemic had, of the ten persons attacked only one has died."[115] Since ample proof that cholera was not communicated by person-to-person contact had accumulated by midcentury, some leading lawmakers and public health officials concluded that sanitary science and hygiene, instead of quarantine, were the key to cholera prevention.

For example, in 1850, as the first reports of a new epidemic were emerging in India and Egypt, the chairman of the Board of Health in Belize contended that cholera was not contagious and therefore saw no sense in the continuation of quarantine procedures for docking ships. He stated that "the Board of Health . . . has . . . declared themselves as opposed to the belief of the contagious character of cholera." Furthermore, the chairman stated that the board recommended "an immediate removal of all quarantine regulations on vessels arriving either from Jamaica or other ports where cholera may have made its appearance, being quite convinced of their ability to prevent the invasion of cholera."[116]

Likewise, in 1854 the Joint Committee on Public Health presented the city of New Orleans with a report concerning several issues related to the spread of disease and required public health measures. Among the New Orleans public health officials, there was an overwhelming consensus that quarantine was not useful in preventing cholera, even though there was no consensus on whether or not cholera was actually a contagious disease. A Dr. Samuel A. Cartwright believed cholera to be contagious, but only among immigrant populations. He explained that "in more than one hundred instances cholera has been checked on plantations by removal of the Negroes, with their bedding and clothing, in the open air. Could not the same results be attained by following the same precautions with emigrant ships." Furthermore, Cartwright attributed the spread of cholera in New Orleans "to the spread of the emigrant or unacclimated population, or that class of people among whom it first appeared in the city."[117]

In this report Cartwright also spoke about the possible connection between outbreaks of cholera in the port city and the traffic of ships, calling into question the received idea about cholera: "Was not the cholera imported into New Orleans by foreign ships, at each and every appearance it made here?" Cartwright explained: "In its [cholera's] first appearance on this continent, in the year 1832; it gradually approached New Orleans from the upper country, and was seen on the steamboats, flatboats and rafts of the Mississippi and the Ohio, several weeks before it made its appearance here, or a single case occurred among the shipping of this port." Later in the same report, Cartwright addressed a possible link between disease prevention and the influx of immigrants to a region, concluding that there was scant evidence to support such a claim. In the end Cartwright concluded that "no quarantine that we have ever had has ever been effective," and they only caused unnecessary "expense, trouble and sundry annoyances to commerce."[118]

In a rebuttal to Dr. Cartwright's comments, a Dr. J. S. McFarlane, also of New Orleans, challenged Cartwright's position regarding immigrants and the propagation of disease. Dr. McFarlane argued that the immigrant population had not imported cholera, but that it was nurtured by the lifestyles of the intemperate laboring classes, who had irregular sleep and feeding schedules, drank liquor, and behaved degenerately.[119] Dr. McFarlane emphasized that the disease was not contagious, nor was it imported by way of ships. Rather, he attributed cholera's emergence in New Orleans to the summer climate and the lack of a real winter during the twelve months preceding the epidemic: "All the cold weather of the preceding season was late in the spring, hence the surrounding country, as well as the city, emerged as it were from midwinter into midsummer; all the usual tenacity acquired by our inhabitants in city or country."[120]

In reality, the termination of quarantine opened up new niches for cholera because it was transmitted in ship water, which was mingled with the dejecta of cholera victims and recirculated, subsequently contaminating food and the individuals who consumed either the water or food on those vessels.[121] In this way cholera spread from New Orleans up the Mississippi by way of boats. Traditional quarantine measures, however, taken in ignorance of the contaminating media in which *Vibrio cholerae* flourished, often concentrated instead on the "bad air" carried by the ships and were designed accordingly. For instance, just one year prior to the outbreak of cholera in the peninsula, on September 18, 1849, the jefe político of Campeche notified the subaltern jefe político of Carmen that they would no longer need to observe ships originating from the port of Campeche.[122] Campeche's Ayuntamiento and Superior Health Council had deemed the observation period unnecessary.[123] Two years later, the first signs of a cholera epidemic were reported near the port of Campeche in the towns of Hopelchén and Hecelchakán.[124]

Mexico was not so different from the European nations in trying to sort through medical conflicts and economic costs to create a rational cholera prevention agenda. The changing agendas of public health officials are seen in the different programs adopted by international conferences about cholera from the Constantinople conference of 1866 to the Venice conference of 1897. The failure of international cooperation to keep cholera from the shores of Europe was blamed by some on the British interest in keeping ships from India from being delayed and, by the British especially, on old-fashioned notions of quarantine rather than sophisticated medical examination of incoming ships.

Mexico was obviously caught up in these controversies, too. Throughout the mid-nineteenth century, medical professionals and laypersons alike found the erratic movements of cholera both puzzling and terrifying.[125] The sporadic nature of the epidemic challenged many traditional medical precepts derived from early smallpox epidemics, which for many doctors at the time were evidence of the different degrees of healthiness of races or classes. But cholera also directed the focus of public health officials to the poor. The very nature of cholera as a disease inseparable from lifestyle made it easy for lawmakers and doctors to agree that its treatment demanded order, cleanliness, and modernization over any lagging traditions possessed by the working class or the peasants. Officials attacked the intemperance and unsanitary habits of the poor, citing them as breeding grounds for pestilence.

Racialized arguments concerning cleanliness and susceptibility served as further evidence for existing preconceptions of the indigenous "other" as vulnerable to disease. Despite cholera's demonstrated ability to infect and kill across race, class, and ethnic boundaries, in the eyes of nineteenth-century policy makers, statesmen, and public health officials, the disease seemed to prey most on those with certain common weaknesses. Among those weaknesses were a poor spiritual and physical constitution, which expressed itself in an intemperate lifestyle filled with such bad habits as the undue consumption of liquor, use of tobacco, spicy foods, and extramarital sex. But the reality of cholera infection in the 1850s could not be concretely tied to any one or more deficiencies in human character.

The medical community continued to wrestle with the meaning of variations in cholera's physical manifestations in the human body, and autopsies on cholera victims showed that the disease ravaged each body slightly differently, begging the question: how could a *true* strain of cholera be distinguished from other variations within the same disease family? And how could that family of choleras be distinguished from other tropical diseases, like yellow fever or malaria?

Certainly, nineteenth-century medical professionals viewed the protean nature of cholera symptoms as intimately intertwined with daily habits and routines. The general belief that cholera tended to lurk in "offensive areas" where dirt and damp persisted encouraged the notion that a lack of personal hygiene or an unkempt home and workplace would result in an "irritation of the bowels." Likewise, advice to ward off the disease called for a quick turnaround in behavior: "If any of these evil habit and neglects . . . exist in yourself or your family, begin to alter such habits and avoid such neglects, without delay . . . there is no disease which can be more readily met than cholera in its premonitory stage."[126]

Routine practices within the medical community also fell under scrutiny during cholera outbreaks. On May 17, 1850, Dr. José M. Reyes wrote to the director of the Superior Health Council in Mexico City in compliance with recent laws requiring physicians to convey all the details of cholera patients under their care. The writings of the medical community were usually not intended for public consumption, but these works reveal a different side of the cholera epidemic. Often these reports used the cold technical language that was becoming common to the professionalizing nineteenth-century medical practice, which was losing its old Galenic vocabulary. Autopsy reports and other medical briefs, such as that of Reyes, give us invaluable insights into the sense-making procedures doctors pursued as they worked out the etiology of cholera.

José M. Reyes's report stated that one of his patients had clearly and rapidly died from Asiatic cholera morbus; in fact, he had succumbed in less than two hours. The patient displayed all the characteristic signs of cholera: cold sweats, cyanosis (bluish color of the skin caused by a lack of oxygen in the blood), and uncontrollable diarrhea. In death, the corpse still displayed its bluish hue, and its fingernails, fingers, hands, and feet were swollen, purple, and still presumably infected. Reyes then explained that such physical manifestations were common in cholera patients due to their rapid dehydration. The doctor also discovered five pockets of dense liquid in another deceased patient's intestines, which Reyes preserved samples of for testing at the Central Health Committee. It was the doctor's judgment that all the signs, including rapidity of death and the manifestation of some unknown "malady" in the intestines, pointed to the cause of death as a true strain of Asiatic cholera.[127]

Reyes's report was not so different from those of other physicians who practiced medicine during Mexico's 1850 cholera epidemic. Frequently, physicians were confronted with symptoms that truly represented cholera as they understood it, along with a number of anomalies—in Reyes's case, the strange liquid in the victim's intestinal tract. Perhaps Reyes's patient did not perish from cholera alone but instead succumbed to a closely related gastrointestinal malady, or even a combination of illnesses. Obviously, even by the standards of the time, diagnosis was not foolproof, and a cursory glance at medical reports from doctors throughout Mexico shows that many doctors still grappled with multiple ambiguities in relation to cholera almost two decades after the first pandemic swept through Mexico. To help identify true cases of Asiatic cholera, Dr. José Reyes outlined physical manifestations distinctive to cholera cadavers and circulated them to colleagues. First, "the victim must have succumbed to the disease in no less than two hours, during which time they sustained chills, vascular cyanosis, and an evacuation of the rectum." Second, "The body maintains a cyanotic state after death evident in the fingernails, fingers, hands and feet [which are] of a dark purple color." Reyes concluded, "The body was consumed by a lack of fluid in the blood."[128]

Evidence of the kind of uncertainties doctors encountered in the field can be found in a case described by a colleague of Reyes, a Dr. Erazo. In a report he submitted to the Superior Health Council, Dr. Erazo described a patient with cholera-like symptoms who, he determined after further examination, did not have true cholera. In Erazo's account, he and Dr. Reyes examined the patient after two other physicians had diagnosed him with cholera. Dr. Reyes and Dr. Erazo did concur that the patient exhibited cholera-like symptoms but lacked the characteristic cyanotic skin color. Additionally, the patient suffered from *manchas* (skin blotches) not typically associated with cholera. Their final diagnosis was that the patient suffered from a well-known and sporadic gastrointestinal problem called *miserere* (misery).[129]

The report is typical insofar as cholera, like many other diseases in the nineteenth century, had to be read from the behaviors and symptoms of the patient's body. After Koch, the diagnosis of cholera would depend upon the presence of the "comma bacillus" in the patient's dejecta. This would require a different kind of medical training, one that would eclipse the whole corpus of medical knowledge that was based, first and foremost, on the patient's appearance to concentrate on microscopic evidence culled from within the patient's body. After Koch, *Vibrio cholerae* was either there in the body, or it was not. Ultimately, cholera challenged the whole system of diagnosing diseases at every step, no matter how assiduously medical professionals practiced their art. For this reason quarantines and medical inspections of ships, brothels, butcher shops, and other matrices of disease propagation so often failed to prevent the disease once it resurfaced.

Yet if the doctors could not understand cholera's physiological trajectory in the human body, they were sure that the strict control of the environment surrounding human bodies would nevertheless prevent it, pointing once again to the truth of Baldwin's dictum that epidemiology and prophylaxis followed different historical courses in relation to cholera. Medical professionals reasoned that personal hygiene and sanitation could, if implemented correctly, prevent disease. Although a solid connection between filth in the environment and illness in humans had yet to be verified by medical science, preliminary correlations had already been established between festering waste and illness. Waste removal, in particular, was seen as a key component in controlling a disease that, until well after the 1850s, was considered to be induced by bad air. Because waste in public spaces emanated putrid odors into the air, it must also serve as ideal breeding grounds for disease. Thus, waste removal had emerged as a key requirement for the prevention of disease during the 1830s cholera epidemic. At the same time, if waste removal resulted, as it often did, in mixing runoff from human waste with the water supply in a given neighborhood, waste removal could actually increase the cholera threat. Like the treatment of patients with drugs that accelerated their dehydration, the absence of a true sense of what cholera was caused by left a shadow on the public health strategies adopted to fight it, and the gains of the thirties in terms of public cleanliness were allowed to slip in the violent decade of the forties.

When cholera once again arrived in Yucatán, Governor Barbachano, who, as we have seen, made himself a sort of adviser to the public on a number of matters in his letters and columns, received hundreds of requests for waste removal funds. Jefes políticos in Campeche and Mérida were the most outspoken.[130] Officials in the urban and rural municipalities emphasized that a lack of funds was keeping them from being able to direct the prompt collection of garbage, which was necessary to good public health.[131] What could Barbachano do? State funds had already been dedicated to vaccination propagation, cemetery maintenance, and salaries for Public Health Committee employees. Thus, funding for waste management continued to shift to municipal governments, who could not afford it. Instead, local officials were forced to adopt a host of creative financing or bookkeeping tactics, such as placing a tariff on imported corn and other grains and dedicating the revenue to public health services. Other expenses—such as payments given to the local cura to perform the rosary; the construction of outhouses; payments to nurses; the purchase of sheets, ether, laudanum, mustard, and beds; fees for burials; plus the cost of maintaining families in quarantine—were randomly plugged into different accounting categories.[132] Mandatory contributions to soldiers fighting in the Caste War were among the expenses sometimes folded under public security or maintenance. Generally, district políticos responded negatively to pleas for more funds. The only exemption honored was the distribution arising out of revenues from mandatory war taxes or church fees.[133]

Throughout the first decade of the Caste War, the Yucatán Public Health Committee focused its attention on preventative measures through civil legislation and enforcement of sanitation codes.[134] Public health officials reasoned that Yucatán should wisely spend its sparse funds on curbing the severity of the disease by taking specific preemptive measures.[135] The council members also claimed to have learned how to track the disease from their experience of twenty years ago; improved means of transportation, such as steamship travel, could allow tighter surveillance so that the level of hysteria and fear experienced during the 1830s outbreak would be sensibly diminished.[136]

In 1855, as the epidemic was intensifying, the communities and regions that had a junta (committee) on public health had to change the title to Delegación de Sanidad (Sanitation Delegation). The name change was symptomatic of the state's merger of health care and sanitation, putting under one roof the administration of hospitals, cemeteries, sanitation and waste removal, distribution of medicines, doctor and nurse training, and licensing of medical professionals. All were centralized under the state government in the 1860s. Theoretically, this meant that every Delegación de Sanidad was under state control, but the amount of work for the unfortunate members of the delegations proved to be too overwhelming in the war-torn, bankrupt regions and communities.

Conclusion

The mid-nineteenth-century cholera crisis in Yucatán significantly reconfigured social interactions between the state and the church, between whites and nonwhites, and even between Caribbean regions. Within an eighteen-year time frame beginning in 1846 and ending in 1865, close to 1,057 pueblos, rural haciendas, and ranches were destroyed. Gone, too, were entire family fortunes and records, documents for properties and inheritances, informal social networks, and the tacit knowledge that flowed through them. War was one reason for this catastrophe, and cholera was the other.[137]

I have emphasized the fact that the state attitude toward the cholera epidemic had a double aspect: On the one hand, state officials, the public health bureaucracy, lawmakers, and politicians genuinely wanted to prevent the disease's spread and find means to treat a vulnerable population. On the other hand, a public health agenda built around asserting control over the manners of private life derived organically from the civilizing mission undertaken by the state from the beginning of the Caste War. In any case, the state knew neither how to treat the sick nor the causes that promoted the sickness, and its handling of the cholera epidemics, rife with inconsistencies and flaws, brought harsh criticism from ordinary Yucatecans, who spared neither medical professionals (divided between different factions) nor state authorities. This provided the background of the dramatic restructuring of public health services in 1882.[138]

In Yucatán, as in the United States and Europe, the ad hoc approach to cholera epidemiology and treatment began to change in the final decades of the nineteenth century as doctors learned that a microorganism, *Vibrio cholerae*, caused the disease, that the microorganism spread through contaminated water, and that rehydration and the "cleaning of the blood," rather than the mass of therapies used throughout most of the century, were the only treatments that addressed the disease. Thus, norms regarding the body, the atmosphere, and how contagion was spread were all dissolved or shown to be essentially flawed due to certain peculiar characteristics of cholera: its high mortality rate, the physiological changes it wrought on its victims, the very messiness of the disease, and the need to safely dispose of victims' dejecta.

Hysteria had attended cholera's path as it crossed and recrossed the peninsula, uprooting people from communities, especially in the southeast. Administering health care in the southeastern portions of the peninsula was close to impossible. Because of the Caste War, transport of essential medical supplies and vaccines to rebel-dominated areas remained a risky endeavor. Train service throughout the southeast was far from comprehensive or reliable in the 1850s. Cargo was often lost to bandits. Fearing for their own lives, medical professionals generally did not want to work in the remote southeast where Maya rebels tended to focus their anger on non-Indians as purveyors of ill will, disease, and deceit. Pueblos were abandoned, indigenous labor pools were compromised, and a decline in subsistence crops plunged Yucatán into an economic crisis some of whose effects still lingered at the turn of the century.

While the state public health commission may well have intended to serve all citizens equally, in fact many rural or poor families confronted with the horrors of disease and death were practically unable to access public health services. Looking back, one could say that this was a blessing in disguise, considering that the treatment offered by the medical establishment usually worsened the disease. But there is more to the medical encounter than simply the utilitarian prescription of cures: much medical advice about sanitation and hygiene was helpful, even if offered from an erroneous set of ideas about the nature of disease. As for the point of view of the rural Maya, who were left to defend their communities against rebel attacks, plant and harvest milpas, and tend to the sick, the benefits of using a hospital located several hundred kilometers from home may have seemed doubtful. In rural Yucatán, as in many peasant societies in Europe, the hospital evoked fear rather than images of care.

The war was an awful drain on the state's capacity to build any kind of public health infrastructure. Just three years after the war's inception, the government in Mexico City cut off subsidies to support the war effort. To raise money on its own, Yucatán auctioned off church jewels and implemented a barrage of new taxes. Noncombatants were ordered to pay additional taxes to the treasury, landowners and merchants even more.[139] Subsequently, the state was hard-pressed to locate adequate revenues to fund public works, including public health commissions, hospitals, doctor training (education), and medicines.[140] The upheaval caused by the cholera crisis cast doubt on the ability of the state's public health councils to effectively cope with future catastrophes.

Although the state worked hard to remove the church from its role as caretaker of the sick and indigent and replace it with state-funded public health councils, the task was too great for a state too poor to cope with both a war and an epidemic. Many rural residents found that a reliance on alternative methods of healing and consultations with nonlicensed practitioners and healers were preferable to long journeys to urban centers to access doctors and medicines that very few could afford anyway.

Given the comparative failure of the state to design and implement a public health service during the cholera epidemic, reform seemed in order. Especially as the war retreated to the southern part of the peninsula, the area controlled by the state in the north was again subject to the whole force of the civilizing agenda of the governing class. Within that agenda, public health care and the attendant changes in public behavior advised by the científicos became important in the aftermath of midcentury cholera episodes and the birth of Yucatán's henequen export industry.

In the next chapter I will examine how revisions made to public health practices affected local health care. In the late 1870s, the political and economic trajectory of the peninsula radically shifted toward full-scale modernization, leaving local communities (outside of the henequen zone) behind as urban areas were sanitized and modernized. In the henequen zone, the henequen haciendas were hugely expanded and required a greater and greater labor pool. The end of the Caste War altered the Yucatecan landscape, too, as national troops were called in to quell the violence in 1902. By the turn of the twentieth century, Yucatán's capital city of Mérida became the gleaming "white city" many elite lawmakers had imagined. Foreign investors and travelers felt safer in the region after the Caste War and the well-publicized campaign against tropical diseases. However, the integrity of Yucatán received one final blow from the national government when it carved the territory of Quintana Roo out of the state in 1902 for colonization and development. For many Yucatecans, particularly soldiers, veterans, and regional leaders, the loss was especially painful as they had fought to protect these communities from rebel attacks but ultimately lost control of the area to the federal government.[141]

In the eyes of outsiders—American and European businessmen, archaeologists, scholars, and travelers—Yucatán was another of the Caribbean polities that was beginning to emerge from the dangers posed by smallpox, yellow fever, and malaria due to modern public health efforts and thus was becoming more habitable and profitable. Yet this modernization occluded the grinding poverty in the countryside and perpetual debt servitude endured by the Maya peasantry laboring on henequen haciendas. This situation finally obtruded itself into the Western consciousness when American muckrakers started bringing the plight of the workers before the world, especially John Kenneth Turner in his 1910 book *Barbarous Mexico* (which inverted the social categories dear to the creole elite by branding *them* as the barbarians). What Turner saw in 1908 was another effect of the end of the Caste War. Some Maya returned from the security of the southeastern forests, where they had sought refuge during the war, to labor on haciendas under conditions ripe for the breeding of disease and work-related injuries. Tuberculosis and other lung-related illnesses increased, as well as nutritional diseases, alongside repeated waves of yellow fever, malaria, and smallpox. Along with a weakened labor pool, a new set of obstacles surfaced for statesmen as they struggled to maintain their vision of a modern, civilized state and generate much-needed income for a state still nursing its wounds from the protracted civil war.

CHAPTER FIVE

MODERNIZING THE PERIPHERY

Henequen, the Caste War, and Yellow Fever

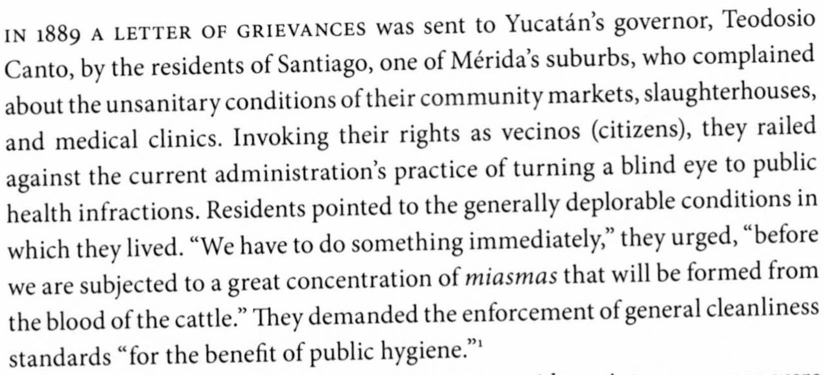

IN 1889 A LETTER OF GRIEVANCES was sent to Yucatán's governor, Teodosio Canto, by the residents of Santiago, one of Mérida's suburbs, who complained about the unsanitary conditions of their community markets, slaughterhouses, and medical clinics. Invoking their rights as vecinos (citizens), they railed against the current administration's practice of turning a blind eye to public health infractions. Residents pointed to the generally deplorable conditions in which they lived. "We have to do something immediately," they urged, "before we are subjected to a great concentration of *miasmas* that will be formed from the blood of the cattle." They demanded the enforcement of general cleanliness standards "for the benefit of public hygiene."[1]

The conditions that had thrown Santiago residents into an uproar were commonplace in late nineteenth-century Mexican urban areas.[2] This rash of objections about unsanitary conditions coincided with a period of profound economic prosperity for Yucatán. As affluence became a distinct possibility for the urban dweller, abuses and conditions that had once been overlooked were now unacceptable. Complaints ranging from the lack of supplies of vaccine to the accumulation of garbage in the streets are woven throughout the Superior Health Council's administrative papers.[3]

In the last chapter, we surveyed Yucatán's health situation in the 1850s, when the countryside lay in ruins due to the civil war, and the state government was, essentially, bankrupt. Twenty years later, the scene had changed dramatically. This was partly due to events that had transpired far outside of the Yucatecan sphere. In the United States, the mechanical reaper invented by Cyrus McCormick in the 1830s had sped up the harvesting of grain but still required workers to tie the grain. To solve that labor problem, a number of reaper-binder prototypes were invented. The most successful one was the Appleby twine binder, which had the advantage over wire binders of adjusting the bind more closely to the diameter of the grain to be bound. After the American Civil War, grain cultivation on the farms of the Midwest took off, and so did the need for twine. These events were directly relevant to Yucatán, as it turned out that the best twine was made from the fibers of an agave plant indigenous to Yucatán.[4] In the late 1870s, this boom in the worldwide demand for cordage had brought into being a henequen plantation economy in the region, which rapidly changed the entire socioeconomic composition of the peninsula.

The success of henequen exports set into motion massive modernization programs. Under President Porfirio Díaz, who ruled over Mexico for close to three decades between 1877 and 1911, the peninsula received a spate of infrastructural projects such as railroad and telegraph construction, expansion of hospital facilities, and the beautification of public spaces. These transformations required a public health system and sanitation services that would be adequate to the massive changes wrought by modernization, and the clear need for an overhaul of health and sanitation services was evident by the number of citizens' complaints.[5] Yet, implementation of public health legislation was anything but swift and comprehensive. The citizens of Santiago were not the only ones who noticed the poor state of sanitation in their neighborhoods and regions. Such was the ad hoc nature of improvement that Yucatán did not enact a comprehensive health and sanitation code until 1891. In this chapter, I will explore two concurrent developments, one Yucatán's transformation from a marginalized indigenous "backwater" into a new economic frontier, and the other the attention being given to the proliferation of diseases such as smallpox and, in particular, the tropical diseases of yellow fever and malaria. My analysis of Yucatán's transformation falls into two stages.

First, I will show how the expansion of the henequen hacienda and Porfirian modernizing projects were key factors in Yucatán's emergence into the national limelight. The revenue generated by the henequen boom permitted the rapid realization of a number of modernization and beautification projects. These projects, I contend, ultimately obscured the real damage being wrought by overlapping smallpox, yellow fever, and malaria episodes that were tied into the expansion of the henequen zone and the consequent disruptions of rural life. The mobilization of rural labor and the expansion of the plantations compromised land ownership, impeded access to public services by the rural workforce, and proved detrimental to the health of a vast swathe of rural and urban residents.

Sanitation posed the most obvious and trickiest problem. Of all public services, the one whose neglect is most obvious is the cleanup of garbage, and the site of conflict between the citizen and the state is immediately located in the citizen's sensorium—eyes, nose, mouth. Thus, as an elevated level of affluence suddenly seemed possible to even working-class people in Mérida, the evidences of the senses became an urgent civic matter, hijacking the civilizing vocabulary employed during the Caste War.

Throughout Caste War–era civilizing campaigns, the goals of the state and its citizens diverged. Citizens' complaints focused on the state's disregard for their well-being. Sporadic garbage pickup, failure to clean up carnage from slaughterhouses, and the inability of local officials to secure enough vaccine and medical assistance all contributed to a state of neglect. In fact, the state's protection of henequen exports and henequen elites fostered discord between citizen and state. Paradoxically, this breakdown in citizen-state relations helped affirm community identity. As residents banded together against what they perceived to be state misrule, community activism strengthened local-level bonds. As state-citizen relations deteriorated, public health services remained overwhelmed, underfunded, and out of touch with citizen needs. Public health administrators scrambled to organize disease prevention campaigns while also trying to supervise burials, remove waste, and conduct inspections, while state authorities myopically focused on ending the Caste War. The accumulation of failures fueled unrest against the Porfirian regime, ultimately leading to revolutionary activity in the early twentieth century.[6]

The second stage of my analysis is focused on the winding down of the Caste War, which is the moment when the civilizing campaigns of the nineteenth century morphed into colonizing projects designed to encourage immigration into and investment in the region, the success of which would ultimately reconfigure Yucatán's economic and demographic future. Colonization took place in two ways. First, as a means to address labor shortages, workers were forcibly deported from northern Mexico to Yucatán to work on henequen haciendas, and second, Yucatán and the federal government brokered a deal to end the Caste War, which required Yucatán to relinquish the southeast and all its profitable natural resources to the national government in return for the use of federal troops to dismantle the last rebel strongholds in this same area, which was realized in 1902. Colonization efforts did little to change the long-term demography of the region, but the thousands of foreigners who came to the region looking for work, investments, or adventure were often the victims of yellow fever and malaria because they were not acclimated to Yucatán's tropical climate and conditions, their immune systems had no previous experiences of these diseases, and they were less aware or wary of hazards that native Yucatecans avoided; thus, they fell prey to tropical maladies more easily than acclimated residents. Combined, these factors challenged public health officials to reconsider how public health services would function in their newly transformed "tropical" periphery.

Expansion of the Henequen Hacienda, Modernizing Projects, and Sanitation

The expansion of profitable export henequen haciendas in the late 1870s literally reshaped the region's terrain, displacing communities, bringing Yucatán firmly into the orbit of its export partner (the United States), and bringing the state to the attention of the Porfirian government in Mexico City. In the 1880s, when henequen exports really took off, Yucatecan landowners and businessmen gathered all their resources to protect their investments in henequen from Caste War activities.[7] Given their new affluence, the war was no longer a matter of the civilizing mission, but had become the defense of modern capitalism itself, in its agricultural guise. The new incentive to crush the rebels, for which new funds were available, was largely successful, and by the final decades of the century, violence from the Caste War had long become a memory for the northern part of the peninsula. Yucatán's boom in henequen fiber transformed the region into a vibrant plantation economy. By 1883 henequen was the second most valuable Mexican export, "behind precious metals."[8] Henequen exports surged more than tenfold within four decades beginning in the 1870s, from 11,000 tons and increasing to 123,000 tons by 1910.[9]

Yucatán's elite class of henequen hacendados governed most of the region's wealth and land with their own self-interest in mind. They created alliances between the state and foreign companies to build railroads, imported henequen rasping machines on a large scale, and when it was possible, fixed the international exchange rate of henequen fiber.[10] Ultimately, these henequeneros brokered the state's relationship with the nation, and other nations, in order to facilitate the growth of their own fortunes.

Modernization was a central component of President Porfirio Díaz's rule; for Porfirian bureaucrats, one of the treasured legacies of the classical liberal era was free trade. Thus, they stressed using exports to accumulate capital for

Mexico's economy, which meant finding a place for Mexico in the world-market order.[11] Between the late 1870s and the 1910s, President Díaz pushed the nation's agricultural zones to expand exports and court foreign investors. In 1910, after the state had succeeded in seizing church and community properties, it sold them, with the result that about 1 percent of rural families owned 85 percent of the nation's land, "one of the largest land grabs in history."[12] In Yucatán, henequen fiber exports dominated the northwest quadrant of the peninsula. (The agave plant, from which henequen fibers are rasped, is indigenous to the Yucatán Peninsula and thrives in the region's thin, porous topsoil.) Almost all of the rasping and operation of machinery was done by Maya and mestizo laborers, who earned a daily wage between fifty and eighty centavos.[13] Harvesting henequen was labor intensive and required several workers to cut, rasp, and bind the twine. Even after the introduction of the henequen rasper in the late 1870s, workers were needed to run the machine and oversee its operation.[14]

The late nineteenth-century American traveler F. A. Ober was a bemused witness of the harvesting process: "Four men are required to attend each machine. . . . The men (always Indians) feed the machine with astonishing rapidity . . . and these poor laborers work mostly at night, from evening until morning, because the heat of the day causes the juice to ferment and irritates the hands, while it also spoils the fiber."[15] A labor-intensive cash crop, henequen required a ready supply of laborers for harvesting. Mechanization in this case did not diminish the intensity and extent of the labor required to harvest the crop, and that single fact changed Yucatán politics and culture, which began to single-mindedly focus on keeping labor cheap and plentiful. The result of the backbreaking labor of henequen harvesting was not attractive. Contact with the tough, spiny plant caused skin irritation that turned into acute eczema, and there was a very high incidence of fractured and broken limbs among the field-workers, who carried huge bundles from the fields in the sweltering tropical heat.[16]

Thus, the broad base of Yucatecan affluence was campesino misery, and only in the urban areas did the henequen boom, in conjunction with Porfirian modernizing efforts, take on a more palatable shape. Massive public works projects, undertaken during the Porfiriato, transformed urban centers like Mérida into gleaming, clean reflections of European cities. Opera houses, national palaces, boulevards lined with monuments, and paved walkways attracted tourists and investors from abroad. Having practically no railroad track to speak of in 1860, the Yucatán railroad system comprised 752 kilometers by 1902.[17] In addition to the construction of railroads, Yucatecans saw the rise of the telegraph system in the 1880s to 1890s, and the peninsula reached second place in the nation by 1892 for telegraph line construction.[18] All of this building established an infrastructure that permitted the importation of mechanized farm equipment. In particular, Yucatán's henequeneros found that the mechanical binder designed by Charles Withington, when used in tandem with Cyrus McCormick's grain harvester, considerably speeded up harvest time.[19] However, the system was still oddly insular. Yucatán was unconnected to the rest of Mexico until 1936 when Southeastern Railways finally linked Yucatecan rail lines with the nation's main lines,[20] and there was no direct link between Mérida and Mexico City until 1962.[21]

Significantly, railroad growth was determined by the henequen business. The first major push took place in the late 1880s, when the railroads connected henequen haciendas to the peninsula's coast. In the 1890s, the peninsula's leaders boasted that the state had extensive railroad lines, more than any other district in the Mexican republic.[22] In 1892 Yucatán was second only to the Federal District in the nation's race to modernize with railroad lines.[23] Railroad construction was defined by the extensive national project designed to connect the internal market economy of Yucatán with its primary port city of Progreso, and other areas remained a considerable distance from the primary Mérida–Progreso line until the period between 1900 and 1913 when the Peto (1900), Ticul (1904), Valladolid (1906), Sotuta (1912), and Tizimín (1913) lines were completed.[24] Subsequently, wealthy hacendados pushed to obtain contracts for construction of more internal lines to connect the peninsula, and henequen, to port cities. Railway and telegraph line construction also left the countryside pocked with embankments and ditches that collected rainwater, increased flooding, and intensified health problems as these reservoirs of stagnant water became ideal breeding grounds for mosquitoes, the vector of malaria and yellow fever infections.[25]

Improvements in steamship travel also facilitated Yucatán's entrance into a world-market economy and quickened the pace of trade in its port. At the height of the henequen boom, between the 1880s and 1890s, the peninsula was ranked third in the country for maritime activity.[26] As the peninsula's henequen haciendas expanded, contact between rural communities in the northwestern henequen zones and export elites created new zones of confrontation in which disputes over land ownership and a confluence of pathogens literally altered the biota and human geography of the countryside. As the northwestern henequen estates pushed into Maya pueblos, the henequeneros launched an intensive campaign to acquire these lands and incorporate residents as provisional, seasonal laborers through a system of debt peonage.[27]

Maya communities were literally absorbed by neighboring henequen haciendas. Urban elites and henequen hacendados allied to create an entrenched system of power revolving around a core group of family dynasties that dominated politics and the economy well into the early twentieth century.

Typically pueblos in such a position were compelled to sell off their *ejidos*, but many villages in the Hunucmá partido resisted, attempting to stand up to the pressure from powerful hacendados.[28] In John Kenneth Turner's classic and controversial polemic on Porfirian Mexico, he provides colorful descriptions of the reigning henequeneros of Yucatán and a sense of the concentration of wealth and power in the region: "Chief among the henequen kings of Yucatán [is] Olegario Molina, former governor of the state and Secretary of Fomento (Public Promotion) of Mexico. Molina's holdings of lands in Yucatán and Quintana Roo aggregate 15,000,000 acres, or 23,000 square miles—a kingdom in itself."[29] Turner described the fifty henequen kings as a cultivated class of people who lived in palatial homes, traveled abroad frequently, and were versed in several languages, "All of Merida and all Yucatan, even all the peninsula of Yucatan, are dependent on the fifty henequen kings."[30] Turner's interview with the secretary of Yucatán's henequen *cámara* (commission), Felipe G. Cantón, provided some insight into elite attitudes about Maya laborers. In a particularly revealing moment, Cantón explained to Turner his rationale for beating workers: "'It is necessary to whip them [the workers] oh, yes, very necessary,' he told me, with a smile, 'for there is no other way to make them do what you wish. What other means is there of enforcing the discipline of the farm? If we did not whip them they would do nothing.'"[31]

In 1897 one member of the powerful Peón dynasty, Joaquin Peón, who owned fincas Nohuayum and Uelilá in the Hunucmá partido, battled with residents in nearby towns to expand his property lines.[32] The town of Hunucmá lay in the way of westward expansion of henequen plantations toward the coast and blocked road and rail construction to the port city of Sisal. The residents surrounding these haciendas in Hunucmá fought encroachments onto their land, and, on occasion, they achieved favorable results that eventually prevented henequeneros from overrunning all of their lands.[33] But such victories could not disguise the changes for the worse that the villagers could see unfolding around their once peaceful pueblos, and social banditry became one method of resistance. An example is the 1895 murder of Hunucmá's jefe político by "known bandits" as he lay in his hammock.[34]

Ultimately, communities in prime henequen country, like Hunucmá, were absorbed into larger political districts that created new zones of contact between aggressive henequeneros and these once isolated communities. Entire pueblos like Hunucmá and Cuzumá were folded into larger districts as henequen haciendas increased in size at the expense of neighboring communities.[35] In March 1879, the state declared that all pueblos and ranchos with less than twenty-five families would become auxiliary properties of the closest city suburb. In return, the city that annexed these small communities had to extend its regular public services to those pueblos and give them a chance to be represented in the public commissary.[36] As communities were reorganized and annexed and access to services, taxation, and loss of land rights became matters of intense dispute, the dockets of district circuit courts were swamped with cases of abuse of authority, murder, and sedition.[37]

Hacienda expansion and railroad construction theoretically brought villagers closer together with rail lines connecting henequen production zones such as Hunucmá, Maxcanú, and Peto to the capital of Mérida, while also of course facilitating the transport of henequen crops from the interior to the port of Progreso.[38] Railroads also put populations vaccinated against smallpox into contact with those who were not, and this may have been one of the causes of the smallpox epidemic of 1897, which killed 127 persons in the Hunucmá partido.[39] The regional publication *Boletín de Higiene* declared that the smallpox epidemic from its center in Hunucmá had spread outward to other communities, escalating the death toll in these small communities to a state of true crisis.[40]

Without meaning to stigmatize Hunucmá in particular, the *Boletín de Higiene*'s article drew unwanted attention to the town. In addition to deaths from smallpox, a mystery illness claimed even more lives.[41] The high death toll in 1897 due to this "unknown illness" set Hunucmá's mortality rate apart from other parts of the peninsula at a time when henequen haciendas were expanding in the area.[42]

The "unknown illness" was possibly linked to the insufficient stock of smallpox vaccine on hand prior to 1897, though the possibility exists that deaths in Hunucmá were misrepresented and simply recorded as "unknown." Whether the illness was misdiagnosed or constituted a real medical anomaly, the convergence of new and old pathogens, using new vectors to infiltrate populations, produced strange physical manifestations that generated confusion and fear among laypersons and medical professionals. While people were certainly familiar with smallpox at this point, it is possible that the physical manifestations of a co-infection of smallpox and syphilis or smallpox and influenza differed enough from a singular infection of smallpox that physicians labeled

Table 2: Deaths Due to "Unknown Illnesses," 1897

Henequen Zone Pueblos and Partidos	Number of Deaths
Dzidzantún	2
Dzilam de Gonzalez	1
Halacho	17
Hocobá	17
Hoctún	7
Homún	4
Hunucmá	183
Izamal	14
Maxcanú[1]	22
Mérida	76
Mocochá	64
Motul	30
Muna	11
Opichén	3
Source: AGEY, PE, Beneficencia, Box 304, Hospicios, Hospitales, Salubridad, 1897.	

1. Maxcanú also suffered marked losses during the 1897 smallpox epidemic (see chapter 2).

the illness "unknown." Ultimately, this confusion drew attention to the incertitude of medical science during a critical juncture in the state's public health and disease prevention campaigns; furthermore, this confluence of pathogens on the frontiers of the henequen expansion zones forced peasants to depend on the hacendados to cover their medical care costs.

One of the most famous abuses of the Porfirian period was the regime of debt servitude enforced upon agricultural laborers, which kept them prisoner to the plantations they worked on. Yucatán was notorious in this regard, with the henequeneros looking for any excuse to seize laboring bodies and put them out in the field. Not surprisingly, they exploited disease in this way. The hacendados obtained the right from the state to reinvoke old debt contracts of peasants discharged from military service.[43] Caste War refugees and army deserters surfaced to work on henequen haciendas where meals and shelter were guaranteed in exchange for their labor.[44] The system of using company stores (*tiendas de raya*) to create debt among the rural workforce also became notorious, and hundreds of thousands of Mayas and mestizos sought work on the hacienda complex, exchanging their labor for the security of food and shelter. Wells and Joseph contend that "by providing a continuous supply of imported corn, beans, and meat at the store and by diminishing the *acasillados*' ability to provide for their families, hacendados ensured they alone controlled the means of subsistence in the henequen zone."[45] The isolation of the region's Maya peasantry on the state's productive henequen haciendas meant that health care and distribution of medicines, including smallpox vaccines, became the responsibility of the henequeneros.

Long seasonal residence in the hacendados' barracks also led to the failure of subsistence milpas.[46] Milpa farming, traditionally the responsibility of male family members, had already been interrupted by the Caste War as the civil insurrection either disabled or killed many young men.[47] As testimony to the weakened state of the male population during the final two decades of the nineteenth century, many men drafted to fight in the final phases of the Caste War simply could not participate due to illness or injuries sustained while fighting. Permanently disabled, and sometimes left as the sole caretakers of young children, many Yucatecan men begged the government for release from military obligations.[48] In essence, the death or crippling of the male family heads and community leaders undermined the family's ability to sustain itself and the community's ability to preserve its integrity.

While henequeneros pushed the boundaries of their agricultural estates and lured workers to their haciendas, Yucatecan state-builders strove to beautify their capital city and reinvent their region's image at home and abroad. Advocates of public works and public health projects were often heralded as heroes, and the press surrounded their names with invocations of patriotism and progress.[49] At the turn of the century, Porfirian-style modernity, from which arose Mexico City's broad and central Paseo de la Reforma and public monuments like the sculpture of the last Aztec ruler, Cuauhtémoc, unveiled in 1887 "to impress foreign capitalists," also found a home in Mérida.[50] There, the construction of the Paseo de Montejo, along which many of the peninsula's henequen royalty bought stately mansions, lent an air of opulence to a city that, forty years before, was struggling with cholera and war amid filth and poverty.

Governor Olegario Molina played a crucial role as *el constructor* (the builder) in laying out a modern Caribbean capital.[51] The Molina family had made their fortune through tobacco farming. Olegario Molina himself was educated in Yucatán and had degrees in law and engineering. He had been involved in bringing about the construction of the railroad from Merida to Progreso in the 1880s, which had given him a taste for grand infrastructural projects.[52] With his solid connections (his family was involved with International Harvester) and his científico views, he convinced wealthy henequeneros to back projects to improve state facilities, including prisons, insane asylums, and the Hospital O'Horan.[53]

Once in power as Yucatán's governor, Molina initiated a task force to prevent *paludismo* (malaria) in 1902. Admitting that it would be a difficult battle, Molina drew upon his up-to-date knowledge of European research to point to the swamps around Progreso as the "germ of death." Molina's concerns about Progreso's swamps stemmed from the close proximity of Mérida to Progreso. Molina feared that ocean breezes would blow the "invisible germ atom" off the swamps and into the capital city. He ordered the swamps dredged, but his fears about invisible menaces destroying the "white city" pervaded.[54] Following his unprecedented re-election in 1905, Governor Molina's massive construction projects gained momentum.[55] Moreover, Molina accelerated his public works programs in anticipation of the first presidential visit to the region scheduled for April 11, 1906.[56] Of paramount importance was the beautification of the state's capital city. At the dawn of the twentieth century, European and American travelers noticed that Mérida had become a modern city. However, in the eyes of both foreigners and urban elites, rural communities were still part of a barbarous past and bastions of superstition, poverty, disease, and filth. Therefore, Molina's efforts for the 1906 presidential visit focused on deflecting attention away from the beleaguered countryside by drawing it to Mérida's grand avenues, monuments, and state buildings.

Foreigners from industrialized nations still assumed that Mexico was "backward" in comparison to European and North American regions. Travelers to Mexico often noted the stark contrasts between the housing of the poor and that of the wealthy.[57] The image of Mexico cultivated for foreign travelers during the Porfiriato, which was spread through business channels, was of Edenic levels of abundance, a country rich in mineral deposits and agricultural goods; travelers were often unprepared for their confrontation with the wretched condition of the nation's poor.[58]

Indeed, despite the construction of grandiose monuments and government buildings, complaints about the foul state of sanitation throughout the peninsula, and in particular the bustling city of Mérida, poured into newspapers and government offices from citizens. Disgusted with conditions in slaughterhouses and cemeteries in particular, citizens complained vociferously that these places were overcrowded, that the slaughterhouses brimmed with diseased, dying, and dead animals, and that the cemeteries were overpopulated with decaying human bodies. The general health was in danger from miasmas that hovered over cesspools of garbage, blood, fecal matter, and decay. The uneven enforcement of sanitation and public health regulations (which seemed to be the result of bribery and string pulling) contrasted with the harsh restrictions and fines routinely levied on individuals simply seeking to bury their kin. As for the general appearance of things beyond the new boulevards, relatively little attention was paid to the basics of waste removal and the maintenance of public spaces.

The U.S. foreign consul in Progreso, Edward Thompson, observed that most of the peninsula's unsanitary conditions could be found in the Maya mud-and-thatch houses and even "under the most favorable of circumstances sanitary decrees are carried into effect among them with the greatest difficulty."[59] But what Thompson failed to discern was that most Maya peasants could not afford to upgrade their living conditions to Euro-Western hygienic standards. In fact, this job, elsewhere, fell naturally to the state. But it is also important to note that despite Mérida's transformation into a modern city, a sanitation code did not even exist until the last decade of the nineteenth century, when civil authorities finally had the power to fine residents and businesses for throwing waste into the streets.[60]

According to the medical community, if one family member failed to utilize lye and calcium in the raking of a dirt floor or did not boil water long enough to clean fruits and vegetables, they alone were responsible for placing their family at risk of disease by not following sanitation recommendations. Officials did routinely inspect taverns, bordellos, restaurants, hotels, granaries, marketplaces, slaughterhouses, and even cemeteries and fined those that failed to pass sanitations standards, forcing them to fumigate as well. The complaints from the public over unsanitary conditions in community spaces rained down upon the administrative arteries of the Superior Health Council in Mérida throughout most of the late nineteenth and early twentieth centuries, indicating that the image of a populace with a lax, tropical attitude toward dirt and sanitation was a far cry from the reality.

The capital city of Mérida failed to implement an effective waste removal program to keep newly paved streets clean. Residents were alarmed that their streets were the site of a continual parade of animals, particularly pigs, that roamed about foraging and defecating.[61] Regulations prohibiting the interment of corpses under church patios and in private homes had not been honored, and in some cases bodies were literally beginning to poke through flooring.[62] In some Yucatecan towns, those traditional sites of miasma, slaughterhouses and markets, were still uncontrolled.[63] In essence, the beautiful facade of Molina's modern and clean periphery was a sort of Potemkin village of the henequen royalty, behind which the population fought perpetual disease epidemics and unsanitary living conditions.

Although the state of Yucatán implemented its first health code in 1891, difficulties implementing new regulations exposed weaknesses in the state apparatus.[64] In many cases, the rather flexible interpretation and application of health code rules by the state's officials unfairly punished some while letting others escape the reach of the law. For example, the illegal burial or exhumation of a body was considered a serious breach of the law. The justification for loading such acts with considerable penalties was the popular belief that exposed corpses effused dangerous agents, germs or miasmas that could compromise the health of the living. Stiff fines and jail time were levied against those found guilty of violating the interment codes. Thus, in 1891 when Marcelina Uc gave birth to "a creature that the *partero* [male midwife] did not even recognize," the partero quickly buried it without a name or a marker. However, the distraught mother apparently disagreed with this decision and exhumed the body, naming it Felipé Varguez y José Dolores Kú. For this act, Marcelina was given her choice of two months, three days, and eighteen hours of jail time or a fee of seventy-six pesos for her freedom. Marcelina choose to pay the fee and promised henceforth to leave the body buried, without an official name in the registry.[65]

In an example of burial law violations from 1905, a laborer and native of Ek Balam, José Concepcion Cano, was charged with burying his stillborn daughter in his pueblo's public cemetery (Tixcuytun) without obtaining the proper permission or filling out the proper paperwork. Pedro Uc, Feliciano Nah, and Marecelino Utzil all helped José bury his little girl, whom they named Nicolasa Cano. All of the members of the funeral party admitted their attendance, but they were not charged. José, on the other hand, was deemed the "author" of the crime by the judge and thus fined a grand total of 140 pesos for his crime, which was reduced by three pesos for the four days he spent in jail. José Cano could have opted to spend thirty-nine days in jail (minus the four as time served) instead of paying his fine. On his plea of poverty and the fact that he had confessed his crime, the judge reduced his fine to 127 pesos. On January 6, 1906, wealthy landowner C. Eusebio Lavin, who had a business interest in seeing the case resolved, paid the fine. In his confession, José Cano said that his wife's labor was "difficult and laborious and that she was in danger with an extremely high fever." He added that he did not know what to do, as his pueblo did not have access to a doctor. Señor Cano then explained that he had sent his son to the town's Registro Civil when his daughter was stillborn, but no one was there. Thus, he decided that he had no choice but to bury the baby without getting official permission.[66]

The record shows a pattern of sporadic enforcements for such violations that increase and then disappear, as though determined by some unspoken quota. Other explanations could be the structural weaknesses in the state judicial system (as, for instance, the lack of personnel in Cano's village's Registro Civil) and the uneven implementation of public health and sanitation codes, which simply expressed other social inequalities in Yucatán. More importantly, though, these violations expose a disjuncture between the policies and realities facing Yucatecan families as they struggled to deal with the death of a loved one.

While despair and loss had certainly been part of the fabric of daily life in Yucatán through the years of war and epidemics, many residents found that the new public health regulations added more to the confusions of everyday life than to their security. Small-business owners like vendors of food and beverages and other working-class residents often underscored the uneven application of fines and penalties for health code infractions in their letters to the governor or the Superior Health Council.[67] Even prostitutes found the new regime less scrutable than the old one. Letters overflow in the files and describe in often nauseating detail the unhealthy conditions still persisting in public spaces, local markets, cemeteries, and boarding houses. According to the letters, blood pooled in the same streets children played in, wild and dangerous packs of dogs could be found scavenging outside the local rastro for scraps, and corpses awaiting burial left a foul stench as they decayed in storage areas near cemeteries. All the letters show a common sense of the right, as if it were self-evident that the state existed to keep neighborhoods and public facilities clean. In fact, the conditions of such places were often foul because there were no regulations applicable to them or their implementation depended on inefficient, corrupt, or negligent local officials and magistrates to oversee the entire process of surveillance, from reporting infractions to enforcing compliance to collecting fines.

However, such regulations complicated matters for those who traveled some distance to sell their livestock. At the slaughterhouse, ranchers had to pay a high fee of eight reals to the local alcabala (boss), in addition to the fee

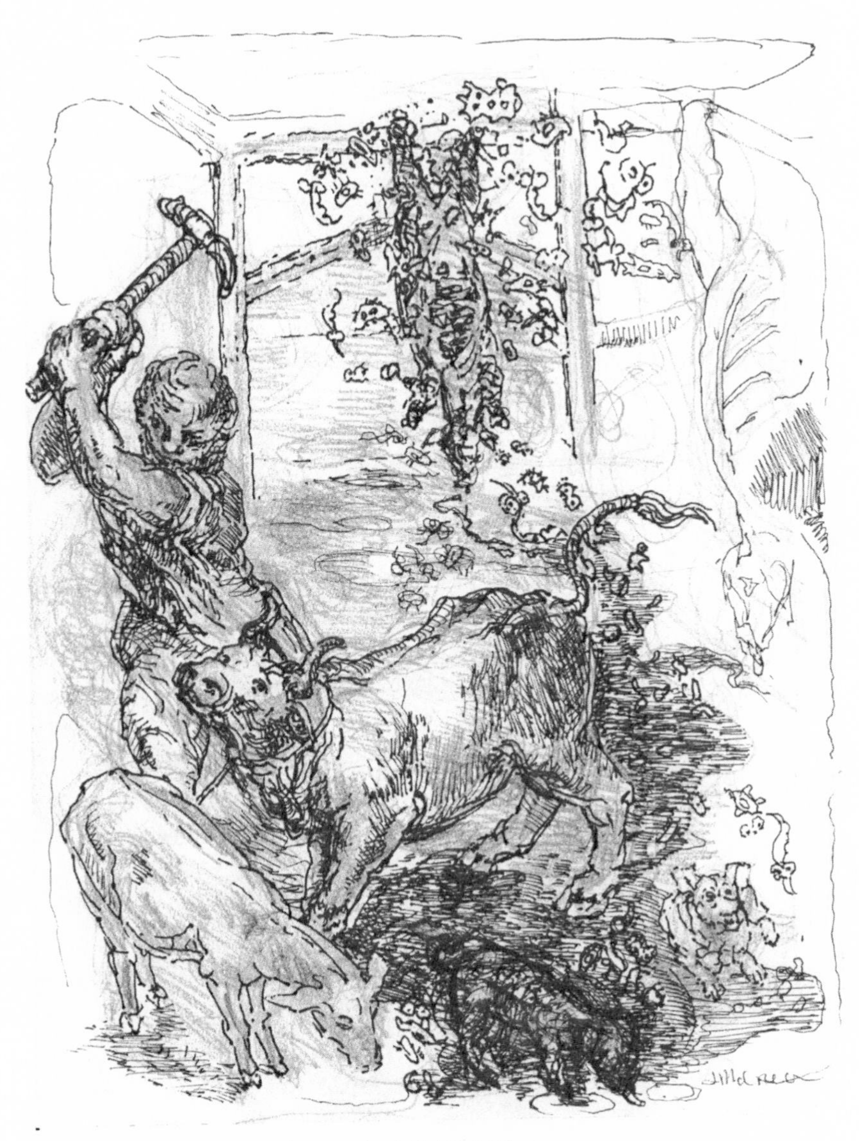

Figure 4: *Las Miasmas en el Rastro* by Judith B. McCrea.

for portioning of meat and use of the facilities, before cattle could be killed. If the rancher could not produce a license for raising and slaughtering livestock, he was liable to be fined for the slaughter and the infraction and charged a fee for rastro use. Under these conditions, we can imagine a scenario wherein the value of the cow itself was equal to or less than the fees and fines applied at the time of slaughter. This put in place a perverse incentive for bribery, which could lead to the transmission of tarnished foodstuff.[68]

Because of this system of restrictive fees, the slaughterhouses were unsavory, and the corruption was massive. Assuredly, the fear of disease and death from unseen "miasmas" (as well as the fear of noxious odors, congestion, and, most likely, lowered property values) compelled residents of Santiago, one of Mérida's suburbs, in 1889 to request that construction cease on a new public rastro just "three blocks from the central plaza."[69] The regulations on sanitary conditions, which had come into force during cholera epidemics in the 1830s and 1850s, were either not enforced or overridden in cities and pueblos throughout the peninsula, up to the promulgation of the new regulations in 1891.[70] The public rastro in Mérida was a notable disgrace, and in 1889 its condition, from complaints in letters and newspaper columns, was laid at the feet of the official in charge of local sanitation, who lacked the competence in veterinary science that would allow him to properly oversee the slaughter of livestock. Animals were usually butchered in the evening and the meat left hanging in the open air until the market opened the following morning, which lured stray dogs and pigs to the site. This in itself was enough to make residents ill, but they were also sickened by the ever-present odor that wafted throughout the neighborhood. Whether butchered for cash and food, or left to scavenge and roam in public places, animals were the moving vectors in the landscape of disease control, the potential bearers of disease. As obstacles to the creation of disease-free environments, animals presented new challenges to public health and municipal officials alike as the focus of disease causation shifted.

Some citizens viewed the presence of animals in their public spaces as living proof that chaos had taken root and the state was incapable of enforcing order. They were absorbing the epidemiological notions that had begun to catch hold in the developed economies, where disease had become associated with controllable environmental factors—clean water, clean air, and the separation of rabid or parasitically infected animals from human habitation. The answer to disease was the decidedly holistic program of interfering in the interaction between environment, animals, and humans. The state's goal of beautifying urban centers and constructing a modern, clean, and healthy community entailed the control of these potential disease vectors.

Urban animal control led by hygiene and sanitation professionals in the late nineteenth and early twentieth centuries blurred the line between public responsibility and private habits as the attempt was made to cull and disperse roaming bands of street creatures. Sanitation crews were polled to determine which neighborhoods were clean and healthy and which were dirty and diseased. In the name of public safety and national pride, an unofficial informant system sprang up in which some citizens were given the power to spot disease-infested animals in their neighborhood and demand aid in purging them.[71] Those residents who were indifferent to loose dogs and swine in public areas not only posed a threat to public health, but also stood in stark and unpatriotic opposition to modernization itself.

The grievances that preceded the 1891 laws were many—garbage-strewn streets, roaming bands of predatory animals feeding on all manner of refuse, rancid slaughterhouse odors, overpopulated cemeteries—and pointed to larger political struggles and weaknesses within the state.[72] Oblique references to these larger problems can be seen in letters to the newspapers, the occasional bandos or announcements circulated in urban locales, and correspondence to the Superior Health Council. Roaming, or unclaimed, animals in particular unleashed moral panic and were often symbols of the continuing barbaric habits of a sector that was undermining the community, the state, and the body politic. In the words of one complainant from a suburb of Mérida, such conditions held the potential to "rot our bodies and our communities to the core."[73]

Ultimately, the public health bureaucracy could no longer hire people with no training to implement policy. The modernizing agenda brought with it the need for input from specialists versed in veterinary medicine, laboratory science, parasitology, and tropical diseases. These specialists in turn required the construction of laboratories, special wings in hospitals devoted to the study of tropical illnesses, information from field-workers about possible vectors and parasites, clinics, and access through journals and books to the mass of scientific information being generated across the globe. Within medicine itself, the responsibilities of the family practitioner had already diverged from the laboratory specialist, with the former often lagging behind current medical science. In the integration of the polity with the medical community, medical professionals envisioned preventive policies to safeguard the populace against disease via vaccines, such as the one for smallpox and ones that were surely in the process of development to ward off such curses of the tropical zone as yellow fever and malaria. Knowing that these and other diseases were carried by mosquitoes, parasites, and other vermin, sanitation specialists could destroy their habitats by overseeing street cleaning, waste removal, and sewer installation and by enforcing standards on all places where humans came together, such as businesses, restaurants, bars, and homes.[74]

The potential to transform Yucatán, through public health legislation, into a modern, clean, and healthful place to live and conduct business appealed to Yucatecan leaders' dreams of glory.[75] In 1894, with these goals in mind, a group of well-known lawmakers, many with medical training like Dr. José Palomeque, the *secretario general* of the governor's office, convened to work out the code and administration of public health. They created various new branches of public works, including sanitary police squads that were to inspect all public facilities (such as rastros, parks, and streets) for violations, provide mandatory compliance dates, and issue fines. They also created, under the direction of Dr. Fernando Casares Martínez de Arredondo, a commission for epidemiology, bacteriology, vaccination, and medical statistics. Dr. José Peón Contreras was appointed the head of sanitary inspection, and Dr. Waldemaro Cantón was placed in charge of controlling communicable diseases in the port of Progreso.[76]

The blueprints illustrating structural connections between politics, public influence, and public health policy are perhaps nowhere else more evident than in turn-of-the-century modernization campaigns. The forces of power that drove change in public health policy were firmly planted in the world of politics and medicine. For instance, Dr. Cantón served as a federal deputy for Yucatán beginning in 1886 and, along with Dr. Peón Contreras and Dr. Waldemaro Cantón, contributed articles to regional medical periodicals such as *La Emulación* and *La Revista Médica*.[77] In 1895 Dr. Casares Martínez de Arredondo founded the publication *Boletín de Higiene*, the principal mode of public communication for Yucatán's Superior Health Council. Later, in 1902, he became the president of the board overseeing the Hospital O'Horan and the Asilo Ayala. Dr. Casares Martínez de Arredondo was also appointed to serve on the national Superior Health Council's special campaign to eradicate yellow fever.[78] Dr. Peón Contreras, renowned for his publication of over sixty works of fiction and nonfiction, theatrical plays, and poetry, also tirelessly served as a physician for the poor, charging only nominal fees for his services.[79] Dr. Peón Contreras and his family acquired shares of railway stock, so much so that by 1902 they owned the majority interest in the Campañía Constructora del Muelle Fiscal de Progreso.[80] Not to be outdone by the Peón Contreras family, the Cantóns were formidable rivals in the railroad industry as well with Waldemaro Cantón serving as the agent in Mexico City for the Mérida-Peto railway, father Rodolfo G. Cantón as the director of railway's board, and brother Olegario G. Cantón serving as chief engineer.[81] Dr. Palomeque's philanthropy helped open the Casa de Maternidad in 1901, and by 1902 he had secured a position on the first advisory commission for Yucatán's rail system.[82] But even with all the power and influence these men possessed, they seemed unable to bring an end to the most problematic obstacle to progress of their generation—the Caste War. The extent of the changes to public health codes and practices was limited, then, by the continuation of the Caste War in the remote pockets of peninsula's southeastern lands.

Brokering the Future of Henequen: Labor, Immigration, and the End of the Caste War

In the last years of the nineteenth century, Porfirio Díaz's plans to pacify Mexico's troublesome frontiers in the northern and the southern peripheries were well under way.[83] Federal troops were dispersed throughout the peninsula's most remote regions with orders to seize all rebel leaders and stop their attacks on haciendas.[84] Some of Mexico's most recalcitrant Indian rebels were defeated, including the cruzob Maya of the south and the Yaquis, Apaches, and Mayos of the northern frontier. In the last spasm of the civilization campaigns that had been waged off and on by Mexico's creole elite, the agenda of breaking ethnically distinct Indian groups dovetailed with the Porfirian project of capitalizing on Mexico's cheap labor to produce agricultural products for export.[85]

Thus, when residents of the Tomochic area of Chihuahua, mostly mestizos and indigenous Tarahumaras, initiated hostilities under the leadership of journalist Catarino Garza, Díaz made it clear to the governor of Chihuahua in 1891 that he "wanted the movement crushed as quickly and quietly as possible and its promoters punished."[86] Control of rebellious Indian groups was an integral part of Díaz's grand plan to entice foreign investment and colonization of the republic's "backlands."[87] But in this last phase of the civilizing movement, pacification had been transformed into extermination. Joseph and Wells argue that the Díaz administration put in place military programs with all the hallmarks of genocidal campaigns.[88] While the elimination of "savages" may have been part of Díaz's nation-building agenda, regional landowners also sought access to pools of indigenous workers, thus they kept a cautious eye on the rebels. Mexican hacendados knew firsthand the destruction that Indian rebels could inflict on their investments, but they were also acutely aware of their dependence on indigenous labor to maintain their export enterprises.

It was pressure from henequeneros that turned the national government's attention to ending the Caste War.[89] The threat Caste War rebels posed to the new wealth garnered by henequen exports had become an embarrassment and an impediment to foreign investment. The lucrative potential henequen held for Yucatán meant that, now more than ever, the Caste War needed to end and the Maya to be "tamed." Under Díaz's rubric of progress, the indigenous Maya had to be tamed once and for all and either mobilized as a cheap labor force or replaced with other sources of cheap wage labor.[90]

By 1898 Yucatán's governor, Francisco Cantón, took decisive action and authorized a final push that would systematically exterminate all rebel leaders.[91] Governor Cantón's bloody-mindedness, however, came up against a natural defense that had saved the Maya rebels before: the unhealthiness of the southern Yucatán landscape to those who had not acculturated to its peculiarities. Many of the soldiers succumbed to malaria; almost four thousand contracted the illness as they approached the rebel headquarters at Chan Santa Cruz.[92] Shortly thereafter, Mexican military leader General Ignacio Bravo captured Chan Santa Cruz, and the territory, which became Quintana Roo in 1902, was marked for federal colonization and resettlement programs.[93] In the end, a handful of land grants were sold to Yucatecan leaders as part of their reward for going along with the partition of Quintana Roo.

The violence and subsequent partitioning of this territory brought in its train the usual disruption of populations, which in turn spread contagions. Many either fled into the interior of Yucatán state or went across the borders into neighboring British Honduras and Guatemala. For decades both rebel and nonrebel Maya had been migrating to British Honduras and Guatemala either to regroup or to avoid the violence of the Caste War.[94] Rebels evaded the punishment of being sold off to Cuban sugar plantations by the Mexican government by finding sanctuary on the other side of the Río Hondo in British Honduras.[95] Refugee communities grew throughout the latter half of the nineteenth century along the Río Hondo, in Corozal, and around Lake Bacalar, while others pushed farther south into the thick rain forests of Guatemala's Petén region.[96] After the Caste War ended in 1902, the new communities remained intact.[97] Migrants found that they could remain independent of the haciendas as they harvested and traded rain forest extracts such as chicle, dyewood, and rubber.[98]

The separation of Yucatán and the territory of Quintana Roo allowed the national government a free hand to colonize the region. In fact, only a few years after the creation of the state of Quintana Roo over "three million hectares of *terrenos nacionales* (national lands) were granted by the federal government to private investors. Of the eleven concessions doled out, only two Yucatecans, Olegario Molina and Rafael Peón Losa . . . received properties."[99]

Quintana Roo's lucrative chicle trade had been completely usurped by English and U.S. companies, largely organized through "Belizean agents and the Chicle Development Company";[100] understandably, Yucatecans were irritated by the loss of such lucrative resources. At the same time, the state of Yucatán simply did not have the resources to put down the Maya rebels by itself. Díaz's federalization of Quintana Roo paid off—at least for the economic elite—and the territory experienced an influx in foreign capital in the years directly following the end of the Caste War.[101]

In an effort to supplement Yucatán's weakened indigenous labor pool, Governor Olegario Molina signed an agreement with the governor of Sonora in 1902 to deport several thousand indigenous Yaquis from Sonora to Yucatán to serve as laborers on henequen estates. Thus began one of the most infamous chapters of the Díaz period in Mexico. Yaqui deportation to Yucatán was a death sentence for many of the Indians, as they could not withstand the abysmal conditions of the transport and died en route. U.S. reporter John Kenneth Turner made their plight known in the United States with reports that later formed part of *Barbarous Mexico*. He based his story on interviews with surviving Yaqui deportees. One elderly Yaqui man from Ures claimed that "'they died on the way like starving cattle. . . . But the cruelest part of the trail was between San Blas and San Marcos. Those women with babies! It was awful! They dropped down in the dust again and again. Two never got up again, and we buried them ourselves there beside the road.'"[102] Those who did survive the journey found themselves in an unfamiliar region, surrounded by "other" Indians who did not speak their language or understand their customs. Disease and heat decimated the Yaqui population in Yucatán. Additionally, their long trip across Mexico helped spread the illnesses they had contracted in their weakened state. In the short term, the additional cheap Indian labor from the north proved helpful to henequen hacendados. But eventually the Yaquis, who in the eyes of some of Mexico's elites "deserved to die," perished or fled, without really bringing down the cost of labor for the henequen plantation owners.[103] The need to maintain the lowest possible labor costs, due to the variability of the world henequen market, was the crux of the injustices for which Yucatán soon became known: the perpetuation of a debt peon system and the virtual enslavement of the Yaqui Indians from northern Mexico on henequen estates. The effort to break even the low wages of the Maya laborer by importing even cheaper labor from the north of Mexico or from Asia reintroduced colonial-era systems that chained the laborer to the land through debts accumulated from the necessities of living, which were always calculated to surpass the laborer's cumulative wage. Thus the laborers became dependent on the henequeneros for their survival, while enduring physical punishment freely doled out by overseers and crowded, dirty work barracks in which they slept and ate.

The state's public health agents averted their eyes from conditions on the haciendas. But in the towns and in Mérida, many politicians saw the end of the Caste War as an opportunity to put in place the projects of which they had always dreamed. Olegario Molina's inhuman side might have been expressed in the role he played in bringing the Yaqui Indians to Yucatán, but his more progressive side was revealed in his term as governor from 1902 to 1906, when the great projects for paving the streets and building a modern sewage and water system were initiated. To pay for it all, Governor Molina did not hesitate to draw upon himself the ire of some of the henequeneros by levying a special tax on henequen to help defray the cost of public works.[104] Acutely concerned about the proliferation of typhus, yellow fever, and malaria throughout region, the government consulted with physicians and public health officials in Mexico City and Galveston, Texas, in order to show that street drainage and sewer construction were needed as public health measures.[105] Molina then awarded a contract to a Philadelphia-based company to construct sewers and improve city byways.[106] During a 1906 visit by Porfirio Díaz to Mérida, the president "enthusiastically concurred that the region was no longer a refractory provincial backwater but an integral part of the rapidly modernizing Mexican nation."[107] By 1910 many of Molina's projects, from the construction of drains to the widening of the streets, had been completed and brought complimentary attention to Mérida.

As much as outsiders praised Mérida's leap into modernity, both natives and foreigners continued to succumb to waves of disease, particularly tropical maladies such as yellow fever, malaria, and typhus. The American anthropologist Frederick Starr wrote in his work *In Indian Mexico* about the risks travelers took with their lives in turn-of-the-century Mérida. Starr observed that despite the wealth brought to Yucatán with the henequen boom, the hotel where he and his companions stayed teemed with dust, dirt, and mosquitoes: "At the hotel we passed a night of horror, suffering from the heat, dust, ill-placed lights, mosquitoes and other insects." Later his party moved to an American-run hotel where management seemed to keep the mosquitoes out and "we had some comfort."[108] Foreigners had good reason to be afraid of contracting illness since yellow fever seemed fond of nonnatives. The first documented case of yellow fever in the Americas dates from 1647, and there are indications that the ancient Maya knew the disease.[109] In the nineteenth century, yellow fever was a well-known plague of the coastal regions. It was known as vómito prieto (black vomit) and was prevalent enough to disrupt international commerce and daily life.[110] Believed to attack those less-acclimated residents such as Mexicans from the valleys or the northern plains and Euro-Western travelers, yellow fever seemed to flourish in immigrant diasporas and port cities where human and commodity traffic accelerated the transference of diseases.

In fact, yellow fever had become endemic not only to the Yucatán Peninsula by the early twentieth century, but also to most "tropical climes" throughout Latin America, the southern United States, Southeast Asia, and Africa. Yellow fever impeded many of the projects of the imperial powers in tropical colonies and in independent countries that were heavily under the thumb of various Western businesses and states.[111] For instance, the French engineer Ferdinand-Marie de Lesseps's efforts to build an isthmian canal in modern-day Panama in 1898 was thwarted in large part by the deaths of thousands of Caribbean blacks and indigenous workers from yellow fever and malaria.[112] Many also died of snakebite, sunstroke, beriberi, typhoid fever, and even smallpox.[113]

Many newcomers to Yucatán, whether they planned to work on henequen plantations or oversee their investments or "discover" ancient Maya ruins, were ill equipped to deal with the rigors of tropical life.[114] Often nonnative Yucatecans found themselves sweating out fevers in the newly updated quarters of the Hospital O'Horan. The records of the hospital are full of exemplary cases of the often disastrous encounter between a human immune system born and bred somewhere else and the fauna and flora of Yucatán. Take Rosa Caffrey, for example, a native of Ireland who had arrived in Mexico's southeastern peninsula some time in 1906 and about eight months later came down with a high fever and vomiting. She was admitted to Hospital O'Horan in late July of 1907 and diagnosed with yellow fever. The day after she was admitted, Caffrey overheard hospital employees discussing the inordinate number of patients admitted with yellow fever symptoms, including high fever, backache, headache, chills, loss of appetite, nausea, and vomiting. The hospital's tropical illness wing was near capacity, and many, like Caffrey, were in unfamiliar surroundings, away from home, and fearful.[115]

Unlike Rose Caffrey though, most of the new patients were male laborers from the Caribbean and northern Mexico. Secundio Gonzalez, a laborer from Spain, had lived in Havana, Cuba, for three years before he traveled to Mérida to look for work on a henequen hacienda at the turn of the century. Contract laborers from as far away as China and Korea as well as northern Mexico were arriving in Yucatán seeking work on the sprawling henequen haciendas during the boom years. Cuba in 1903, when Gonzales first saw it, had become the epicenter of the fight against yellow fever, led by Walter Reed and Cuban doctor Carlos Finlay, well known for being the first scientist to understand the link between the mosquito and the disease.[116] The American army of occupation had made ridding Havana of yellow fever a priority, with a resulting drop in the incidence of the disease, which was globally publicized. Gonzalez's move to Yucatán, then, removed him from the zone in which yellow fever had been successfully fought to a zone in which it was still endemic. Within a few weeks he fell ill with a high fever and unending vomiting. Juan Huacamca, a native of the northern state of Sonora, convalesced in his own home for several days before seeking medical assistance at the hospital for his fever and chills. Similar stories are noted for laborers, *jornaleros*, and foreigners visiting the peninsula in the late nineteenth and early twentieth centuries.[117]

In November of 1900, several American workers from New York died from yellow fever while working on telegraph lines in Motul, Yucatán.[118] Since yellow fever epidemics tended to coincide with the sweltering conditions of the rainy season, generally June through October or November in Yucatán, it was considered unusual that these workers contracted the disease in late November. According to U.S. Consul Thompson, June through October constituted "the sickly season" in Yucatán, when "under any condition the climate of Yucatán is most trying to foreigners."[119] As the representative in Yucatán of the U.S. State Department, Thompson was charged with the unpleasant task of informing the families of the deceased Motul workers that Yucatecan public health sanctions required diseased corpses to be buried within two hours after death, thus depriving family members of the right to bury their loved ones at home.[120] In one death report for a draftsman and surveyor from New Jersey, Thompson assured his superiors that not everyone who came to Yucatán fell prey to yellow fever, explaining that "persons of unhealthy habits simply court their death by coming down here expecting to work and continue in their accustomed way. The climate and country, *per se* is not unhealthy, *as tropic countries go* but, to people accustomed to the northern temperature, the utmost temperance of all things should be carried out."[121]

Thompson's opinions on maintaining health in the tropics were commonplace and shared throughout the Spanish Caribbean. The notion that disease attacked those who had "degenerate" habits was going through a vogue in Europe as well, where it fit with a popularized version of Darwinism that mixed up ideas about "degeneracy" with pre-Darwinian notions about inheriting acquired traits. Degenerates, in this dogma, inherited their vices and constitutional weaknesses from their parents. Thus, medicine neatly backed morality. In Europe and the United States, doctors advised foreigners from higher latitudes to become acclimated to the islands of the Caribbean by abstaining from "'excesses in drinking, romantic pleasures, insomnia, violent or depressing passions, exposures to the cold, and eating.'"[122] Studies of immigrant communities in the Spanish Caribbean show that yellow fever killed more foreigners than natives from the mid- to late nineteenth century in Havana, Cuba.[123] For his dissertation on vómito prieto (yellow fever), Dr. Eduardo Arceo Zumárraga based his findings on research he conducted at Mérida's Hospital O'Horan between 1909 and 1910 and concluded, "The white race is more prone, as for the constitution of the individual it has no importance on the species; the adults are generally attacked, followed by the women and on a smaller scale the elderly and children, where ever yellow fever is born it is said to make orphans."[124]

Between 1900 and 1909, the intake records for the Hospital O'Horan detail an abundance of cases of malaria (paludismo) and vómito prieto among mostly nonnative Yucatecans, which reached a height during the summer months of June, July, and August.[125] Yaqui laborers were admitted to the Hospital O'Horan and diagnosed with yellow fever, one of the diseases that decimated the deportees. Hospital O'Horan's admissions books are exceptionally useful in reconstructing patterns of illness. Buried beneath the statistics and the diagnoses are stories that tell us who paid the hospital bill and the age of the patients, their hometowns, and their current jobs. However, these records are also filled with flaws that require awareness on the part of researchers. Indeed, the pattern of flaws also tells us a lot about routines and attitudes that were folded into the state of medicine at the time. Often doctors, or more likely hospital administrators, recorded the ailment from which they believed the patient suffered from the patient's own testimony of what was wrong. On occasion, there is no diagnosis for a patient, or an ailment may have been entered based on superficial observations, such as grippe or a cold, when in reality the patient suffered from a completely different illness. Similarly, if the patient entered with grippe and contracted a streptococcus infection during their stay at the hospital, institutional records would not reflect this occurrence, just death or discharge.

The voices of those who suffered from illness outside of the confines of public health clinics or hospitals are absent from the written record. The stories of those who chose to nurse themselves or their loved ones at home are not evident unless for some reason they were discovered by authorities, in which case their stories appear in judicial and penal records. In the files we can find the voices of the common people as they defended themselves from charges of violating civil and military codes, which gives us a sense of the everyday experience of sanitation, illness, death, and folk treatments. Infractions included flight from military duty due to personal or family illness, attempts to conduct a burial at home without permission, practicing medicine or midwifery without a license, and violation of sanitary codes by street vendors selling food or at slaughterhouses, drinking taverns, or cemeteries.

"House inspection" sometimes led to the discovery of those who chose not to go to a hospital or clinic for their yellow fever or malaria symptoms; these sick people were escorted to a quarantine station and their diagnosis reported to the nearest public health council. House inspection became mandatory in 1902. Health officials had the authority to inspect a home, hotel, or boarding house if they suspected residents were infected with yellow fever. According to the new health code, all persons with confirmed cases of yellow fever must receive medical attention. The new health code also instructed that "the sick be immediately and rigorously isolated . . . and the location of isolation well designated by the Junta Superior de Sanidad."[126] Such was the case after Luciano López died of yellow fever on September 5, 1900, which concerned the Municipal Medic of the port of Progreso. That office dispatched a team to fumigate and disinfect all the objects López touched during his illness. Afraid to reveal their illnesses and compromise privacy, many more must have died in their own homes, their passing completely unknown to public health officials. Carlos Honer of Frankfurt, Germany, who had traveled throughout Mexico and most recently passed through Coatzacoalcos, was found by a home inspection visit. He was incapacitated, having been "attacked" by yellow fever, and suffering from acute cerebral spasms. He was promptly transferred to the Hospital O'Horan for treatment.[127] Dr. Augusto Molina, working with the public health service, located what he called a "focus of infection" at a home on Forty-seventh Street in Mérida, where a large number of Spaniards were found convalescing from yellow fever. At least four cases were confirmed, and the house was immediately evacuated and disinfected.[128]

While authorities in Mérida were finding that foreigners traveling to the Caribbean region easily succumbed to yellow fever, the staffs of military units had long found the same thing to be true of the regional and national military regiments scattered throughout the peninsula.[129] Both regional and national troops trekked throughout the Yucatán Peninsula for more than half a century, contracting and unwittingly spreading diseases wherever they were stationed. Military troops bivouacked in unsanitary conditions most of the time, slept in crowded quarters, had limited access to freshwater and medical assistance, ate rotting provisions, and suffered from scant stocks of medicines and a lack of sterilizing agents. The connection between the military and the proliferation of diseases throughout the peninsula can also be seen in foreign health reports. In October 1901 Henry Goldthwaite, the executive officer of health in charge of evaluating the peninsula's conditions, informed the U.S. surgeon-general that a military presence had likely contributed to yellow fever proliferation: "I was informed that this disease [yellow fever] prevailing among the Yucatecan Indians has been contracted by the Mexican troops sent to fight them, and in that way spread afar."[130] Certainly, the end of the Caste War brought to a close the endless proliferation of diseases in Yucatán's former rebel territories, but even in the years following warfare, Yucatán witnessed simultaneous outbreaks of smallpox and hepatitis in 1905 and yellow fever and smallpox in 1906.

Yellow fever had already flared up throughout the peninsula several times in the nineteenth century: outbreaks are recorded in 1825, 1855 through 1858, 1878, 1879, and 1881. But not until the 1906 epidemic did Yucatán's public health officials organize a campaign specifically to target yellow fever.[131] Yucatán's public health authorities looked to Cuba for a model in forming an official anti–yellow fever campaign. With Yucatán geographically oriented more toward the Caribbean, Yucatán's medical professionals rationalized that adaptation of Cuban methods to combat yellow fever could be implemented with relative ease throughout the peninsula.[132] During a visit to Yucatán in June of 1902, Cuban physician Juan Santos Fernández noted, "The state of Yucatán is situated at the same latitude as Cuba and has an identical pathology." Dr. Fernández also concluded that yellow fever was endemic in both Caribbean regions and therein afforded native residents with an apparent immunity to the disease.[133]

The Mexican republic began its first official campaign to combat yellow fever in 1903, just three years prior to the formation of Yucatán's campaign. The federal program concentrated on populations in port cities such as Veracruz and Tampico; in the Yucatán Peninsula, Campeche, Sisal, and Progreso were targeted.[134] Former head of the national Superior Health Council in Mexico City Dr. Fernando Casares, also a native Yucatecan, headed up the Yucatecan anti–yellow fever campaign. Working with Danish scientist Harad Seidelin, the director of laboratory science at the Hospital O'Horan, an entire cadre of public health officials, inspectors, and medical professionals worked to eradicate diseases in Yucatán.

The publicity accorded the campaigns against yellow fever and malaria in Cuba and Panama had invigorated a lively interest in tropical diseases in the United States and in Caribbean countries. Finlay's work linking the mosquito *Aedes aegypti* to yellow fever had, for the first time, given doctors a real tool to fight the disease. That tool lay outside of palliatives or medicine and consisted simply in exterminating mosquitoes and destroying their breeding habitats. That quinine could hold off malaria had been known since the seventeenth century in Europe. Many public health officials continued to utilize traditional measures to combat disease, such as quarantine (employed, as we have seen, by the house inspectors in Mérida) and modifications to diet and sexual behavior.

In the first decade of the twentieth century, two simultaneous medical discoveries finally became the orthodoxy in public health: one was that the causative factor in disease was germs; and the other was that environmental factors could determine the germ landscape. The first pointed toward research in finding cures; the second pointed toward programs to alter the disease landscape in such a way as to favor human beings. These discoveries resulted in the overhaul of the state sanitary code in 1910.[135] They also pointed to the future, in which the state would seek to intervene in the vectors of disease. The fruit of this transformation of the medical paradigm was the Rockefeller Foundation's International Board of Health program to eradicate yellow fever and malaria from the Gulf Coast of Mexico, which was effected by a strange alliance between a revolutionary government and a foundation funded by the world's most renowned capitalist.[136]

Conclusion

The end of the Caste War and the affluence flowing from the henequen boom brought Yucatecans railroads, better roads, telegraph lines, a "white" and gleaming capital city, and sanitation reforms. The cost to the state was the loss of the southeast to the federal government as payment for their assistance in ending the Caste War. The cost to the people was higher. Maya communities were absorbed into larger political divisions as the population scattered onto henequen estates or fled into the forests of Guatemala and British Honduras. Maya smallholders, inducted into the life of the henequen hacienda worker, faced never-ending abuse, penitentiary-like living conditions, and debt peonage that was almost indistinguishable from slavery. The conflation of communities and the state's complicity in expanding henequen haciendas compromised the Maya peasantry's ability to effectively file grievances or get a fair hearing. Likewise, distance from public health facilities meant that they continued to rely on their own methods for healing, hence undermining the state's investment in institutional medicine and public health services. By the early twentieth century, most of the peninsula's Maya population lived either in the enforced isolation of the henequen estates or in the forests of the southeast or in isolated rural communities. Cut off from the rest of Mexico, they were latecomers to the early phases of the Mexican Revolution of 1910. But that revolution, by shattering the Porfirian system, did ultimately resonate in their lives.

The new sanitary code of 1910, which ambitiously outlined public health practices that had proved their worth in other Caribbean sites, proved difficult to enforce. While some political unrest in Yucatán was evident during the early years of the Mexican Revolution, revolutionary ideals and violence generally arrived late in southeastern Mexico. The most logical reason that states such as Chiapas, Yucatán, and Tabasco experienced a delayed version of the revolution has to do with each region's unique sociopolitical framework.

In the case of Yucatán, the state's peculiar history of internecine struggles between different factions and the revolving door of acting state governors created an impediment to tying politics there to the politics of revolution elsewhere. By the time the Mexican Revolution reached Yucatán in 1915, yellow fever and malaria episodes along with a resurgence of smallpox cases compelled the newly inaugurated revolutionary state under the command of General Salvador Alvarado to rethink Yucatán's approach to health care and, in particular, the role of the public in fostering a disease-free environment.[137]

CHAPTER SIX

DISEASE PREVENTION, THE ROCKEFELLER FOUNDATION, AND REVOLUTION IN YUCATÁN, 1915–1924

THE NATIONAL REVOLUTION ARRIVED LATE in Yucatán, almost four years after dictator Porfirio Díaz fled Mexico in 1911 and revolutionaries had seized the central and northern parts of the country. When revolutionary activism began in Yucatán in 1915, it assumed a distinctly socialist form in comparison to revolutionary activities throughout the rest of Mexico. In 1914, before socialist leader General Salvador Alvarado's arrival on the scene, the titular head of Mexico's Constitionalist Party and interim president Venustiano Carranza placed Colonel Eleuterio Avila y Valdós in control of Yucatán with the mandate to oversee the implementation of Carranza's revolutionary reforms there and to garner support among Yucatecans, particularly the powerful henequeneros, to help secure his leadership as Mexico's president.[1] During Colonel Avila's brief stint as governor, the legislature decreed the liberation of the henequen workers from their obligations to henequeneros.[2]

Published in Maya and Spanish, the legislation known as a "liberation decree" outlined the ills that had befallen Yucatán's Maya peasantry under the oppression of the despotic governments of the past.[3] Anticipating retaliation from the henequeneros for passing the "liberation decree," Avila attempted to make them happy by resisting Carranza's levy of new taxes on the Yucatecan planters. However, Carranza's supporters, the Carrancistas, felt that the richest state in Mexico should do its share to fund the war against Carranza's revolutionary opponents, the Villistas and Zapatistas. Consequently, an irritated Carranza replaced Avila with a leader more willing to do his bidding,

Coahuilan native General Toribio de los Santos. Santos immediately began to strong-arm the region's henequeneros into compliance with Carranza's tax requirements.[4] In response, Yucatán's *casta divina* (the pejorative name given to the thirty to forty richest henequen plantation owners) initiated plans for a coup. Carranza anticipated the henequeneros' plotting and quickly removed Santos before they could mount their attack, ordering Sonoran native General Alvarado to quell the henequen elite's bickering and bring Yucatán into the national revolutionary framework.[5]

When General Alvarado arrived in October 1915 and assumed military and political control over Yucatán, his predecessor Santos had barely served one month in office. While Alvarado's seven-thousand-man troop of experienced fighters from the north quickly overpowered Yucatecan forces, public expectations for Alvarado's long-term survival in the governor's chair were low. Alvarado's entrance onto Yucatán's political stage was forced and largely unwelcome by the state's powerful henequen elites for good reason, as they feared increasing taxes and decreasing political power. Alvarado (anticlerical and unabashedly socialist) did little to endear the powerful henequen kings to him. Almost immediately after taking office, Alvarado rolled back the structure of the henequen monopoly brokered between Yucatán's Porfirian governor Olegario Molina and the U.S. International Harvester Company.[6] Ironically, many of the henequen plantation owners had chafed, too, at International Harvester's power to set its own prices for henequen fiber.

International Harvester's influence and power extended beyond price-fixing. The relationships forged between Yucatán's henequen elite, International Harvester, and international banking conglomerates teetered on the edge of violating U.S. antitrust legislation. The U.S. State Department investigated some of these alliances and found them "dangerous." In particular, the head of International Harvester, John McCormick, was also the son-in-law of John D. Rockefeller, who held considerable stock in his son-in-law's company. Rockefeller also sat on the board of the banking firm Equitable Trust Company, which backed International Harvester's investment in Yucatán's cordage industry. This comingling of family relations with international trade investments compelled the U.S. State Department to seriously question International Harvester's ability to *not* monopolize the cordage industry and influence bank policy.[7] The ties between henequen elites, powerful U.S. businessmen, and politicians helped sustain Yucatán's export industry. The wealth generated from the henequen industry in turn built a modern capital city where regional and foreign elites felt relatively comfortable.

Thus, in 1915 when General Alvarado overthrew the forces of what he called the casta divina—the leading henequen plantation owners—he inherited an urban area that had advanced to the public health level of such leading Caribbean cities as Havana and New Orleans. As we saw in the last chapter, yellow fever and malaria had been two of the major targets in the public health agenda promoted by Governor Molina, which resulted in his reshaping of the city of Mérida. On the other hand, conditions in the countryside were abysmal. Within this political landscape, public health reforms and disease prevention campaigns served their traditional role, simultaneously aiming to curb the proliferation of diseases such as yellow fever and malaria and at the same time advance the state's agenda—which happened, this time, to be a revolutionary one. A close examination of public health reforms during Yucatán's revolution reveals that Yucatecans utilized the destabilizing forces of revolutionary upheaval and disease epidemics to reconfigure their relationship with the state. This renegotiation of resident-state relations fostered conditions that made possible the introduction of foreign philanthropy to assist with disease eradication.[8]

Although it seems paradoxical that a socialist revolution, vividly denounced by the U.S. press, politicians, and businessmen, should be more open to U.S. philanthropy, in reality there were underlying affinities between Alvarado's socialism and many of the programs implemented by the progressives in the United States under Theodore Roosevelt and later Woodrow Wilson. In particular, there was the shared goal of civic uplift, and this required a healthy and clean citizenry.[9] In this chapter, I will relate the seemingly contradictory relationship between the U.S.-based philanthropic Rockefeller Foundation and the socialist revolutionary governments of General Alvarado and his successor, Felipe Carrillo Puerto, drawing upon research among the archives of the foundation along with the papers of Yucatán's state government.

General Alvarado, the Revolution, and Public Health Services

In August 1915, Yucatán's governor, General Salvador Alvarado, declared a "tremendous economic crisis" in the state, which prevented many citizens from obtaining "articles of primary necessity." Governor Alvarado pronounced, "Many of the poor and disabled could not obtain effective assistance and medicines to cure the most lamentable cases of illnesses." Alvarado invoked the ideas of the Mexican Revolution by calling for an uprooting of all vestiges of the "barbary" that had perpetuated poverty over the course of the Díaz dictatorship.[10] Alvarado also decried the fact that the condition of Yucatán's indigenous Maya peasantry had undergone little to no improvement since the "age of slavery."[11] Alvarado's claims intersected with the portrait of greedy elites and Porfirian-era profiteers painted by U.S. sensationalist journalists in such works as Jonathan Turner's *Barbarous Mexico* and John Reed's *Insurgent Mexico*.[12] Alvarado, of course, capitalized on these images of oppression in designing his socialist-minded reforms for Yucatán. Cognizant of Yucatán's international reputation as a "backward" Mexican periphery where abuses against Indians went unchecked, Alvarado redesigned social programs with an eye toward modernization of the countryside and so, underneath a rhetoric of revolution, established a continuity of purpose with the liberals of the nineteenth century. What was different about the revolutionary agenda was that this time, the enemy was not the Maya, but the wealth and privilege of an elite group of henequeneros who kept Yucatán in isolation for their own purposes. Although Alvarado aimed to address poverty and improve the lives of the rural peasantry, he also understood he would gain nothing without the support of the state's powerful henequen elites. To ensure support of his reforms Alvarado needed to secure uninterrupted production of henequen by designing reforms that deftly maneuvered around the henequeneros.[13]

Designing these reforms would be a difficult task given that one of the principal goals of the 1915 revolution involved dismantling the tight connection between the state and the henequen agro-industry, which tended to squeeze out any other areas of development. General Salvador Alvarado had intervened in Yucatán in the first place to crush a henequeneros-backed independence movement that broke out in 1915 after General Carranza ordered Yucatán's rich plantation owners to loan the new government money. The general Carranza turned to, Salvador Alvarado, had originally trained as a pharmacist's assistant in Guyamas and later owned his own pharmacy in Cananea. His career as a revolutionary began also in Cananea where he participated in one of the first strikes of the prerevolutionary period with the Partido Liberal Mexicano of Ricardo Flores Magón.[14]

Coming from the outside, the new governor was unencumbered by alliances with Yucatecan factions but was at the same time ignorant of the situation on the ground in the peninsula. The consolidation of power in the hands of a few powerful henequeneros who wielded control and influence throughout the region and beyond presented a monumental challenge for the general from northern Mexico. Of course, Alvarado was aware of the black legend of the henequeneros, who amassed their fortunes on the backs of a Maya peasantry trapped within the debilitating cycle of perpetual debt servitude.[15] Attempts to rectify the imbalances deeply imbedded in Yucatecan communities would, Alvarado soon saw, require a complete reorganization of the state apparatus. Alvarado's condemnation of the living and working conditions of the Maya laborers toiling on henequen haciendas extended from his stalwart belief that the state must abolish such deplorable circumstances as debt peonage, give equal access to social services, and bring the benefits of public health and disease prevention to the entire population.[16] The latter initiative was a priority. Perhaps it helped that Alvarado, before he had become a revolutionary, had been trained as a pharmacist's assistant and thus was disposed to be sensitive to medical matters.[17]

Alvarado's reforms in Yucatán moved beyond rectifying the inequities of the "old regime" of the Porfiriato and dismantling the henequen monopoly. His leadership served to link Mexico's southeastern peninsula to Carranza's revolutionary machinery in central Mexico. But the revolutionary doctrine and goals espoused by Carranza's Constitutionalist Party were not seamlessly grafted onto Yucatán's political architecture. Instead, Yucatán's revolutionary faction tailored the objectives of the revolution, as they saw them, to fit the region's own distinct socioeconomic conditions. These included the enormous wealth produced by the entrenched henequen monopoly, a state population largely composed of a long-marginalized indigenous and mostly poor peasantry, and vulnerability to waves of crushing disease epidemics, as well as endemic tropical diseases. Yucatán's revolutionary-era governors General Alvarado and Yucatecan Socialist Party leader Felipe Carrillo Puerto understood that while henequen exports garnered significant profits for the region and Mexico as a whole, the henequen business depended for its profit on an unsustainable and unethical debt peonage system.[18] Beyond the abuses of the henequen plantations, there was also dire need for reforming the condition of the Maya peasantry in terms of education and health.[19]

Alvarado's vision of annulling entrenched abuses and using the power of the state to make life better for its citizens was expressed in community-level efforts to revamp agrarian, educational, and health services, especially for the Maya peasantry who had not benefited from Yucatán's prosperity—or had even been reduced to a lower quality of life by the expansions of the henequen zone. On numerous occasions throughout his first year as governor, Alvarado spoke publicly about the "Indian" problem in Yucatán, claiming that "the Indian of Yucatán had lived with respect for the hacendado" and endured "an unequal relationship and a highly disproportionate level of submission."

According to Alvarado, the abuse of special privileges gave rise to this repugnant condition, creating a race of peoples afraid of being crushed under the very laws their ancestors helped to forge.[20]

Alvarado first sought to rectify these abuses by initiating agrarian reforms in 1915, which he touted as the most drastic "outside of the government of New Zealand."[21] He demanded respect for the "*pequena propiedad*," the small family farm, which he defined as individuals possessing no more than fifty hectares of cultivated land. Liberation, Alvarado reminded large landowners, required sacrifice, so that the "revolution will sweep away for us all difficulties."[22] For Alvarado, all revolutionary reforms—land, public health, and education—required Yucatecans to sacrifice personal needs for the good of the commonwealth; only then, he argued, would a stronger, more stable state emerge.[23] As has been pointed out recently by historians of the period (like Sterling Evans and Gilbert M. Joseph), the land reform effort was aimed at food-cultivating smallholders, whereas Alvarado viewed the henequen plantations as essential for the economy. "In fact, with the exception of Olegario Molina, who had fled, most of the land-holding henequeneros or 'Casta Divina' learned to work with the new governor and benefited economically and politically from their new alliance with him. Most even became avid members of the political party, the Socialist Party of the Southeast (Partido Socialista del Sureste, known by its Spanish acronym PSS), that Alvarado established in Yucatán."[24]

Continuing with his sweeping reforms, Alvarado developed the "Five Sisters Plan," which was meant to mark a complete break from Yucatán's past of slavery, secession, and nepotism.[25] In the eloquent words of one "impartial and anonymous socialist foreigner," Yucatán's image from the outside was "marked by a political regime producing an inferno of chaos and horror. For addicts it [Yucatán] is an Edenic marvel. For the passersby from other states, Yucatán is a crater of perpetual fire, a Sahara of petrified rocks, a planet with few friendly people and henequen dominance."[26] These metaphors of upheaval reflected one fact that both the left and right could agree upon: that there was indeed a revolution occurring in Yucatán. Rhetorically, at least, the veritable "crater of perpetual fire" was being transformed by radical measures into an Eden. In ordinary life, however, the radical land, education, and public works reforms also brought instability, confusion, and misunderstandings. Populations that had once remained relatively isolated from one another, and had even fled one another during the long Caste War, were now in communication with each other as revolutionary brigades and troops implemented new policies throughout the peninsula. Such physical communication inadvertently spread disease, just as cholera had been spread by the military during the Caste War of the 1850s. Shortly after the arrival of Alvarado's troops in 1915, a violent outbreak of smallpox and yellow fever enveloped the peninsula. Rumor blamed Alvarado and his men for the spread of the disease; Alvarado, in response, proved he well understood the power of containment. He initiated emergency legislation, including mandatory quarantines for the infected to combat the existing outbreaks and curb the potential for future occurrences.[27]

Alvarado also called for the immediate establishment of free, state-financed clinics in all the older suburbs of the capital city of Mérida. Each clinic would be staffed with at least one medical doctor, have a pharmacy attached to it, and would dispense medicines free of charge.[28] Governor Alvarado's pharmacy training helped him to understand the power medical science held over ailing and fearful populations, and he seized the opportunity brought about by disease epidemics to transform Yucatán's public health services.[29] Alvarado's short- and long-term public health reforms were unopposed by the elites, who continued to believe that the great cause of disease and underdevelopment lay in the barbarism of the backlands and small rural pueblos inhabited by an illiterate and superstitious peasantry serviced by witches, quack doctors, and untrained midwives.[30] Alvarado's approach to reform through public health and medical science borrowed elements from the civilizing missions of past administrations and was animated by an attitude that was continuous with the científico project of development. The ideological celebration of the Indian, so often found in the revolutionary rhetoric and images of the period, did not extend to tolerance for the traditional forms of healing often found in indigenous communities.[31]

During the early years of Yucatán's revolution, Alvarado sought to prevent and suppress illness by focusing on hygiene and sanitation, fining and even jailing residents who hid or failed to report illnesses or contributed to unhealthy environmental conditions.[32] Just as we saw in the last chapter with the Molina administration's health code, the new public health legislation made individuals responsible for living up to state-set health norms by requiring residents to submit to quarantine if infected with certain diseases and to inform on those who harbored ill family members, thus initiating a system that pitted residents against one another.[33] In order to implement quarantine mandates during epidemics, Alvarado used military police, who also often doubled as government spies.[34]

Overall, General Alvarado's overhaul of Yucatán's medical services derived from the traditional development agenda of socialist-leaning state-building projects. In distinction from his Porfirian predecessors, Alvarado's regime sought to increase access to public resources, universalize education, increase the number of local clinics, and encourage sanitary brigades, pharmacies, and additional vaccination sites through state financial and moral support.[35] His reforms contained a distinct blend of socialism and modernization theory tinged with moral reformism common among early twentieth-century bourgeois reformers.[36]

By the end of Alvarado's term as Yucatán's governor in 1917, the newly reordered public health services branch was called the General Directorate for Health and Hygiene. The agency for the state of Yucatán included a broad array of services and responsibilities including the regulation of unlicensed dogs; gynecologic checkups for prostitutes; the maintenance of sanitation standards for taverns, markets, slaughterhouses, cemeteries, and garbage collection; as well as the production, distribution, and application of vaccines.[37] In particular, the inspection of taverns took on special importance as temperance movements rallied to shut down drinking establishments. Jailing drunks became a full-time job for local police, but the health consequences of the drinker's deeds seemed to elude reform, as alcohol-related illnesses remained predominant as a chief cause of death, especially among men.[38]

Alcoholism was a flash point. The United States went through prohibition in the twenties. General Alvarado had tried to close many of the bars of Mérida, being a temperance man himself. Members of the local Feminist Leagues in Yucatán complained vociferously about drunken men in their communities and pressed to have alcoholism recognized as a public health issue, since it caused wife beating, impoverished and broke up families, led to public brawls, and encouraged any number of crimes.[39] In the early 1920s, over fifty-six thousand Yucatecan women, distributed across forty-five registered Feminist Resistance and Socialist Leagues, cornered the attention of regional leaders as they clamored for the closure of cantinas and brothels by describing the damage caused to their families by alcoholism and sexually transmitted diseases. Feminists lobbied for prohibition beginning in 1918, and by 1922, at least seven villages had implemented an alcohol ban.[40] Alcoholism, in their estimation, constituted the bane of their communities (and they were not entirely wrong), with men spending their hard-earned wages on alcohol that literally pickled their bodies from the inside out through necrosis of the liver and left just as many widows and orphans as did war.[41]

Visits to brothels, and in particular consort with unregistered prostitutes in clandestine locations and on the street, brought the spectacle of sexual commerce into public spaces. Moralizing about the sexual habits of men who frequented brothels led to conclusions about the proliferation of sexually transmitted diseases and the disintegration of family life. Blamed for infecting their wives with syphilis and causing birth defects and childhood learning disabilities among their offspring, Mexico's men were the target of the campaign to combat sexually transmitted diseases through social reform and condemnation of prostitution.[42] The Feminist Leagues of Yucatán's emphasis on alcoholism, prostitution, sexually transmitted diseases, and childhood illnesses successfully redirected the focus of public health services and education throughout the peninsula.

While Yucatecan Feminist Leagues rallied successfully for social reforms throughout their communities, the General Directorate for Health and Hygiene seemed unable to fulfill its goals. Although intended to bring a more beneficent order to Yucatán, the General Directorate brought instability to the private lives of many Yucatecans who endured the fumigations of sanitary brigades, sometimes had to evacuate condemned structures, dealt with quarantines that separated families, and faced the fines that could be levied for infractions. In the five years between 1915 and 1920, many lost confidence in the benefits that were supposed to be brought about by revolutionary health reforms.[43] The result was an erosion of state-resident relations. Ironically, this atmosphere of suspicion and fear proved to be the ideal condition for the intervention of an outside organization, the New York–based Rockefeller Foundation, which initiated an anti–yellow fever and malaria program in Yucatán in 1919. This campaign offered Yucatecans an alternative source for public health assistance outside of mandated quarantines, fines, and penalties enforced by the revolutionary state.

Combating Yellow Fever with the Rockefeller Foundation and Socialism

By 1919, many Yucatecans were already accustomed to the intensified scrutiny of their private lives, which had unfolded as the socialist regime combined public health surveillance and such obligatory health measures as smallpox vaccination, and so would not be unduly disturbed by the methods chosen by the Rockefeller Foundation's International Health Board (IHB) to combat yellow fever and malaria.

The Rockefeller Foundation began their philanthropic work in Mexico specifically to combat yellow fever, malaria, and hookworm. Founded in 1913 with an incredible (for the time) endowment of fifty million dollars, the IHB, under the direction of physician Wickliffe Rose, drafted proposals to take the work of their sanitary commissions for the eradication of hookworm, malaria, and yellow fever abroad. The Rockefeller Foundation's interest in Latin America peaked with the opening of the Panama Canal in 1914, which brought with it concerns about the spread of tropical maladies such as yellow fever and malaria throughout the Caribbean and Latin America.[44] By and large the Rockefeller Foundation's health program in Mexico infused funds, expertise, and energy into national and state public health branches severely depleted by the costs of civil war.

The IHB drew upon their experiences with anti-hookworm campaigns in British Guiana (1914) and the U.S. South (1915 in Arkansas and Mississippi) in developing their health programs in Mexico. As early as 1914, the IHB initiated negotiations with Carranza's government to launch anti-hookworm, anti–yellow fever, and anti-malaria campaigns.

However, the political climate surrounding revolutionary activity in central and northern Mexico presented severe challenges.[45] The U.S. Marine Corps occupation of Veracruz in 1914 did little to engender trust between the two nations. In fact, fear that the United States would march inland from Veracruz to Mexico City to force President Victoriano Huerta (1913–14) out of office only served to solidify anti-*yanqui* sentiments and swell the ranks of the national military with young men anxious to protect Mexican sovereignty.[46] As a result, the Rockefeller Foundation's efforts to secure a contract from the Mexican government took time. The threat revolutionary fighting posed to the stability of the IHB's health program, and to Americans working in Mexico, surfaced as a critical concern for the foundation, and the fear of violence was renewed when revolutionary leader Francisco "Pancho" Villa raided Columbus, New Mexico, in March of 1916, killing several innocent civilians. In response, U.S. president Woodrow Wilson sent Commander John J. "Black Jack" Pershing to Mexico to capture Villa. In the end, Pershing's failure to capture Villa, plus the defeat of a detachment of American troops at Carrizal, emboldened the Mexican government and signaled that Mexico's revolution could not be overthrown externally.[47] As the United States entered the World War in 1917, American attention shifted away from Mexico, while the Carranza government tried to establish itself as the only legal government of Mexico. As it would turn out, Carranza's missteps alienated the Sonoran generals, including Obregon and Alvarado. But civil war did not resume until 1920. Meanwhile, full-scale implementation of the Rockefeller Foundation's activities finally could begin throughout Mexico and Yucatán in late 1919.

While revolutionary violence clearly posed a threat to residents along the U.S.-Mexico border, fear that deadly diseases could cross the border undetected further exacerbated U.S.-Mexican relations. During World War I and immediately afterward, U.S. employers utilized Mexican laborers extensively to make up for manpower shortages. In particular, southern California agribusiness owners had come to depend on inexpensive Mexican labor to supplement the dwindling American domestic workforce but faced the problem of the popular perception of Mexican migrant workers, which was that they posed a health threat, contaminated as they were with typhus and other diseases.[48] So if the Rockefeller Foundation seems to us extraordinarily altruistic in its work in Mexico, there were also American business leaders who promoted sanitizing the United States' neighbor to the south in order to ensure an orderly supply of cheap, healthy Mexican labor.[49]

The 1918–19 influenza epidemic, which killed almost fifty million people worldwide, also contributed to the fear of the mobility of diseases during wartime.[50] Throughout Mexico, the influenza pandemic crippled national and state public health resources. Regional public health units in particular struggled to address the devastating pandemic while performing smallpox vaccination duties, routine hygiene inspections for public establishments, and routine sanitation maintenance.[51]

The IHB doctors needed assurances from Mexico's President Carranza before they could initiate their disease eradication campaigns, but Carranza proved difficult to approach as he was busy heading off threats to his administration, especially from his former generals. IHB doctors found dealing with the Carranza administration to be a highly frustrating experience, which was underlined by the meeting that the IHB representative, retired U.S. Army colonel and medical corps physician Theodore C. Lyster, finally arranged with Carranza on December 9, 1919. As a physician appointed to combat yellow fever and malaria in Central America, Dr. Lyster understood the intricacies involved in working with foreign governments. During his work in Central America, Dr. Lyster had witnessed firsthand what he deemed to be the transformative power of hygiene and medical science in regions deeply afflicted by tropical maladies such as malaria and yellow fever.[52] However, he was also weary of waiting and anxious to begin work under an official contract with the Mexican government.

Lyster noted in his officer's log that an agreement between the Rockefeller Foundation and Carranza would bring Mexico into a global "campaign for humanity."[53] When Dr. Lyster finally met with Carranza and outlined the

Rockefeller Foundation's anti–yellow fever and anti-malaria plan, he described the inclusion of a new yellow fever vaccine and curative serum developed by Japanese scientist Dr. Hideyo Noguchi, who was already available to start work in Yucatán later that month.[54] But President Carranza expressed far more interest in combating syphilis than yellow fever or malaria. Subsequent conversations with Mexico's National Health Board personnel revealed that the Carranza administration and the IHB held divergent visions about what constituted a healthy Mexican citizenry. In particular, concerns about which diseases deserved the most attention conflicted; yellow fever and malaria were top priorities for the Rockefeller Foundation, while syphilis and other sexually transmitted diseases were much higher on the list for Mexico's leaders. President Carranza asked Dr. Lyster to bring wax models, films, and other educational materials to assist with a campaign to educate Mexicans about syphilis.[55] In the end, the Carranza administration failed to sign off on an agreement with the IHB for a national yellow fever and malaria campaign. Undeterred by the absence of an agreement with the Carranza administration, the Rockefeller Foundation turned to regional invitations from public health administrators, medical schools, and health boards in dire need of assistance.

From a U.S. diplomatic standpoint, adding Mexico to the regions benefiting from the Rockefeller Foundation's philanthropy meant the cultivation of a healthy neighbor without committing U.S. tax dollars.[56] In general, three broad factors dominated America's interest in Mexico between 1910 and the late 1920s. First, Americans worried about suppressing the violence unleashed by the Mexican Revolution. Second, in the years directly following the end of WWI, Americans were in a moral panic about subversives, communists, socialists, and anarchists within their communities and thus looked at the revolutionary rhetoric of the Mexican government, and their penchant for giving refuge to radicals, as a threat. Third and most important was protecting American investment in Mexico, particularly after the inclusion of Article 27 in the 1917 Constitution, which prohibited foreign ownership of land and subsoil rights. Also, oil companies had a large stake in Mexico by this time. Within this context, Rockefeller Foundation administrators worked diligently to maintain neutrality in such affairs.

Throughout anti–yellow fever and anti-malaria campaigns, the Rockefeller Foundation administrators asserted their desire to distance themselves from national- and regional-level politics, stressing that elimination of yellow fever was a "campaign for humanity" and the "foundation recognized no race or nation, only a united fight against a common enemy of humanity."[57] However, the reality of the IHB's work in Mexico was that it needed cooperation with local physicians, communities, and medical school staff, making the IHB partners, whether the administrators admitted it or not, with local governments.[58] Furthermore, concerns echoed by Americans about the infiltration of violence and dissident ideologies into their homeland, as well as a need to protect U.S. investments in Mexico, indelibly shaped the attitudes and behaviors of those involved in the Rockefeller Foundation's anti–yellow fever and anti-malaria campaigns in Mexico.

For the Rockefeller Foundation, Mexico posed a particularly interesting set of potential outcomes. It was a testing ground for the proposition that diseases such as yellow fever and malaria could be eradicated. This would not only open up Mexico to modernization, improve trade relations with the United States and other nations, and expand foreign investment opportunities, but it would provide a program that could be replicated in other tropical countries. In fact, Mexico's tropical zones offered particularly fertile terrain for combating tropical maladies such as yellow fever and malaria, while also improving relations between the United States and Mexico—particularly among regions along the rich oil-laden Gulf Coast.[59] Thus, Mexico fit neatly into the Rockefeller Foundation's mission for the IHB. The rich natural resources of Mexico—especially oil—could be unlocked for international trade as the postwar Western economies rapidly adopted the automobile and the highway as the new dominant form of transportation.[60] The Rockefeller Foundation had numerous ties with the foreign community that held investments in and promoted commerce with Mexico. General J. A. Ryan of the Texas Company began work in Mexico following the ratification of Mexico's 1917 Constitution to settle disputes between U.S. oil investors and the Mexican government.[61] General Ryan believed the work of the Rockefeller Foundation in Mexico did more to bring about lasting peace and a close commercial union with the United States than anything oil lobbyists had done.[62] Improved relations with the United States may have been a welcome consequence of the Rockefeller Foundation's work in Mexico. But for those living in states along Mexico's tropical corridor like Veracruz, Tampico, Campeche, and Yucatán, the arrival of the Rockefeller Foundation's IHB physicians on their soil resonated on another level. Many residents along Mexico's Gulf Coast sought primarily to eradicate diseases like yellow fever and malaria as a means to improve their life spans and quality of life.

The entrance of the Rockefeller Foundation's IHB into Yucatán's diseased landscape also emboldened national, regional, and local efforts to control and order populations amidst revolutionary turmoil.[63] Under the revolutionary government in Yucatán, the implementation of public health projects designed to benefit the formerly excluded population of rural peons and the urban proletariat was also a means of extending the power of the state, especially as its agenda was contested by powerful forces in the Caribbean region. New technology and funding sustained broader social reform programs aimed at modernizing the region by securing a healthy labor force, which would thus attract international investors. To realize such an ambitious health agenda on its own was beyond the capabilities of the Yucatán government. The IHB, however, had one of the biggest endowments in the world and could employ famous scientists like Hideyo Noguchi, introduce new methods for disease detection, set up laboratories to explore preventative vaccines for yellow fever, and organize the control of mosquito proliferation through spraying.

The socialist government and the IHB could collaborate on antidisease and hygiene campaigns even if they were operating based on different incentives. By 1915, Yucatán's image had become considerably better, due to the construction of a progressive urban infrastructure in Mérida in the 1910s. When, in 1910, the annual report of the U.S. Public Health Service was published, the expert on yellow fever who was sent to Yucatán reported that "the general condition of Mérida as to cleanliness of streets, sidewalks, etc. was remarkably good," although he also found that "the sewer system was . . . incomplete," thus providing a niche for mosquito-borne and other parasitic diseases. Still, in comparison to Campeche (which was found to be "vastly inferior" to Mérida), the city came off well.[64] Yet most of the peninsula still labored under the reputation of being "backward," "traditional," and "unhealthy." It is in this context that we can understand the seemingly paradoxical collaboration of the revolutionary socialist state and the Rockefeller Foundation, which occurred in Yucatán under the leadership of governors General Salvador Alvarado, between 1915 and 1917, and Felipe Carrillo Puerto, between 1922 and 1924.

The simultaneous yellow fever and malaria epidemics combined with political turbulence throughout the peninsula caused by the takeover of the state government by General Alvarado reshaped the landscape of disease prevention in Yucatán by empowering local-level socialist leagues, brigades, and residents to take action against disease by targeting insect vectors and disease-causing filth. Household hygiene and personal cleaning rituals increasingly came under the scrutiny of village and countryside activists as disease prevention campaigns underscored the major role played by poor hygiene in disease proliferation. Public health experts analyzed all aspects of everyday life including the marketplace, the slaughterhouse, rooming houses, brothels, cemeteries, schools, and private residences. Those suffering under the crushing burdens of poverty, warfare, disease, and unsanitary living conditions drew upon the power of the revolution's promises of equality to secure access to state services for cleaning up their communities.[65]

Along these lines, the IHB's goal to work with local communities and provide them with training to run the program in the future, without the IHB, complemented revolution-minded reforms incredibly well. The IHB worked with regional health groups abroad to provoke change through the implementation of modern medical practices and public health education. IHB field physicians supplemented state programs by reiterating their desire to teach small-town populations and rural doctors "modern bacteriological methods." The fact that Mexico's medical schools lacked laboratories and microscopes inspired the Rockefeller Foundation to offer fellowships and establish a cooperative system with different state universities to install medical technology and train young physicians throughout Mexico.[66] Thus, a diverse set of interests were being served when Hideyo Noguchi disembarked in Progreso in 1920. The Rockefeller Foundation's programs to improve Yucatán by combating debilitating tropical illness may well have been intertwined with Yucatán's revolutionary reforms, but the Rockefeller Foundation's own aims, including the desire to test developing medical technologies, were also being served.

For instance, by being granted the permission to test Noguchi's anti–yellow fever vaccine in Yucatán, the Rockefeller Foundation obtained a living laboratory to further study the efficacy of the fluid in humans.[67] Prior to its use in Mexico, Noguchi's vaccine research focused on isolating a microorganism (*Leptospira icteroides*) in guinea pigs while he worked in Guayaquil, Ecuador, in 1918.[68] Thus, the vaccine and serum Noguchi developed had had virtually no field trials beyond animal specimens when they were introduced to the residents of Mexico. Unfortunately, the vaccine did not live up to expectations. Problems with the amount of agar (a gelatinous substance derived from red marine algae) preservative and a lack of communication and training on behalf of local vaccination teams contributed to its failure in Yucatán as an effective yellow fever preventative.[69]

Even more worrisome for the IHB were reports of vaccine reactions. Some complaints simply pointed to the vaccine's ineffectiveness, principally the contraction of yellow fever after vaccination, while others noted mild side effects such as the formation of abscesses at the vaccination site, and a few observed severe complications like swelling of limbs and infection after receiving the vaccine.[70] Several IHB field physicians witnessed adverse physical reactions to the

Noguchi yellow fever vaccine after application.[71] As news about the Noguchi vaccine circulated, the Rockefeller Foundation reconsidered its usefulness for the Mexico campaign. Regional health officials and International Health Board physicians concurred that since distribution of the vaccine required injection of the fluid into human bodies, public fear of the vaccine held the potential to undermine the entire campaign.[72] Mexican physicians and public health administrators in Yucatán pointed to complications with the distribution and application of smallpox vaccination in the past, which led local physicians and Rockefeller Foundation employees to conclude that enforcing obligatory preventative vaccination for yellow fever would be nearly impossible.[73]

Not wanting to risk failure, the IHB doctors tried a new tactic by focusing entirely on the elimination of mosquito larvae. This decision proved to be tremendously successful. In eliminating vaccination as a preventative measure against yellow fever, IHB doctors effectively shifted the burden of disease prevention from the human body to the mosquito vector and its environment.[74]

The IHB's shift from vaccine prevention to mosquito control also paralleled major political upheaval on the national front. In the wake of President Carranza's assassination in 1920, a Sonoran comrade of General Alvarado, Alvaro Obregón, assumed Mexico's presidential post. According to IHB physician T. C. Lyster, President Obregón was more eager to conquer epidemics that posed a transnational threat and less obsessed with syphilis than his predecessor. Thus, under Obregón the Rockefeller Foundation received the assurances they had long desired with official approval of the campaign extended to the Rockefeller Foundation in January of 1921.[75]

With official recognition of the Rockefeller Foundation's anti–yellow fever and anti-malaria campaign in Mexico now in hand, the IHB workers began to fan out along the tropical coastline of Mexico, educating local health units in effective mosquito elimination tactics, diagnostics of parasite-borne diseases, and therapeutics. Field physicians stressed control over the environment as vital in preventing mosquito-borne diseases, which caused stresses at the community level and raised the question of responsibility for any unsanitary conditions, from the household kitchen to the pigsty. The public health literature was dominated by tropes of filth and the contrast between civilized and barbaric human-animal interactions; these tropes seeped into the fabric of daily life, creating fears about the very soil Yucatecans tilled and the air they breathed, on the off chance that these harbored disease.[76]

IHB doctors coordinated with regional health brigades to administer door-to-door home inspections, while training specialized local eradication teams.

At the same time, public health brigades dispersed throughout the peninsula on bicycles, allocating considerable time and effort to acquiring screens and tight-fitting lids for water tanks, placing mosquito larvae–eating fish in water reservoirs, and "oiling" or "bombing" cisterns, tanks, and cenotes to kill mosquito larvae.[77] Whether disease and illness lingered at a busy commercial port or in one's private home, the acknowledged link between disease and the environment completed, in this period, the reconfiguration of the architecture of disease eradication that had begun in the Caribbean in Havana during the 1890s, but under the aegis of the revolution rather than that of top-down scientific management.

Concentration on vector eradication led to a demand for experts in laboratory research and scientists who intimately understood the reproductive and feeding habits of mosquitoes.[78] The IHB medical personnel could draw upon a literature already rich in concerns about climatic conditions, sanitation, personal hygiene, waste disposal, soil quality, and the health of domesticated pets and livestock, and they added to it as they took advantage of the instrument provided by the state to enter into the private realm to alter or eradicate conditions deemed unsanitary.[79] In turn, Yucatán's socialists organized voluntary networks in the form of socialist brigades and leagues to assist the IHB with the eradication of disease. This grassroots organization was the key difference between the revolutionary epoch and Molina's Porfirian reforms. IHB physicians and administrators utilized the energies of socialist youth brigades, medical student collectives, and local health leagues (juntas) to implement an aggressive mosquito eradication project throughout Yucatán. Concurrently, socialist resistance leagues assumed control of public services including vaccination of schoolchildren and distribution of medicines. This very success put the Rockefeller Foundation's goal of neutrality in doubt: the IHB and the revolution's socialist leagues must have been hard to separate for the average citizen. The populist effect of the program was that citizens became much bolder in demanding access to state services. Requests for the construction of new roads and schools, increases in teacher salaries, construction supplies, assistance in fighting off infestations of locusts and maintaining order, access to licensed doctors and medicines, and improved public sanitation dominated league-state correspondence throughout the revolution.[80]

In May 1921 Mérida's *liga* president, Liborio Felto, sent members of his chapter to haciendas outside the capital city to help rural landowners fight off a plague of locusts that was destroying crops.[81] One year later in May of 1922, liga members were sent to maintain order in the town of Calotumul after a spate of drunken gun battles wreaked havoc in the town. Frightened residents

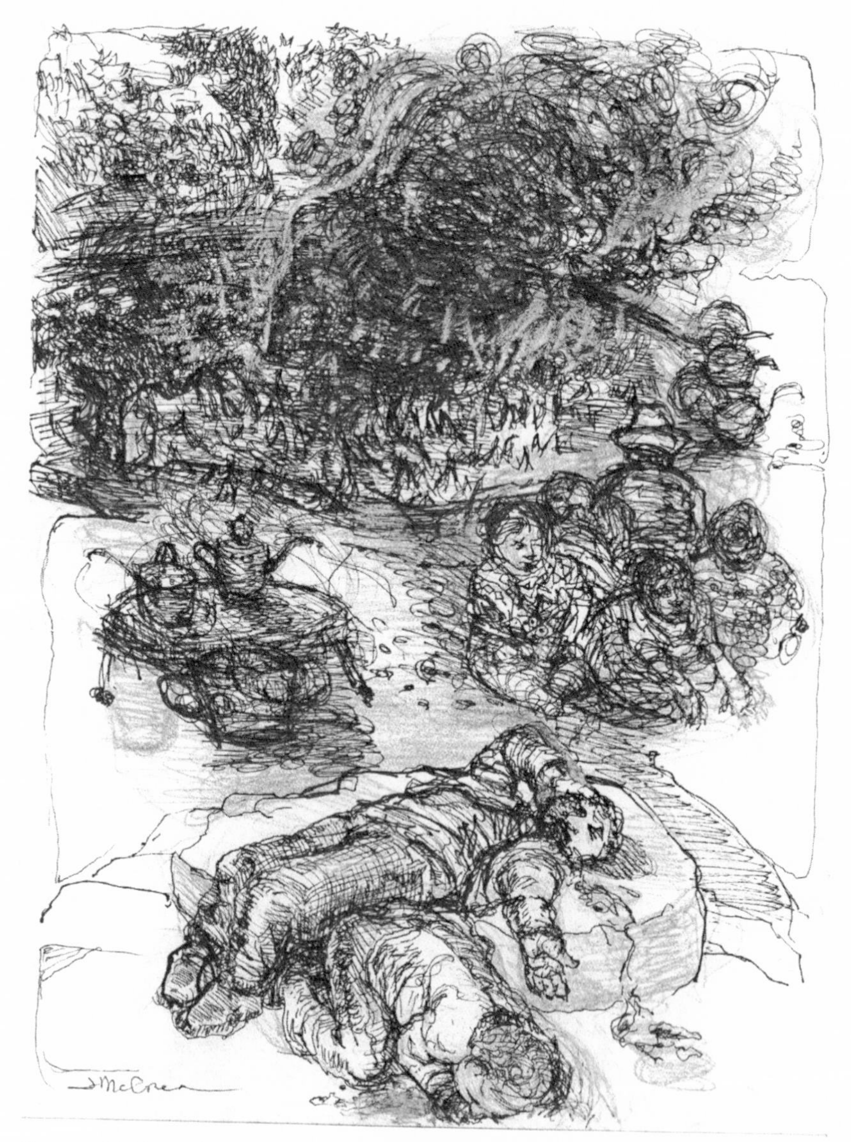

Figure 5: *El Vómito Prieto* by Judith B. McCrea.

sequestered themselves in their homes, afraid they would be trampled while intoxicated men rode their horses through town. Also, Calotumul residents called upon liga members to protect them because they did not have enough funding to pay a police force to maintain order.[82] In an effort to combat what many medical professionals viewed as the stubborn use of unlicensed healers in small towns, the president of Yucatán's Superior Health Council, Dr. Miguel Castillo Torres, began a campaign to purge the region of these practitioners. In April 1922, Dr. Torres wrote to the governor outlining his plan to rid Mérida of "spiritualists." To make his point clear about the danger "spiritualists" brought to Yucatán, Dr. Torres referred to them by their "true and vulgar" names, "sorcerers, witches, fortune tellers, herbalists, and bonesetters." In fact, Yucatán's Sanitary Code, passed in 1909, required all medical professionals to register with the Superior Health Council and provide evidence of degrees earned.[83] Dr. Torres attached a detailed list of victims who suffered offenses at the hands of "vile and cruel" quacks along with their home addresses.

Using the assistance of the ligas to help locate the offenders, officials began a purge on unregistered and unlicensed healers in November of 1922. The hunt for these "quacks" soon extended beyond Mérida. For instance, the municipal head of Peto wrote to Yucatán's governor to complain about "three curanderos whose only occupation is to exploit the town and they are not competent." The governor's office responded by having the Superior Health Council send a medical student and a liga representative to Peto to conduct a search for the curanderos.[84] Felipe Carrillo Puerto credited the ligas with helping every Indian village. "It is this organization that has garnered the fruits of the Revolution," he wrote, "and saved them for the Indians." Carrillo Puerto listed the accomplishments of the eighty-thousand-member ligas as building schools, beautifying towns, and advocating against drunkenness. The influence of the ligas appears to have been quite pervasive, extending into art and leisure time as well. "Each Liga has a band or orchestra—that is compulsory—for our people are far too sad and must learn to sing and dance," he said, "they have been slaves so long they have forgotten how to play."[85]

Revolutionary philosophies celebrated the end of the days of slavery but also reinforced the link between control over one's own household and the health and security of the community. Anti-malaria and anti–yellow fever campaigns capitalized on the revolutionary government's program to inspire compliance. Inevitably, some residents found the incursions into their daily routines, coupled with household inspections and fines, irritating.[86] Complaints from householders to public health officials usually addressed what they viewed to be excessive and abusive applications of the law for public health infractions. Public grievances regarding failure to meet public health and safety standards often focused on high fines and unfair inspections.[87] The oppressive fines, interruptions to daily life, and interferences with the operation of small businesses provoked a backlash against state-sponsored public health services and officials.[88] Rather than willingly make sacrifices for the public good, letters from residents brimmed with questions regarding the role of the state versus individual and community responsibility. After the first wave of enthusiasm, citizens raised questions about the compromises of individual privacy in the name of the health and safety of the population. The result was resistance to state legislation. Ironically, however, the struggle between resident and state authorities also legitimated state authority. In fact, avoidance of state policies oftentimes only served to motivate state programs to redouble their efforts to track, quarantine, and fine residents who evaded public health mandates.[89]

But whatever resistance existed on the grassroots level, on the level of governance, the revolutionary state's continuing ability to advance an anti-disease agenda was codified in the passage of the Yellow Fever Vigilance Law of September 1921, requiring residents to open their homes to public health agents for inspections.[90] In no small way, the Yellow Fever Vigilance Law facilitated success for the Rockefeller Foundation's anti–yellow fever campaign in Yucatán. In the end, Yucatán's success in the battle against yellow fever became a model that was followed in other tropical regions plagued with persistent malaria and yellow fever cycles. The 1921 declaration that yellow fever had been eradicated in the Yucatán—a goal that had eluded Díaz-era modernizers—seemed to crown the IHB and Socialist Party program.[91] As irritating as some residents may have found the inspections and fines, they were successful.

With yellow fever eradicated by 1921, some small towns sought to redirect the state's attention toward other health issues largely ignored during the height of the anti–yellow fever campaign. In the town of Umán, located about thirty kilometers southwest of Mérida, residents were overcome by pandemic influenza in early 1919. In a state of frenzy, municipal heads pleaded for assistance. The government responded by sending medical students and a sanitary brigade to help the community, but they did not stay beyond the immediate threat.[92] By 1921, the town was desperate for medical personnel. Umán's residents then appealed to the Central League of Resistance of the PSS for permission to allow local, unlicensed healer Eduardo Peniche to practice without legal repercussions. Claiming that the public health junta of Umán contained no staff or supplies, residents wanted the state public health council to grant Peniche authority to practice medicine. The president of the Superior Health Council, Dr. Castillo Torres, denied the request, stating that Peniche took advantage of "simple and ignorant people."[93] But rural towns spanning the peninsula made similar requests, and towns like Peto and Tizimín also requested veterinarian

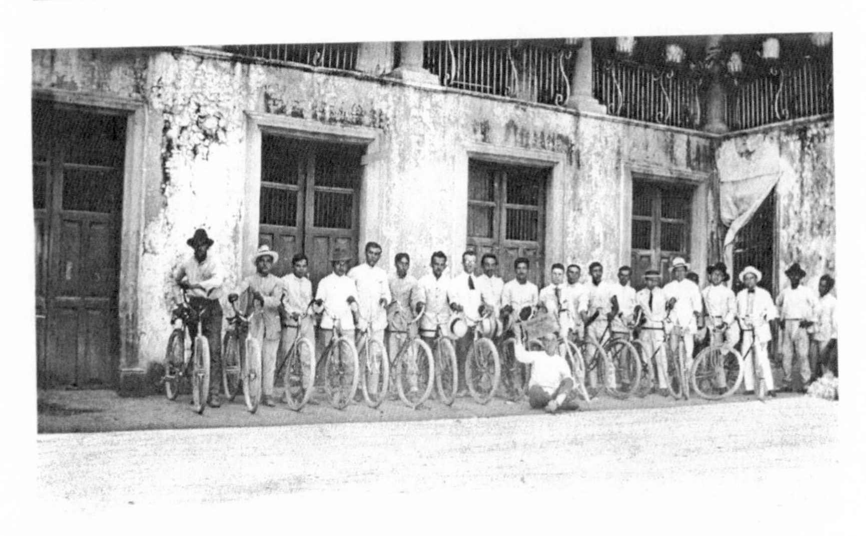

Photo 1: Yellow Fever Service in Mérida, 1923. Owned by the men who used them, the bicycles were used in their same districts (RAC, RFA, Photograph Collection, RF Collection, Series 323 O, Yellow Fever, Folder 1, 10573, Connor April 30, 1923). Thank you to the Rockefeller Archive Center for permission to print this image.

expertise for outbreaks of animal-borne diseases (like "bad red," which afflicted pigs), access to smallpox vaccine, and fumigation supplies.[94]

In some towns like Peto, local leaders expressed relatively little need for the IHB and the state's yellow fever eradication campaign. Located deep in the peninsula's south near Quintana Roo, the town attracted many laborers who came to the area to extract sap from the massive zapote trees to make chicle (a latex or sticky substance used as a bonding agent). According to Dr. Connor, the *chicleros* were "organized as workers" and enacted a strict policy to protect everyone from yellow fever. Contractors were obliged to transport every sick worker from the zapote forests back to Peto immediately. If the entire family traveled with a sick worker, then the whole family accompanied the sick employee back to town and were isolated. Many of the workers carried supplies of quinine and diligently enforced the return of sick workers to Peto. As a result, Peto had not recorded one case of yellow fever since 1917. Dr. Connor attributed the low incidence of yellow fever in Peto to a combination of factors: immunity among the workers to yellow fever, careful planning to remove and quarantine sick workers, and the preventative use of quinine.[95]

In other parts of the peninsula, nearly one year had passed without any reported cases of yellow fever since the eradication declaration of 1921, an unprecedented achievement. IHB suggested that the region be surveyed to ensure that preventative measures remained in place. In this capacity, the IHB's Dr. Connor disembarked in Progreso in early February 1921, accompanied by Dr. Lyster. They were met in Mérida by the chief of the Superior Health Council for the capital city, Dr. Gil Rojas, who gave the doctors bad news: yellow fever prevention in the region had slowed to a crawl. Necessary public health services and the stock of such resources as oil to bomb the cisterns were being cut back due to funding shortfalls. The Department of Health in Mérida was relying primarily on volunteer brigades (*brigadas volantes*) to conduct "sweeps" throughout Mérida looking for mosquito larvae reservoirs and bombing mosquito nests with oil. Without the money for the oil, the volunteer brigades obviously could not assist in mosquito eradication. Rojas explained to Lyster and Connor that the irregular funding from the Mexican government (Obregón's government, as the general had replaced the assassinated Carranza) hampered the struggle against yellow fever and malaria, concerns that were echoed in the report Lyster turned in to the Rockefeller Foundation with a plea for supplemental funding.[96] But with a yellow fever eradication statement already in circulation, members of the Yellow Fever Commission remained divided about the issue of continued funding. Field physicians generally advocated for no change in the intensity of the campaign, while others, in particular administrators, argued that the decline in the incidence of yellow fever should lead to a reduction in services to regular surveillance and inspection only.[97] Rockefeller board members reminded commission members that the Rockefeller Foundation's program explicitly laid out its intention at inception that the project "eventually stand on its own financial feet."[98]

Despite Connor and Lyster's discovery that the yellow fever prevention campaign was lagging in Mérida, the Rockefeller Foundation and the press hailed the success of the anti–yellow fever campaign in Yucatán in press releases and papers at international conferences; the IHB's success in Yucatán became the official, triumphal story in both the public mind and among the international community of scientists. Dr. Connor noted in the *American Journal of Tropical Medicine* in a report dated June 19, 1922, that the last recorded case of yellow fever occurred in Talisman on December 20, 1920, while also noting that there may have been milder cases in some areas since then. At the second Convention of the Special Commission for Yellow Fever held in Mexico City in August of 1922, Rockefeller Foundation physicians presented their findings detailing extensive mosquito eradication efforts. With nearly a year free of yellow fever in Yucatán, the topic of conversation at the convention shifted from eradication to prevention efforts. IHB doctors cautioned that the danger of a yellow fever reappearance depended on whether the Mexicans could "combat inertia in a country where it has been an age-long ideal to do as little work as possible."[99] Furthermore, those involved in public health education for the Rockefeller Foundation observed that Mexicans would often write reports that made their services look much better on paper than they were in reality.[100] Ultimately, the convention approved a plan for graduated reductions in eradication work in accordance with recommendations made by field doctors Lyster and Connor. Much of the reasoning behind the plan stemmed from the belief that Yucatán was no longer the center of disease in Central America, which had shifted to San Salvador.[101]

Just two short years after the Rockefeller Foundation's IHB officially began work in Yucatán, the subdirector for the national Campaign against Yellow Fever declared that yellow fever no longer threatened Mexico as whole. In the end, the Yellow Fever Commission in Mexico City concluded that despite some problems with the side effects and efficacy of Dr. Noguchi's *Leptospira icteroides* vaccine, the groundwork had been laid here, too, for the use of the vaccine as a prophylactic against yellow fever. The decrease in the intensity of the national campaign against yellow fever was charted in the commission's reports, which correlated the rapid decline of yellow fever incidence against the work of the IHB in Yucatán. The newly appointed director of the special Yellow Fever Commission in Mexico, Dr. White, worked with his IHB colleague Dr. Scannell to compile a final report indicating improvements. Their report showed that yellow fever infection declined from 115 reported cases and 53 deaths in 1921 to only 41 cases and 25 deaths in 1922, and by 1923, the subdirector of the anti–yellow fever campaign in Mexico confirmed that not one case of yellow fever had been reported throughout the entire republic since 1922.[102] This report consequently led to additional reductions in the Rockefeller Foundation's contributions to Mexico's national anti–yellow fever campaign, leaving only squadrons of workers assigned to anti-larvae maintenance and surveillance of allegedly endemic zones.[103] By the mid-1920s malaria and yellow fever prevention had faded into the landscape as reports of low to zero infection rates continued between late 1921 and 1923.[104]

If the high point of científico public health policy came with Molina's construction of a modern urban infrastructure in Mérida, reflecting the technocratic, top-down process of public health policy favored by the elites, the IHB-PSS struggle against yellow fever from 1919 to 1921 was surely the high point of the revolutionary grassroots-led health policy. The IHB physicians in 1922 were becoming increasingly frustrated with the political climate in postrevolutionary Yucatán. After the election of Socialist Party leader Felipe Carrillo Puerto to the governor's seat in 1922, public health was identified ever more firmly with the Socialist Party, further compromising the Rockefeller Foundation's already tenuous neutrality. Felipe Carrillo Puerto's program was built around unlocking the membership of the PSS and the Socialist Action League (Liga de Acción Social) to serve as brigades that could implement his education, public health, agrarian, temperance, and labor reforms. A consequence of Carrillo Puerto's use of political party brigades to implement reforms was that public works in the region were more often than not linked to socialism.[105] Under the leadership of Felipe Carrillo Puerto, the PSS organized approximately eight hundred regional resistance leagues (ligas de resistencia).[106] Undoubtedly, channeling socialist reforms through these resistance leagues facilitated the implementation of new legislation at a community level.[107] The IHB, relying on foreign doctors, had no natural support in the communities, which meant that its doctors tended to focus their attention on education and supervision in urban locales, and the anti–yellow fever campaign had depended on socialist brigades in the countryside. As the threat of mosquito-borne disease diminished, the political costs of allying with socialists, communists, and "Bolsheviks" became harder to bear for the IHB. According to Rockefeller physician Dr. Russell, conditions were still "disturbed," transportation spotty, bandits everywhere, and in the oil regions along the Gulf Coast he declared, "There is a good deal of Bolshevism."[108]

Political turmoil in Yucatán reached a frenzied pitch in early 1924 with the assassination of Governor Felipe Carrillo Puerto, the circumstances of which are fraught with controversy to the present day.[109] Many scholars contend Carrillo Puerto was killed by federal troops who used former interim Mexican president Adolfo de la Huerta's (June 1920 to November 1920) revolt to cloak their own counterrevolutionary movement, while others discern the hand of disgruntled and powerful henequen elites behind his capture and murder.[110]

Carrillo Puerto's party, the PSS, canonized Carrillo Puerto after his death as a revolutionary hero alongside other revolutionary martyrs like Emiliano Zapata and Pancho Villa.[111] Carrillo Puerto's obsequies included messages from U.S. supporters, one of whom claimed he was "a man of unusual abilities. . . . He was adoringly loved by his own people, the Maya Indians, and was respected and admired by white people."[112] In the aftermath of Carrillo Puerto's murder, the PSS was irrevocably split, and under Governor José María Iturralde Traconis (1924–26) political enfranchisement for women ceased, agrarian reforms were rolled back, and public works for the peninsula took a backseat to improvements to Iturralde Traconis's birth city Valladolid, located in southeastern Yucatán.[113]

These events took their toll on public health initiatives. Health services suffered as the dissolution of the PSS and socialist resistance leagues removed the volunteers who had made all the difference in the yellow fever eradication campaign. In an attempt to sustain preventative measures against yellow fever resurgence, Mérida's director of the Superior Health Council proposed new legislation in January of 1924. The legislation proposed state-operated household inspections to control household hygiene (Ley para la Higienización de las Casas). The household hygiene legislation evoked the ideals of the revolution by calling into question the rights of individuals to compromise the well-being of others. It mandated measures that, as we have seen, went back to the first public health program in Yucatán, including home inspections and fines, along with mandatory fumigations, all with the idea of halting disease at the doorstep of the resident's home. The director for the Superior Health Council in Mérida declared that "the rights of the individual end where those of another begin"; furthermore, he preached it would be irresponsible of the state to allow individuals enough liberty to govern their homes for their own convenience if those methods damaged the members of the collective. The director added, "How many epidemics must be tolerated due to the carelessness of those who traipse over our lands . . . ignorant of the teachings of hygiene!"[114]

Unfortunately, the death of Carrillo Puerto and the scattering of socialist brigades made it impossible to implement the Household Hygiene Law. Furthermore, general household hygiene inspections were completely impossible to sustain long term without continued funding from an outside source such as the Rockefeller Foundation and a tactical end defined for the work. While Yucatán was the wealthiest Mexican state in 1914, by the twenties, the boom days of the henequen industry in the peninsula had passed, and the state's financing was precarious. The world market now had other sources of henequen, namely British colonies in Africa.[115] Given the decrease in resources, the decline in the infection rates for yellow fever and malaria softened support for funding household inspections. In 1925 a survey of regions throughout Mexico considered to be the most prone to yellow fever resurgence reported no cases of the disease.[116] The focus of the Mexican public health campaign in the twenties shifted to the anti-hookworm program. IHB physicians regularly found themselves pleading with the Rockefeller administrators for more money, claiming that local governments were not "sufficiently moralized" to ensure payments to maintain local public health services.[117]

Meanwhile, the Rockefeller Foundation's work throughout the globe enjoyed growing accolades. In the eyes of the international community, the cooperative efforts of the Mexican states and the Rockefeller Foundation's IHB had facilitated the emergence of a healthful Mexico by the mid-1920s.[118] By 1926, the Rockefeller Foundation had given over nine million dollars for projects in eighteen different countries.[119] A *New York Times* article from November 1929 declared the Rockefeller Foundation had spent $21,690,738 in 1928 to improve public health throughout the globe. Much of the work throughout the Caribbean and Latin America included "intensive work against malaria."[120]

The withdrawal of the Rockefeller Foundation from the Mexican healthcare scene—whether an effect of the success of their programs or an effect of the political chaos in postrevolutionary Mexico—coincided with a shift in Yucatán and the Mexican republic as a whole from a focus on malaria and yellow fever to a focus on syphilis, alcoholism, and rabies prevention by the mid-1920s. In Yucatán, the shift demoralized Yucatecan public health officials, leading to the resignations of several key individuals as well as medical student strikes.[121] The withdrawal of administrators and physicians from public health services points to a severely weakened public health branch struggling to carry out the multiple tasks folded into its realm during the revolution. The Superior Health Council formed under the revolutionary state scrambled to manage health and hygiene education, vaccination production and administration, health inspections, licensing of medical specialists, and operation and maintenance of hospitals, clinics, pharmacies, laboratories, insane asylums, and cemeteries.[122]

During and after Iturralde Traconis's governorship, antidisease campaigns shed the socialist brigade structure and devolved into standard operating procedures for police units and sanitary brigades, oftentimes without the presence of a knowledgeable official for oversight. Low on funds and consumed by paperwork covering a wide range of minor infractions, the Superior Health Council of Yucatán concerned themselves primarily with enforcement. Funding issues prompted more fines for public spitting and urination, failure to comply with canine rabies inspections, and alleged noncompliance among prostitutes to appear for mandatory gynecological exams.[123] In fact, in a landscape no longer dominated by epidemic diseases, rabies and canine control became a major concern. So did sexually transmitted diseases, along with the control of alcohol—two concerns that converged in the agenda of controlling prostitution and brothels.[124] Looking back we can see that the high point in the epidemic-defined public health agenda was the cooperation of various socialist governments and the IHB. Afterward, public health campaigns would focus on newly threatening social ills including alcoholism and sexually transmitted diseases, while keeping an eye on household and personal hygiene.

Conclusion

The yellow fever and malaria eradication campaign in revolutionary Yucatán drew together unlikely partners—foreign philanthropists funded by American capitalists and Mexican revolutionaries. Yet, they proved to be symbiotically matched: while the foundations provided the money and the model, the revolutionaries could provide the manpower and the spirit. While seeming to break with the prerevolutionary paradigm of ignoring the poor or imposing upon them civilizing programs, in the end, the Yucatecan state continued to extend its authority into the private realm. The state was more successful at creating a popular health ethos, effectively linking personal responsibility for maintaining a hygienic household, business, and body to the well-being of a state that presented itself as a product of the popular will. The state emphasized that individuals' responsibility for sanitizing their homes, gardens, patios, and water cisterns contributed to clean homes, communities, and state. Fighting disease during the revolution dovetailed neatly into larger revolutionary arcs focused on extracting Yucatán from its "backward" past. Moreover, the overlapping of endemic tropical diseases and the socialist revolution in Yucatán provided an ideal laboratory in which to study vanguard therapeutics and preventatives such as the Noguchi vaccine. However, the appeal of efforts to eradicate disease, improve public health for all residents, and provoke social reform could not overcome the fact that the revolutionaries needed institutional support and cooperation in order to advance their cause. In order for disease eradication campaigns to work, foreign philanthropists and revolutionaries had to work within the very structures that designed contradictory policies, implemented legislation in uneven ways, and summarily punished the very people it claimed to help.

Yucatán's revolutionary socialist state also provided a structure through which its revolutionary ideas could be transformed into concrete projects by way of community socialist leagues and brigades. Brigades spread throughout the capital city of Mérida and the countryside with checklists for household inspections and equipment to kill mosquitoes, and they were connected, in urban areas, to the physicians of the Rockefeller Foundation's IHB. Within a relatively short period of time IHB physicians enjoyed success in Yucatán, and as a result, Yucatán became a yellow fever–free peninsula by the early 1920s.

By the time the Rockefeller Foundation initiated cutbacks to their anti–yellow fever and anti-malaria work in Mexico, the whole of the Mexican republic had shifted attention toward new menaces like syphilis and other diseases of lifestyle, notably sexual lifestyles.

In summary, the Rockefeller Foundation's success in Yucatán was based on a number of factors: the lack of a war, the presence of a motivated popular movement, and finally, the foundation's ability to carefully scout out and select regions for philanthropic activity. In fact, the Rockefeller Foundation tended to launch campaigns only in places overseas where regional elites and scientists would most easily accept their methods.[125]

As Yucatán's socialist revolution came to an end, the goals of regional public health officials and the Rockefeller Foundation diverged. Interestingly, once yellow fever threats dissipated a rise in deaths attributed to "unknown illnesses" occurred in state hospitals, giving rise to concerns that perhaps yellow fever and malaria had only ceded the stage to a more nefarious and elusive malady.[126] This unknown malady attracted little attention from the Rockefeller Foundation or the nation. Although the Mexican government made overtures to the Rockefeller Foundation for assistance with other diseases, namely syphilis (an obsession of the revolutionary elite), the Rockefeller Foundation could not imagine itself designing a campaign to reform sexual behaviors. With the yellow fever project already deemed a success within international scientific communities, the Rockefeller Foundation remained only marginally involved in Yucatán's public health apparatus after the revolution, offering training and scholarly exchanges.

In the end, the promises of Yucatán's socialist revolution far outpaced structural capabilities on the ground level. Alvarado's desire to rectify the ills of the past and increase access to improved public facilities certainly fit within the parameters of revolutionary reforms. However, maintenance of public health, land, and education reforms after the revolution concluded proved difficult, especially after Carrillo Puerto's assassination in 1924. Socialist brigades and leagues dissolved after the death of Governor Carrillo Puerto, taking with them the vigor and operational tactics that public health programs required.

CONCLUSION

Outsiders, Disease, and Public Health in Modern Yucatán, Mexico

IN *COLONIAL PATHOLOGIES*, Warwick Anderson has shown how an intersection of interests between the Rockefeller Foundation doctors and American officials in the American colony of the Philippines brought about the "medical exoneration of the tropical environment as a directly pathogenic agent."[1] Anderson claims that the medical exoneration was relative to a racial ideal—the optimum health landscape for a white male—but Mexican history is not driven by the same dynamics as U.S. history, and in Mexico there is no binary opposition between whites and blacks.

However, as I have shown, Mexico's development since independence does illustrate another binary that is especially pertinent to Yucatán and its public health policy: the civilized versus the barbarian. From the perspective of this dominant cultural opposition, we can see that the goal of public health policy in Yucatán was to create the optimum health-care landscape for the civilized man. Although different regimes held power in Yucatán over the century we have surveyed, regimes that were animated by very different ideologies, even the most populist of them, operated on behalf of "civilization" and against "barbarism." The idea that the tropical environment could be subdued by the power and to the benefit of the civilized man justified some of the great successes of the public health programs implemented in Yucatán, from smallpox inoculation campaigns to the cleanup of Mérida's streets and the purification of its water system. But this public health perspective also identified illness and barbarism—and under this guise it justified a massive effort to change the lifestyles of the Maya villagers and the working class. It sought to segregate human and animal space, terminate old and binding funerary rituals, and crush popular medicine as "superstitious," although as we have seen, until the coming of germ theory, the medical establishment was often wildly wrong about the cause of and cure for epidemic and tropical diseases.

In the last chapter, we saw the introduction of a foreign medical body to Yucatán. Although Yucatán was often in the path of diseases that originated elsewhere, this time the foreign body carried cures rather than illnesses. The goal of the Rockefeller Foundation's International Health Board in the early twentieth century was to "export U.S.-style public health theory and practice to dozens of countries around the world," and it served as a model for future international agencies to construct public health and disease eradication programs in Mexico.[2] However, underneath the model of "U.S.-style public health" and the successes of disease eradication campaigns in Yucatán lies a more ambiguous story, one in which the Mexican government's brief participation in grassroots public health programs was aborted in favor of the top-down administration of public health and its restoration to the hands of technical "experts." The disembedding of international, national, regional, and local public health services from Yucatecan daily life is a notable social fact that crops up again and again in my history of the region's experiences with epidemic cholera, smallpox, and yellow fever in the nineteenth and twentieth centuries.

The reason for the alienation between the doctors and the people, to put it crudely, was not primarily the greater education and expertise of the former. Of course, that education generated a viewpoint and vocabulary different from the viewpoint and vocabulary of the population, but as the brief transition in health programs between 1918 and 1923 showed, such differences could be bridged. Rather, from the beginning Yucatán's public health officials and the foreign medical professionals who came to aid the region were involved in elite infighting, first between the church and state during the Reforma, then between Yucatán and Mexico City or Yucatán and Campeche during the mid-nineteenth century, and finally in the disputes between the hacendados and the revolutionaries in the 1915–25 period. Undoubtedly, the Yucatecan state seized the occasions offered by the incidence of disease epidemics to develop state-building and modernizing projects under the guise of ensuring public safety. In doing so, the governing class often came up against residents' long-held practices and rituals for treating and preventing illness in chaotic moments of social disorganization, which extended even to funereal practices. Furthermore, it was just at these disease moments that the state was most determined to quell rebellion, civilize indigenous populations, stabilize investments, or—after 1915—spread revolutionary doctrine. These ideological programs invariably overrode the goals of optimum public health or of a medical community seeking to advance medical trials and employ new technologies while maintaining their political neutrality.

In my chapter on the smallpox epidemic, I noted the trip made by Dr. José M. Domínguez in the 1850s to take advantage of a connection he had in New Orleans to ship more smallpox vaccine to Yucatán. What in theory seemed to be an unobjectionable idea in practice aroused a lot of resistance because the method Domínguez chose to transport the vaccine was the *brazo á brazo* method, which meant inoculating an orphan with a cowpox germ and then scratching his or her arm to communicate it to another orphan, in this way using human vessels to preserve the pus. Such actions rang every alarm with an indigenous population that did not, for good reason, trust the creole elite. It seemed to lend validity to the rumor that the children of the poor could be poached for medical experimentation.[3]

If distrust (and even war) existed between the classes and ethnicities in Yucatán, foreign medical intervention up to the end of the nineteenth century was paltry and dependent on the chance visitation of foreigners. For instance, the U.S. consuls in Mérida and Progreso played a role in facilitating the importation of medical technologies and advice from foreign countries. In times of crises they disseminated information from foreign doctors regarding procedures for burying diseased bodies and new ways to prevent the spread of cholera.[4] Some of that advice, which represented the general medical opinion of the time, turned out to be much worse than native practices, as, for instance, the prescription of purgatives and emetics for cholera victims. Regional periodicals translated and printed columns of advice based on the practices of foreign doctors like Dr. Quin.[5] French archaeologist Augustus Le Plongeon and his wife, Alice, distributed vaccine in the Yucatecan countryside as they worked on their archaeological excavations at Chichén Itzá.[6] Travel writer John Lloyd Stephens and his friend Dr. Cabot arrived in the mid-1840s and began operating on several residents in rural towns to correct their crossed eyes (*biscos*). Dr. Cabot also left behind medical instruments and instructions for local doctors to follow.[7]

Although relatively small-scale interventions like this may have been well intentioned, residents must have wondered about making life-altering choices for themselves and their families about treatments that pitted known curatives, which fit within a broad body of religio-medical knowledge, against unfamiliar treatments that were recommended solely by the authority of the foreign adviser or doctor. In fact, until the development of germ theory in the late nineteenth century, there were few really successful cures in the Western medical system—smallpox vaccines were at the outer boundary of the possible—and it was not so much in the discovery of specific medicines or procedures but in the organization of cleaner environments that Western public health in the nineteenth century scored its biggest successes.

Thus, along with the perceived willingness of Yucatecans to accept outside assistance, noted by some Rockefeller Foundation physicians, we should emphasize that the history of stresses in a century of diseased moments, along with the sheer struggle to survive, had taught the working class and campesinos the arts of evading legislation, clandestinely burying the dead to avoid fees, and consulting with non-state-licensed medical professionals who were trained in local ways of healing either unacknowledged or condemned by Western medicine.

Broadly speaking, outside of the pain and grief locals experienced within diseased moments, the purveyors of medical services, politicians, and powerful citizens used them as opportunities to move communities in the desired direction of "civilization." Whether orchestrating preventative measures to contain contagion during cholera epidemics and simultaneously collecting information on rebels during the Caste War or propagandizing for the revolution and eradicating yellow fever- and malaria-bearing mosquitoes, public health units became indelibly intertwined at the international, national, regional, and local levels.

In the 1930s, toward the end of the Rockefeller Foundation's public health work in Yucatán, a group of American scholars (Harvard University professor of tropical medicine George Cheever Shattuck, anthropologist Robert Redfield of Chicago University, and Katheryn McKay, a registered nurse and midwife from the Carnegie Institute) conducted an extensive investigation assessing disease tendencies and public health facilities among the Maya of Yucatán.[8] Their findings highlighted the "sovereign remedies" that the Maya had used for centuries to cure illnesses and injuries such as snakebite, hookworm, and other parasites.[9] The team also found that the medicine man (shaman) "among the Maya [was] still a personage of distinction" and that the medicine man was also sometimes considered a "doctor, *yerbatero* or *curandero*, but he may claim descent from the priests of former times and may have inherited a certain priestly knowledge which is recognized and respected by his people."[10] The U.S. researchers also called on other scholars to conduct future investigations into the indigenous plants and herbs that these men knew how to use before their information died with them. Although this team did not overtly say so, they were, in a sense, closing the curtain on the old opposition between the civilized human versus the barbarian, which had long underwritten the ideology of public health care in Yucatán.

The team's analysis also revealed that the top causes of mortality in the peninsula were intestinal problems (including parasites), fevers (*calenturas*), malaria, pulmonary illnesses (excluding tuberculosis), pellagra, tuberculosis, and leprosy. Many of the illnesses emerging onto the epidemiological scene at the turn of the century, such as malaria, tuberculosis, and pellagra, became the region's principal causes of death at midcentury. The team of specialists also found that considerably more persons died from malaria and pellagra in rural areas such as Dzitás and Ticul than those living in urban centers like Mérida.[11] These findings show the effect of the process of marginalizing the Maya population that began in the nineteenth century and resulted in keeping the Maya away from health services intended for the civilized, or the creole elite.

Shattuck, Redfield, and McKay concluded that more industries needed to be developed in Yucatán to provide employment for those Yucatecans who, in the 1930s, found themselves without a stable salary or resources due to the continuing decline in henequen fiber production, an industry that was a victim of international competition and a faulty attempt by the government to inflate the wholesale price in the 1920s. The authors were ahead of their time in suggesting that tourism, then in its infancy, be built up and encouraged in order to provide capital for a region where "the rich are losing money, the poor are getting poorer, and a very large proportion of the population is now living on a scale dangerously near to the lowest subsistence level that is compatible with health."[12]

This advice, however, was probably not the reason that tourism became one of the biggest moneymakers for the states of Yucatán and Quintana Roo in the late twentieth century. The whole Caribbean region had, by this time, become a huge site for tourism and vacationing. Recently, Quintana Roo's state governor claimed that 34 percent of the nation's tourist profits came from the state and that the hotel zone has more hotels than the Dominican Republic.[13] Travel brochures entice foreigners to experience the "Mystery of the Maya" by visiting ancient monuments like Chichén Itzá, Uxmal, and Tulum and to sun themselves on the Caribbean beaches, now known as the "Maya Riviera." In the small towns surrounding Mérida, many of the eldest residents now care for their grandchildren while their mothers and fathers make the long commute, usually by bus, to the "Maya Riviera" to work in the low-wage service sector in the vast stretch of hotels in Cancún known as the "hotel zone" (*zona hotelera*).

The cycle of boom and bust that was once a feature of the henequen industry, along with the exploitation of Maya labor, has reemerged in the tourist industry, which, more than ever, attaches this seemingly peripheral region to the health of the world's developed economies.[14] Having survived more than a century of being identified with the literal and figurative ills afflicting Yucatán, the Maya are now surviving both their inflation as markers of cultural capital and their exploitation as a source of cheap labor for the tourist industry. One of many examples demonstrating the ability of Maya communities to harness capital from tourism and follow contemporary trends in environmental conservation can be seen in the organization of ancient Maya sites into community-run ecotourism parks.[15]

Thus far, however, the booming tourism industry has not generated revenues to enhance the public health landscape.[16] If anything, critics of tourism in developing nations like Mexico have noted an overall degradation of the native landscape and increased energy expenditure.[17] The consequences are seen in poor air quality in tourist zones; an increasingly tainted water supply system; rising numbers of malaria, diarrhea, and asthma cases; and other markers of environmental destruction.[18] Though the old civilization/barbarism opposition no longer holds as much rhetorical power, precious little is allocated or subsidized for those who need public services the most. Hence, assistance from outside Yucatán continues as international philanthropic organizations and nonprofits work to eradicate disease, hunger, infant mortality, malnutrition, and other illness associated with rural and poor populations worldwide.[19]

As much as outside assistance may be needed, oftentimes the disjuncture between institutional objectives and the needs of the local populations produces a host of unintended complications. For instance, in the 1970s CNEP (National Commission for the Eradication of Paludism) initiated a malaria eradication campaign in Mexico, focusing on the Gulf Coast, including Yucatán. CNEP's work throughout Yucatán and Mexico included the use of dangerous chemicals such as DDT (dichloro-diphenyl-trichloro-ethane), malathion, and HCH (hexachlorocyclohexane) to eradicate mosquito vectors. Their application caused a host of physical maladies from mild headaches and dizziness to more severe symptoms including seizures and difficulty breathing.[20]

In the 1960s, the use of DDT and HCH as standard preventatives against mosquito-borne diseases appeared to benefit communities by killing mosquitoes and their larvae over large tracts of land in a short period of time. But the effects of DDT on the human population and on the environment were disastrous. Well-documented consequences of DDT use include premature births, birth defects, contamination of livestock and crops, and mortality among domestic animals.[21] Moreover, the continued application of DDT, a chief agent of mosquito eradication programs throughout the world, caused mosquitoes to develop resistance to the poison. Laboratory tests showed that some mosquitoes (such as *Anopheles sacharovi* and *A. albimanus*) had adapted to the presence of DDT in the environment by learning to avoid surfaces sprayed with the chemical.[22] With DDT-resistant mosquitoes thriving in their chemical landscape, malaria gradually resurfaced in the 1960s and 1970s.[23]

Banned from use in Mexico in 2000, DDT is no longer sprayed to prevent malaria or other mosquito-borne diseases. Nonetheless, the recent emergence of dengue fever in Mexico's tropical Gulf Coast has compelled some public health officials to revisit the use of chemical spraying as a preventative.[24] Dengue fever, transmitted by the *Aedes aegypti* mosquito, has now become endemic throughout the peninsular states of Yucatán, Quintana Roo, and Campeche. Although rarely is the disease fatal, it has mutated into a deadly form of hemorrhagic dengue or dengue shock syndrome.[25] The dengue now concentrated along the peninsula's coastline bears many of same characteristics of the tropical diseases that brought about the great nineteenth- and early twentieth-century campaigns to combat their vectors through a focus on endemic zones, the use of environmental and vector controls, and the targeting of at-risk populations for public health and hygiene education.[26]

Notably, one common feature of the yellow fever campaigns of the early twentieth century and contemporary programs targeting dengue in Yucatán can be seen in the quandary public health officials confront as to how to eliminate mosquito vectors safely. Fumigations, bombing of cisterns, and the application of chemicals all have adverse side effects on the landscape and the human relationships with the environment. A consequence of these practices can be seen in the emergence of new strains of the dengue that are resistant to most treatments, demonstrating just how unpredictable diseases are and how quickly their vectors can adapt to survive.[27] Such occurrences beg the question: are preventative technologies and methods for disease eradication reinvigorating old maladies or creating new ones?[28]

The infrastructural reality of coping with disease and illness still bears the impress of the old urban/rural pattern, as modern-day citizens of the Yucatán countryside and coast must weigh the benefits and costs of traveling to the General Hospital Agustin O'Horan in Mérida or staying at home to utilize local options such as small clinics, pharmacies, and herbalists. For many of the peninsula's poor, access to a major hospital, a team of experts, pharmaceuticals, and technology can only be realized at the Hospital O'Horan. The Hospital O'Horan is the largest public hospital in the region, servicing approximately one hundred persons daily in their emergency facilities alone, and the administration boasts that the facility provides services to residents of Campeche, Quintana Roo, Tabasco, Chiapas, and Belize.[29] The main building is situated at the center of a bustling complex of state facilities including the Archivo General del Estado de Yucatán (AGEY) and the state's school of nursing. A bust of Hideyo Noguchi stands on the eastern periphery of the Hospital O'Horan compound as testimony to Yucatán's role in what evolved into a global fight against yellow fever and the development of what later became a useful preventative vaccine.[30]

Today, the Hospital O'Horan functions under the state's Servicios de Salud (SSY) department, which was formed in 1996 and encompasses a wide range of public services including mobile health units and campaigns to fight tuberculosis, SIDA (AIDS), and dengue fever.[31] The Hospital O'Horan is the oldest of fifteen medical facilities located in the Mérida metropolitan area. Middle-class and wealthy residents tend to frequent the private-run clinics such as Clínica Mérida or the foreign-run facilities such as the Medical Centre of the Americas, affiliated with Mercy Hospital in Miami, Florida. Since the Hospital O'Horan is state run and funded, it provides service primarily to the region's poorer classes. Because many residents travel to utilize the services offered at the Hospital O'Horan, its surrounding grounds serve as a public gathering place for literally thousands of peninsular residents who often make annual pilgrimages to the facility.

Even with an impressive level of public health services coordinated through international organizations, national campaigns, and regional outreach, many Yucatecans rely on a combination of tenuous options available to them to meet their medical needs. In particular, those who reside in Yucatán's countryside continue to consult Maya physicians and homeopaths in conjunction with mainstream health care. Recently, a group of five hundred Maya traditional healers condemned the state Commission on Human Rights (Comisión de Derechos Humanos del Estado de Yucatán, CODHEY) for failing to respect their work. The traditional healers are part of the Organization of Indigenous Maya Physicians for the Yucatán Peninsula (Organización de Médicos Indígenas Mayas de la Península de Yucatán, OMIMPY). OMIMPY members provide residents in Yucatán, Campeche, and Quintana Roo with traditional Maya medical services including consultation with midwives (*parteros*), herbalists (*yerbateros*), bone setters (*hueseros*), and prayer practitioners (*rezadores*). The president of OMIMPY, Carmitó Ek Catzín, complained that recent accommodations provided for the organization in the city of Mérida did not meet the promises extended by ex-governor Patricio Patrón Laviada. Ek Catzín vowed to make the current governor meet those expectations.[32]

Considering the historical tensions between state-licensed medical professionals and practitioners of traditional medicine, Yucatán's governor, Ivonne Ortega Pacheco, has a difficult task in front of her. Her allocation of 1.2 million pesos to the state's Program to Assist Community Culture (El Programa de Apoyo a las Culturas Municipales y Comunitarias, PACMYC) in January of 2009 would seem to indicate that Governor Pacheco is cognizant of the need to extend funds to promote Maya culture. But the state's classification of traditional medicine as a cultural endeavor, along with crafts, painting, literature, and Yucatecan cuisine, would seem to suggest that the respect members of OMIMPY desire as legitimate health practitioners remains out of reach.[33]

AFTERWORD

H1N1 and the Legacy of Uncertainty

IN APRIL 2009, a new strain of influenza virus called H1N1, also known as "swine flu," began to spread throughout Mexico (reported first in the state of Veracruz) with such alarming rapidity that in less than one month, over four hundred Mexicans had been infected and nineteen had died from the virus.[1] Schools were closed, sporting events cancelled, and businesses shuttered. As of this writing, there have been 70,665 confirmed cases of H1N1 across thirty-two Mexican states and 1,052 deaths.[2] On a global level, international organizations warned that this particular strain of influenza could morph into something worse than the 1918 Spanish influenza pandemic that killed at least fifty million people worldwide.[3] H1N1 was dubbed "swine flu" since it was at first thought to be a respiratory disease that usually infects pigs; however, further study revealed that this "novel form of influenza" contained two flu viruses that circulate in Europe and North America among pigs, birds, and humans.[4] The latest estimates from the WHO (World Health Organization) now place worldwide deaths from H1N1 at 18,366.[5]

In the relatively short span of time in which the news about the virus broke, the damage to Mexico was nothing short of stunning. Within days, the international news media had located and focused on the small community of La Gloria in the Gulf Coast state of Veracruz as "ground zero" for H1N1.[6] This obsession with the origination of the virus cast Mexico on the world stage as a principal harbinger.[7] As *Newsweek* noted at the time, "Fingers are now pointing, either at the entire pig species *Sus domestica*, or at the nation of Mexico."[8] On April 25, 2009, the WHO announced that H1N1 constituted a "public health emergency of international concern,"[9] and by June, the WHO declared H1N1 pandemic. Responses to the H1N1 pandemic ran the gamut from officially enacted trade restrictions on Mexican agricultural exports to travel bans, while at the same time the media generated a broad stigmatization of peoples associated with viral epicenters both at home and abroad. Tourism, Mexico's third most profitable national industry, sustained a decline of 0.3 to 0.5 percent in just a few weeks.[10] Mexican tourists traveling abroad and Mexican immigrants working in the United States suffered detainment and discrimination. These reactions are part of a phenomenon that Georgetown professor of global health law Lawrence O. Gostin categorizes as "social distancing."[11]

Some of these reactions are similar to those we have seen in the context of nineteenth-century pandemics and bear the familiar imprint of paranoia, fear, and overreaction. As we have seen, the relationships of people and animals—the spaces we share, the treatment animals are accorded, their "dirtiness" or "cleanliness"—suddenly become visible in a disease moment. Our old habits of accusing the "other" of harboring or spreading infection tend to resurface at this point, and official reactions employ "social distancing" to regulate various international flows of goods and people, as the presence of Mexican goods and the presence of Mexican people are linked by state regulators and some sectors of public opinion to the disease.

Most people understand that influenza spreads from person to person. Thus, fear and uncertainty about persons from regions known to have an active outbreak of influenza or those exhibiting signs of illness often provoke overreaction. China and Hong Kong implemented some of the most aggressive measures to control the spread of H1N1 by quarantining travelers from Mexico, Canada, and the United States during the epidemic.[12] Singapore summarily isolated anyone who had recently visited Mexico, and in northeastern China twenty-two Canadian university students were quarantined at their hotel in Changchun despite the fact they exhibited no signs of the flu.[13] Taxi drivers, restaurants, and other small businesses denied Mexican tourists in Argentina out of fear for their own health.[14]

Israel's deputy health minister decided to rename swine flu the "Mexican flu" because of its reference to an "unkosher" animal.[15] Although this unintentional "slip of the tongue" made by the Israeli minister stemmed from his affiliation with a fervently religious party, scientists in Israel conceded that renaming the epidemic could stigmatize Mexico.[16] Shortly after Israel's announcement about the renaming of the swine flu, Mexican ambassador to Israel Frederico Salas stated he was "offended" by the term.[17] The renaming of the virus never happened, but isolating Mexico as the origination point for the malady had already caused irrevocable damage.

In July 2009, public health leaders from around the world met in Cancún, Mexico, to discuss the influenza pandemic. At the summit, Mexican president Felipe Calderón admonished countries not to discriminate against Mexicans by closing their borders during the influenza epidemic. As a remedy, Calderón suggested that nations communicate better to avoid "the generation of misunderstanding, distortion or discrimination, as we have suffered."[18]

As we have noticed in the history of public health in Yucatán, disease moments lay bare the intricate relationship between an epistemologically justified set of norms, like public health, and cultural norms that stratify and categorize groups within the social whole. The threat of the pandemic struck Mexico at a time in which the nation was extremely politically polarized, due to the tensions that resulted from the election of Calderón in July 2006. Furthermore, Mexico, and indeed the world, was shocked by the violence resulting from the government's attempt to suppress the narcotics cartels. Thus, this disease moment threatened to realize apprehensions of anarchy that were already floating around in Mexican public opinion.

These conditions certainly bore on the action of Mexico's *secretario de salud* (secretary of health). As did his compatriots in most nations around the world, he immediately disseminated recommendations to the public to help avoid the spread of H1N1 and listed the standard preventatives, including the consumption of fruits and vegetables rich in vitamin A, frequent hand washing, and avoidance of dramatic temperature changes and exposure to environmental contaminants such as cigarette smoke. Children, the elderly, and those with compromised immune systems were singled out as especially vulnerable. If symptoms appeared, the secretario advised against self-medication—advice that goes back, as we have seen, to the popular fear of being stigmatized and punished, with quarantines or forced treatment, after allowing the official medical establishment to "see" one's disease. "Physical methods" and acetaminophen were recommended for controlling a fever; if the fever persisted, a physician should be consulted.[19] But getting to a hospital or a doctor in Mexico can be difficult. The government-run health system does not cover everyone. Public clinics charge modest fees, but many still cannot afford to pay the fees, take time off from work, or even pay for over-the-counter medicines.[20]

While on the surface many of the secretario's recommendations appear reasonable, we know that rationality is relative to the social conditions in which such recommendations can be enacted. The stress of daily life and the demands of therapy are often in conflict. In Mexico City, H1N1 spread particularly fast, probably because avoidance of overcrowded places is virtually impossible in a metropolitan area where the population hovers close to twenty million.[21] Moreover, since Mexico City is one of the most polluted cities in the world, with three hundred bad ozone or smog days per year,[22] it was practically impossible to avoid airborne contaminants or illness related to pollution, regardless of whether one smoked.[23]

In some situations, the strong motivation to attend religious or sporting events superseded the fear of contracting H1N1. In Yucatán, over three thousand people traveled to the church of Cristo Rey in Pacabtún to celebrate Divino Niño at the height of the H1N1 epidemic. Devotees traveled from Veracruz, Chiapas, Tabasco, Campeche, and Quintana Roo. PAN (Partido Acción Nacional or the National Action Party), the ruling party, is particularly close to the church, especially for a Mexican political party, and was in no position to confront it, which may be why one ministry coordinator, answering a question about canceling the event, responded, "There are many people and everyone participating washes their hands and uses antibacterial gel." A parishioner noted that even though she took precautions and washed her hands frequently, "we are in the hands of God."[24]

In circumstances similar to those surrounding nineteenth- and early twentieth-century disease outbreaks, families in Mexico struggled to interpret a barrage of information about a virus that the medical community scarcely understood.[25] To cope, many physicians established communication platforms to exchange information about how the disease spread, effective therapeutics, and what sectors of the population seemed to be the most vulnerable, and they exchanged information at a pace and with a scope that was impossible for their nineteenth-century forebears, or even for doctors in 1980. Without a doubt, the Internet facilitated timely access to important information about H1N1. Information traveled in real time throughout cyberspace via e-mail and social networking sites like Facebook, Twitter, and MySpace as well as various blog sites, instantly providing all kinds of information—some true, some not so true, some plainly false, and some clearly leading to hysteria and paranoia. The predecessor of these medical communication networks can be plainly seen in the modes of communication Yucatecan policy makers and doctors established during the nineteenth century with medical communities in the United States, Belize, and Cuba in their efforts to cope with smallpox, cholera, and yellow fever outbreaks.

As we have seen during nineteenth- and early twentieth-century disease epidemics, public health officials and physicians in Yucatán were also faced with the problem of misinformation and misunderstandings that ultimately compromised state public health campaigns, even though those same officials, in the era before germ theory, were as often the spreaders of misinformation—for example, in recommending cholera therapies that contributed to victims' dehydration. (But where cures were available, the story was different.) Certainly, Dr. Monsreal meant no harm when he answered a call to tend to smallpox victims in the small rural town of Halachó. But Monsreal found that residents were hesitant if not resistant to seeking medical assistance. Indeed, the residents of Halachó did not seem to trust urban doctors and their methods. Monsreal found the Flores family of Halachó unwilling to submit to treatments they did not understand and endure isolation (see chapter 2). Interestingly, the same distrust has emerged today about the H1N1 vaccine, which has cast a dark shadow of suspicion over vaccine manufacturers. Deliberations about who should receive priority when limited stores of the vaccine are distributed have sparked debates much like the ones generated during smallpox vaccination campaigns in nineteenth-century Yucatán. Regardless of the epidemic or the vaccine, worries about availability of vaccines, false vaccines, vaccine efficacy, and vaccine side effects remain as relevant today as they were over hundred years ago and are often cast in the same terms and tropes, that is, as a struggle between "rationality" and "superstition."[26]

Similarly, misinformation and misunderstandings about H1N1 have provoked hysteria and paranoia. Despite the fact that there is no scientific evidence to support a link between eating pork and contracting influenza, twenty countries banned meat from Mexico, Canada, and the United States.[27] In Mexico, the major pork-producing states of Michoacán, Yucatán, México, Zacatecas, Sonora, and Morelos suffered significant setbacks to their economies during the ban that began in April 2009. Annually, up to 1.6 million tons of pork are produced in these Mexican states. During the ban on Mexican pork sales, the industry declined between 60 and 80 percent. With over forty million Mexican families dependent on the pork industry in Mexico, the restrictions left many households devastated.[28]

Amid the fears about H1N1, Yucatán's director for the Center for Regional Studies at the Universidad Autónoma de Yucatán reminded Yucatecans to not forget that "there are other silent threats like Chagas and Dengue."[29] In fact, the early twentieth-century focus in Mexico on yellow fever and malaria eradication took up the resources and interest that could have been employed for other disease prevention efforts. These costs were not negligible; for instance, when public health policy turned to combating mosquito-borne illness in Mexico's tropics, other public health concerns were eclipsed, the result of which was the resurgence in 1905 and 1906 of highly preventable smallpox outbreaks. Similarly, measures to deal with syphilis and alcohol-related illnesses lagged in the teens and twenties.

The mechanism by which public health threats are weighed is another social fact that becomes visible in disease moments, as we have seen. Legacies of uncertainty and paranoia are clearly part of the H1N1 pandemic of today as they were in the diseased moments of Mexico's past. As a public health menace, H1N1 has thus far eluded eradication. The prevention of person-to-person transference requires strict containment of victims, a preventative that does not mesh well with busy work schedules and the need to earn a living, travel, and pursue an education. The consequences of an epidemic reach beyond binaries of life and death: anxiety, depression, fear, and social distancing remain long after an epidemic subsides.

For Mexicans, the identification of their nation as an epicenter for H1N1 meant the world's spotlight was directed at their overburdened health-care system, households, industries, and schools. On occasion, life under the critical eye of "first world" nations entailed a level of scrutiny and judgment reminiscent of those nineteenth-century civilizing campaigns that codified "indios" and rebels as obstacles to progress and identified as "intemperate" those who spread filth and disease. In responding to threats to public health and security, such as H1N1, people with a specific political agenda to fulfill both in Mexico and outside its borders often revive antiquated, stereotypical, and damaging images of the Mexican people.[30] As unproductive as these accusations are, the most dangerous element of such xenophobia remains the inability to recognize that disease knows no national boundaries. And as modernization has triumphed, with its interlocking mechanisms of increased communication and trade, intensified working routines, larger populations, and greater stress on the natural environment, new vulnerabilities appear. Modern technocratic civilization will surely shape its own ecology of disease just as much as past civilizations did.

NOTES

Chapter 1

1. For a discussion of soil, see Gómez-Pompa, *Lowland Maya Area*, 118.
2. De Kruif, *Microbe Hunters*, 303.
3. Koch, *Essays;* Snow, *Snow on Cholera;* Debré, *Louis Pasteur*.
4. For more information on the terms *batab*, *hidalgo*, *pacíficos*, *indio*, *cruzob*, and *bárbaro*, see Rugeley, *Yucatán's Maya Peasantry*.
5. Scott, *Moral Economy*.
6. Taussig, "Peasant Economics," 64.
7. Scott, *Moral Economy*, 193, ellipsis in original.
8. Rosenberg, *Cholera Years*.
9. Stephens, *Incidents of Travel*, 42.
10. Villasenor, *El separatismo*, 148–49.
11. Bricker, *Indian Christ*, 90.
12. Ibid.
13. For more on the secessionist movements, see Rugeley, *Rebellion Now*, 55; Remmers, "Henequén, the Caste War and Economy of Yucatán," 157–59; Rugeley, "The Maya Elites," 482–84.
14. Ancona, *Historia de Yucatán*, 46; Lira, "Justo Sierra," 24.
15. Díaz Zermeño, *Cancerbero del traidor*, 35–36.
16. Arrom, *Containing the Poor*, 208.
17. Brading, *First America*, 656.
18. Ibid., 648, 653.
19. Morrison, "The Life and Times."
20. Moseley and Delpar, "Yucatán's Prelude," 25.
21. Beezley, *Judas*, 9.
22. Agostoni, *Monuments of Progress*.

23. Wells and Joseph, *Summer of Discontent*, 131.
24. Joseph, *Revolution from Without*, 66.
25. Snook, "Sustaining Harvests," 62.
26. Turner, *Barbarous Mexico*.
27. Creelman, "President Díaz."
28. Knight, *Mexican Revolution*, 1:59–62.
29. "Big Vote for Diaz," *New York Times*, June 27, 1910.
30. Gonzales, *Mexican Revolution*, 73–74.
31. Koth, *Waking the Dictator*, 83–84.
32. "Diaz Flees from Mexico City to Spain: Deposed President Steals Away in the Night on Narrow-Gauge Road," *Pittsburgh Post-Gazette*, May 26, 1911; "Diaz Resigns; de la Barra In, Rioters Shot: Mexican Capital Wild with Joy When President, Denying Faults, Surrenders Power," *New York Times*, May 26, 1911.
33. Carey, *Mexican Revolution*, 24.
34. McLynn, *Villa and Zapata*, 162–63.
35. Henderson, *In the Absence*, 206.
36. Hart, *Revolutionary Mexico*, 293.
37. Wolf, *Peasant Wars*, 40–41.
38. Gonzales, *Mexican Revolution*, 169–70.
39. Huntington, *Climactic Factor*, 177.
40. An exception to this generalization would be the neighboring Isthmus of Tehuantepec region that contains the busy port of Veracruz and has a reputation as a particularly unhealthy zone. See Knaut, "Disease."
41. Espinosa Rendon and Carrillo Ancona, eds., *El repertorio pintoresco*, 11.
42. Joseph, "The United States." Joseph contends that the "Yucatán has always been more naturally oriented toward the United States, Central America, and the Caribbean islands than toward the remainder of the Mexican Republic" (176).
43. Some works on tropical medicine: Delaporte, *The History of Yellow;* Curtin, *Death by Migration;* Cueto, ed., *Missionaries of Science;* Rosenberg, *Cholera Years;* Jiménez and Palmer, *La voluntad radiante*.
44. Mayer, *Mexico;* Knox, *The Boy Travellers*.
45. Evans, *Bound in Twine*.
46. Pomeranz and Topik, *The World*, 139.
47. *El Siglo XIX: Boletín Oficial del Gobierno de Yucatán* (Mérida), June 3, 1850, no. 263, 3–4.
48. *La Unión Liberal*, March 28, 1856, 4–5, Colección de Biblioteca Menéndez. *Las Garantías Sociales* (Mérida), April 2, 1856, no. 80, 3. Justo Sierra O'Reilly, "Crónica del estado," *Union Liberal* (Campeche), March 28. Another way public health officials acquired vaccine was through the donations of philanthropic world travelers. In 1856 Sr. Francisco Clausell sent, from England to a friend in the Yucatán, a box that contained a portion of the precious vaccination fluid in vials and tubes along with some "lino" and lancets. Notification of Sr. Clausell's good deed was advertised in the periodical *La Union Liberal* and in *Las Garantías Sociales*. The article applauds Sr. Clausell's generosity. The publicizing of Clausell's gesture in official newspapers set an example for other travelers who also might desire exposure for similar acts of philanthropy.
49. Echeverría V., *¡Nos llevó el tren!*, 12.
50. Wells, *Yucatán's Gilded Age;* Evans, *Bound in Twine*.

51. Wells and Joseph, *Summer of Discontent*, 44.
52. Farriss, *Maya Society*.
53. Clendinnen, *Ambivalent Conquests*.
54. Cline, "Civil Congregations"; Cline, Appendix C, "Remarks on a Selected Bibliography"; Redfield, *A Village*; Redfield, *The Little Community*.
55. Among some of the most notable contemporary histories of the Caste War period is Rugeley, "The Maya Elites," 478. For a reexamination of the Caste War, see Rugeley, "Origins of the Caste War." More traditional accounts of the Caste War are Reed, *The Caste War of Yucatán*; Navarro, *Raza y tierra*; Bricker, *Indian Christ*.
56. Cline, "Remarks on a Selected Bibliography," and Rojas, *The Maya*; Baqueiro, *Renseña geográfica*. Nelson Reed's book remains one of the most popular and highly criticized narratives of the Caste War authored by a Western scholar. His compelling narrative style reminds us that the loss of a *story* in historical accounts denies the reader a certain proximity to the events and people. However, Reed's work has been criticized because he relies almost entirely on nineteenth-century Yucatecan author Serapio Baqueiro's account of the Caste War.
57. Wells, "Forgotten Chapters." For instance, in the 1950s and 1960s studies of the Yucatán and the Maya by Robert Redfield and Alfonso Villa Rojas emphasized the "closed community" and the steps of "progress" within a single village, Chan Kom, in southern Mexico. The groundbreaking ethnography produced from these studies established an important base of analysis and data for future studies. Howard Cline's article in the appendix of Villa Rojas's *The Maya of East Central Quintana Roo* (1944) is an instrumental work of the previously mentioned genre. Cline criticized provincial interpretations of the Maya and the Caste War and challenged scholars to consider "the social, economic, and cultural phases of Yucatecan life" that led to the Caste War (169). Cline also argued that politics did not provoke the Maya to rebel in 1847, but rather other cumulative social economic forces did.
58. Brannon and Joseph, Review of *Land, Labor, and Capital*. According to Thomas Benjamin, works by Gilbert Joseph, Robert Patch, José Arturo Güémez Pineda, and others are important because they "analyze how national and global forces of change impinged upon Yucatán and shaped land tenure and production, labor conditions and utilization, and the power and employment of capital" (Brannon and Joseph, Review of *Land, Labor, and Capital*, 630).
59. Some studies that focus on the subaltern and regional economies are Van Young, *Hacienda and Market*; Mallon, "Peasants and State Formation"; Stern, ed., *Resistance, Rebellion, and Consciousness*; Hu-DeHart, *Yaqui Resistance and Survival*; Larson and Harris, eds., *Ethnicity, Markets, and Migration*.
60. The following is only a sampling of the peasant and area studies scholarship that particularly informed this study: Scott, *Weapons of the Weak*; Scott, *Moral Economy*; Wachtel, *Gods and Vampires*; Van Young, "To See Someone Not Seeing"; Mallon, "Peasants and State Formation"; Stern, ed., *Resistance, Rebellion, and Consciousness*; Hu-DeHart, *Yaqui Resistance and Survival*; Larson and Harris, eds., *Ethnicity, Markets, and Migration*.
61. Van Young, "To See Someone Not Seeing."
62. Some social histories that examine issues of race, ethnicity, state-building, and imperialism through the lens of medicine, disease, or public health are as follows: Kraut, *Silent Travelers*; Lindenbaum and Lock, eds., *Knowledge, Power,*

and Practice; Crandon-Malamud, *From the Fat of Our Souls;* Chen, *Medicine in Rural China;* Anderson, "Disease, Race, and Empire"; Anderson, "Immunities of Empire"; Harrison, "The Tender Frame of Man"; Anderson, *Colonial Pathologies;* Pineo and Baer, eds., *Cities of Hope* (and in particular see Parker, "Civilizing the City of Kings"; Pineo, "Public Health Care"; and Adamo, "The Sick and the Dead"); Florescano and Malvido, eds., *Ensayos sobre la historia;* Cueto, ed., *Missionaries of Science;* Grandin, *Blood of Guatemala*, 82–98; Peard, *Race, Place, and Medicine.*

63. See, for instance, Harris, "Voices of Disaster"; Herring, "There Were Young People"; Schwarz, "The Explanatory and Predictive Power of History"; Cook and Lovell, "The Civilization of the American Indian Series"; Montellano, *Aztec Medicine.* On American slave societies see Numbers and Savitt, eds., *Science and Medicine*, especially the following essays: Patterson, "Disease Environments of the Antebellum South"; Keeney, "Unless Powerful Sick"; Warner, "Public Health in the Old South"; Gorn, "Black Magic." See also Crosby, *Columbian Exchange;* Cook, *Born to Die.* Philip D. Curtin's work on the migration of British army troops throughout the Caribbean and India provides exhaustive demographics concerning the contraction of infectious diseases such as typhoid, typhus, malaria, cholera, smallpox, and tuberculosis. Cook's work, like Alfred Crosby's *The Columbian Exchange*, demonstrates the mobility of disease and its varied effects on native and foreign populations. For works on Mexico and disease, see Cooper, *Epidemic Disease in Mexico City;* Crandon-Malamud, *From the Fat of Our Souls;* Oliver Sánchez, *Un verano mortal;* and Oliver Sánchez, "Una nueva forma de morir." Marcus Cueto, Armando Solorzano, Nancy Leys Stepan, David Sowell, Libbet Crandon-Malamud, and Julyan Peard have authored works on the nature of health, illness, and medical science in different regions throughout Latin America, showing the links between medical science, public health, nation-building, and imperialism. See, for instance, Cueto, "The Rockefeller Foundation's Medical Policy"; Solorzano, "The Rockefeller Foundation"; Stepan, *"The Hour of Eugenics"*; Stepan, *Picturing Tropical Nature;* Sowell, *The Tale of Healer Miguel Perdomo Neira;* Peard, *Race, Place, and Medicine;* Palmer and Molina Jiménez, *Educando a Costa Rica.*

64. Anderson, "Disease, Race, and Empire"; Anderson, "Immunities of Empire"; Harrison, "The Tender Frame of Man."

65. Anderson, "Immunities of Empire," 63.

Chapter 2

1. All translations—Spanish and Maya—are my own unless otherwise indicated.
2. Estado de Yucatán, *Monografía*, 90. Subvacunadores were generally those medical professionals placed in the field to oversee vaccination efforts in rural districts. Not all subvacunadores had medical training, however: some were laypersons who had been taught how to give a vaccination by a member of the council.
3. AGEY, Poder Ejecutivo (PE), Gobernación, Box 98, "Petición del cargo de director de vacuna," Mérida, December 2, 1852. Manuel Campos, a medical surgeon, resigns as director of vaccination in Campeche. In his resignation Dr. Campos states that after some years in this position of vaccinator, he has become weary from watching so many die of viruela and he cannot possibly attend to

them all adequately. The position went vacant for two years, until the governor finally appointed Lic. D. Juan Perez Espinola to the post. For more information on the administrative efforts to appoint vacunadores in the Yucatán, see CAIHY, Manuscripts collection (MC), Books 60, 63, and 31, Mérida, 1842–53.

4. AGEY, PE, Gobernación, Box 98, "Petición del cargo de director de vacuna," Mérida, 1854.
5. For more information on the administrative efforts to appoint vacunadores in Yucatán, see CAIHY, MC, Books 60, 63, and 31, Mérida, 1842–53.
6. Pérez Galaz, ed., "Situación estadística de Yucatán," 438.
7. Reed, *The Caste War of Yucatán;* Bricker, *Indian Christ;* Navarro, *Raza y tierra;* Cline, "Civil Congregations"; Cline, "Remarks on a Selected Bibliography"; Remmers, "Henequén, the Caste War and Economy of Yucatán"; Patch, "Decolonization."
8. Estado de Yucatán, *Monografía*, 42. Also see Cook, *Born to Die*. Cook places smallpox epidemics in Mesoamerica between 1519 and 1521 and again in 1576 through 1580 (132, table 3.2) and again in 1613 through 1617 (170, table 5.2). While mortality statistics for each colonial epidemic are almost non-existent outside of church records and Spanish chronicles, Cook addresses broad implications of the devastation of Amerindian populations due to disease. According to Cook, "More than 90 percent of the Amerindians were killed by foreign infection," including measles, smallpox, and influenza initially, followed by typhus and much later the plague, yellow fever, and cholera (206). Also, see Crosby, *The Columbian Exchange*. Crosby explains that the Spanish term for smallpox (*viruelas*) was used as a general descriptive in the sixteenth century to refer to a host of pustular maladies such as measles, chickenpox, or typhus. However, by the nineteenth century, the use of the term *viruelas* in literature and print media was clearly associated with smallpox. This logic is also in tune with Crosby's methodology, which argues that smallpox was the "most important disease of the first pandemic in the recorded history of the Americas" (43).
9. Coatsworth, "Indispensible Railroads in a Backwards Economy." On railroads in Yucatán, see also Wells, "Forgotten Chapters," 210.
10. Reclus, *The Earth and Its Inhabitants*, 164–65; Heller, *Alone in Mexico*, 152. Upon arrival by steamship to the port of Campeche in 1846, Heller commented, "The sea is so shallow in the small inlet that lighter vessels must weigh anchor two to three nautical miles away from the land."
11. Echeverría V., *¡Nos llevó el tren!*, 14–16.
12. See, for instance, Williams, "The Resurgent North and Contemporary Mexican Regionalism"; Cline, *The United States and Mexico;* Martinez, *Troublesome Border;* and Turner, *The Dynamic of Mexican Nationalism*.
13. AGN, Gobernación, Sin Sección, Box 363, 7, 1849. The states of Colima, Guerrero, and Nuevo León and the Distrito Federal requested more vaccine; AGN, Gobernación, Legajo 992, 2, Epidemias, 1854 (over two hundred pages of requests from various territories in the Mexican republic requesting vaccine shipments).
14. See Alan Knight's description of the separatist roots of northern Mexico and the evolution of the Serrano rebellions in this area during the Mexican Revolution of 1910. Knight, *The Mexican Revolution*, 1:368.

15. Barbachano, "La salud pública," 56. According to the 1813 count of the peninsula's population, out of a total of 500,000 inhabitants, 70,000 were of European ancestry or considered creoles, 55,000 were mestizos, and 375,000 indigenous.
16. AGEY, PE, Gobernación, Box 79, Secretaria General de Gobierno, Milicia Local, Varios Lugares, February 10, 1850.
17. Priestley, *José de Gálvez*, 202.
18. Dumond, *The Machete and the Cross*, 19–20.
19. For more information on the colonial roots of rivalry and the sisal port, see Dumond, *The Machete and the Cross*, 19–20. In 1871 a single-gauge railroad was constructed between Progreso and Mérida, after which Sisal declined. See monthly consular and trade reports, *United States*, 473.
20. Dumond, *The Machete and the Cross*, 66.
21. Among the publications that outlined the rivalry between Méridanos and Campechanos published in the mid- to late nineteenth century were Baquiero, *Ensayo histórico*, 5:65, and O'Reilly, *Los Indios de Yucatán*. O'Reilly's work was originally published in the Campeche periodical *El Fénix* between 1848 and 1857; see chapter 12 in particular, "La situación de Campeche."
22. Aznar Barbachano y Juan Carbó (diputados al congreso de la unión por el nuevo estado de Campeche), *Memoria sobre la conveniencia*, 88. For a contemporary summary of the rivalry between Campechano and Méridano elites, see Wells, "Forgotten Chapters," 207–15.
23. AGEY, PE, Sección, Gobernación, Box 139, Serie Consulado de S.M.B. in Mérida and Sisal, Ayuntamiento de Hunucmá, 1864.
24. Tekax is located in eastern Yucatán (southeast of Mérida). It prospered for many years before independence with the sugar industry and had sixty-six pueblos, 188 haciendas, and 705 ranchos. See Estado de Yucatán, *Estadística de Yucatán*, 255.
25. AGEY, PE, Gobernación, Box 101, Prefectura del Distrito de Tekax, April 11, 1855.
26. Pérez Galaz, ed., "Situación estadística de Yucatán," 456.
27. Ibid., 460.
28. Pérez, "Medidas para la conservación y propagación del fluido vacuno," 373–74.
29. *Las Garantías Sociales* (Mérida), July 11, 1856, no. 123.
30. The name "Superior Health Council" is used throughout this book to refer to the myriad of titles applied to the state of Yucatán's health services branch. Between 1832 and 1930, the title for state health services in Yucatán changed no less than seven times. In the 1830s, "Junta General de Sanidad del Estado" was used; by 1855 the name changed to "Junta Superior de Sanidad," which endured until 1894 when "Consejo Superior de Salubridad" was adopted. By 1912 the name changed back to the 1855 version, "Junta Superior de Sanidad." In 1917 "La Dirección General de Salubridad é Higiene Público" was used, and then by 1926 the name was changed back again to "Junta Superior de Sanidad." Finally in 1930 the name reverted to a very similar version of the 1830 name, "Departamento de Sanidad del Estado."
31. AGEY, PE, Gobernación, Box 100, Secretaria del Estado y Despacho de Gobernación, Mexico, July 17, 1855.
32. Remmers, "Henequen, the Caste War." Remmers's research also illustrates the Yucatán's dependency on trade with the Caribbean and the United States: "Between 1868 and 1871 . . . Yucatán sold 854,057 pesos worth of goods to Mexico but bought products valued at 1,716,370 pesos. Yucatán paid for these goods with drafts from henequen sales in New York and Cuba" (715).

33. AGEY, PE, Gobernación, Box 101, Prefectura del Distrito de Mérida, February 23, 1855.
34. Kiple, ed., *The Cambridge World History of Human Disease*, 449, 1010–11. Variolation has a long folk history in Asian and African medicine. In some instances the fluid from an active smallpox pustule was extracted, dried, and either swallowed or inhaled in powdered form through the nasal cavity.
35. Experimentation with animals may have occurred before the 1770s but without publication or notoriety.
36. Hibbard (late vaccine physician to the New York dispensary), *A Treatise on Cow-Pox*, 15–16.
37. For a discussion on the introduction of smallpox vaccination campaigns in India, see Arnold, "Smallpox and Colonial Medicine."
38. The texts that contain some information concerning medicinal cures can be found in Roys's *The Book of Chilam Balam of Chumayel*. Additionally, one of the largest sources of Maya medicinal practices during the nineteenth century is "Yerbas y hechicerías"; a manuscript is located at the Latin American Library at Tulane University's William Gates Collection (TULALWGC). Also *El libro del Judío* can be found at the Harvard Peabody Museum, Cambridge, Massachusetts. Sections of *El libro del Judío* have been published in edited form, see Barrera Vasquez (presentation and revision), *El libro del Judío;* Zapata, *El libro del Judío ó medicina doméstica*.
39. Roys, *Ritual of the Bacabs*, xxii.
40. Ibid.
41. Ibid., xi. "The manuscript the *Ritual of the Bacabs* was named by William Gates, because of its frequent mention of these deities. . . . Nearly all the incantations are written in a single hand, which could well be the last half of the eighteenth century, but this is not certain" (vii).
42. Walton, Beeson, and Scott, eds., *The Oxford Companion to Medicine*, 1:567.
43. For a contemporary view of Maya understandings of "hot" and "cold," see Adams and Hawkins, *Health Care in Maya Guatemala*, 76–77.
44. Zapata, *El libro del Judío ó medicina doméstica*.
45. Ibid., 98–99.
46. Le Plongeon, *Here and There in Yucatán*, 16.
47. Manzano and Sansores, eds., *Diccionario maya*, 364. For the purposes of this study, I have only utilized definitions that the editors indicated are derived from the nineteenth-century dictionary publications by Juan Pío Pérez. Pío Pérez's manuscript was first sent to the press in 1867, but for various reasons it did not see the light of day until almost eleven years later (see editors' notes 28a–30a). Pío Pérez, *Diccionario de la lengua maya*, see page 56a for his other publications. Throughout the Manzano and Sansores edition, the referent number 8 is used to indicate derivation from Pío Pérez; unless otherwise indicated, only those definitions that are referenced by the number 8 are included in this analysis.
48. Manzano and Sansores, eds., *Diccionario maya*, 364. One of the definitions for *k'ak'il* that is not from the nineteenth-century Pío Pérez source states that the illness was a "great fire like pestilence that ordinarily afflicts the indios."
49. Ibid., 665. The part of the definition that goes beyond a general reference to viruelas to include *gruesas* is not from Pío Pérez, but from a colonial source, see

30a for details. The colonial source is Swadesh, Álvarez, and Manzano, compilers, *Diccionario de elementos del Maya Yucateco colonial.*

50. Manzano and Sansores, eds., *Diccionario maya*, 844.
51. Confluence in smallpox occurs when an individual's pustules group together to form a rash or mass of pustules. The rash then pulls the outer layer of skin away from the underlying flesh. Confluent smallpox has a higher mortality rate than nonconfluent forms. Black smallpox is another name for hemorrhagic or flat smallpox. Black smallpox derives its name from the bleeding that occurs under the skin, making the "skin look charred and black." Hemorrhagic smallpox is the most severe of all forms of smallpox. Extensive bleeding "into the skin, mucous membranes, and gastrointestinal tract" makes this form the most deadly. Hemorrhagic smallpox does not produce the telltale rash or pustules—hence the term *flat smallpox*—and the skin remains smooth while the bleeding occurs under the skin. See Rotz and Atkinson, "Clinical Features."
52. Manzano and Sansores, eds., *Diccionario maya*, 151.
53. A disease that was particularly prevalent in infants, diphtheria obstructs the victim's airway as the larynx swells shut from an invasion of exotoxins. Generally speaking, diphtheria was seen as a disease of poverty but was not considered dangerous in the way cholera, smallpox, and yellow fever were, and even periodic peaks in diphtheria mortality received little to no attention from physicians.
54. Fallaw, *Cárdenas Compromised*, 89–90.
55. Scott, *Domination and the Arts of Resistance*, 215–16.
56. For more on Balmis's travels and training of local populations in variolation, see Jannetta, *The Vaccinators*, 43–44.
57. A number of sources testify that the expedition left on November 30, 1803. It returned in 1806. Contemporary accounts—like the *Madrid Gaceta*—are clear about the dates and the number of orphans (a handful, or more than twenty) used for propagation. According to historian Sheldon Watts, the expedition was organized in 1803 and used twenty-two orphan boys "and two of them vaccinated seriatim every six or eight days using the arm-to-arm method to keep the vaccine fresh during the long voyage across the Atlantic" (*Epidemics and History*, 118). Also see Rigau-Pérez, *The Introduction of Smallpox Vaccine*, 395–96. But see also the translation of the account in the *Madrid Gaceta*, October 14, 1806, published in the *Edinburg Medical and Surgical Journal* (1807): 376–79.
58. For more information on Balmis's time in Yucatán, see Barbachano, *La escuela de medicina*, 23. Dr. Alejo Fancourt vaccinated in Mérida while Dr. Cipriano Blanco vaccinated in Campeche (Estado de Yucatán, *Monografía*, 46).
59. Smith, "The 'Real Expedición Marítima de la Vacuna,'" 31.
60. Servín Massieu, *Microbiología, vacunas y el rezago científico*, 57.
61. Smith, "The 'Real Expedición Marítima de la Vacuna,'" 32.
62. *Gaceta Médica, Periódico Academia N. de Medicina de México* (Mexico: Imprenta del Gobierno Federal en el Ex-Arzobispado) 21, no. 3 (January 1, 1894): 60.
63. McCaa, "Revisioning Smallpox in Mexico Tenochtitlán," 459.
64. See Dr. Eduardo Liceaga's article about humanized vaccine, "A Century of Arm to Arm Vaccination in Mexico." Dr. Liceaga explains the process for preservation of fluid: "First—In Mexico, the inoculations from arm to arm, after having carefully selected a vacciniferous child quite unobjectionably, have been nearly exclusively employed since 1804 up to the present date. Second—The preservation of the

vaccine virus in the City of Mexico has been entrusted to only five physicians in a whole century. . . . Fourth—The central office in the City of Mexico gathers the lymph from the children who are not under the slightest suspicion of being able to transmit some infectious disease. The tubes with the gathered virus having been closed by means of the alcohol lamp, the official sends them to the capitals of each of the States, those towns forming now secondary distributing centers, where the same rules we have just spoken of are strictly adhered to" (290).

65. Thompson, "To Save the Children," 444.
66. AGEY, PE, Gobernación, Box 101, Prefectura del Distrito de Mérida, April 24, 1855.
67. AHAY, PE, Gobernación, Box 113, Vol. 1, No. 55, "Vacuna," 1857.
68. The vaccine was propagated in cattle udders and then transferred in pus form to a preservation receptacle (usually a glass vial, or sometimes a thread of fabric).
69. For laws regarding the raising of ganado vacunado, see Pérez, "Law of December 11, 1849," 303.
70. *Ganado vacuno* should not be confused with *ganado vacunado*. *Ganado vacuno* referred to bovines (that is, cattle), whereas *ganado vacunado* (vaccine cattle) and "*la cría de ganado vacunado*" referred to cattle used especially for vaccine production. Cattle were not "vaccinated" against diseases in the Americas until the early twentieth century. Hence, *ganado vacunado* in the context of nineteenth-century Mexico should not be confused with *vaccinated cattle*. See Aparecida de S. Lopes, "Revolución y ganadería en el norte de México."
71. ANEY, Volume: Writings of 1852, Book no. 12, Section 1, 144. The original appeal by Nicolas Piste to the Republic of Indians is written in Yucatec Maya, March 24, 1818. The response to D. Correa's request is in the same book, pages 151–52, dated May 22, 1852.
72. Rugeley, *Yucatán's Maya Peasantry*, 125.
73. Pérez, *Colección de leyes*, 73–74.
74. Ibid., 373–74.
75. Ibid.
76. Rugeley, *Of Wonders and Wise Men*, 55.
77. O'Reilly, *Los indios de Yucatán: Consideraciones*, 187. This collection was originally published in serial form in *El Fénix* throughout the 1840s and 1850s. See Wells, "Forgotten Chapters," 202.
78. Estado de Yucatán, *Monografía*, 64. On smallpox in Yucatán also see Restall, *Maya Conquistador*, 6–7.
79. Estado de Yucatán, *Monografía*, 64.
80. AGEY, PE, Gobernación, Box 101, Prefectura del Distrito de Mérida, February 23, 1855.
81. Ibid. He argued that the welfare of many recently born babies relied on their timely vaccination since they were the most vulnerable to the smallpox virus. He deduced that the loss of the vaccine in the peninsula could not have been related to any sort of negligence on the part of those who oversaw vaccine conservation, nor could the lack of vaccine have anything to do with the ongoing Caste War.
82. *Las Garantías Sociales* (Mérida), July 11, 1856, no. 123, 4.
83. AGEY, PE, Gobernación, Box 101, Prefectura del Distrito de Mérida, February 23, 1855.
84. Dudgeon, "Development of Smallpox Vaccine," 1370.

85. Tomes, *The Gospel of Germs*, 33. For more information on Robert Koch's work on cholera and other diseases, see Carter, *Essays of Robert Koch*, 171–86.
86. Dudgeon, "Development of Smallpox Vaccine," 1371.
87. AHSS, Salud Pública (SP), IV, Box 3, 1920–22, Work of José María Oropeza, "Apuntas para la historia de la vacuna en México," Casa de Oswaldo Cruz (COC), Rockefeller Documents (RD), Doc. 010, Dr. Torres, "Sanitary Campaign in Brazil," 16.
88. Koplow, *Smallpox*, 20.
89. Similar methods were utilized throughout Spain in the early nineteenth century. "Commissioners" were sent to pry foundlings who had not experienced smallpox away from their foster families for propagation; see Rigau-Pérez, *The Introduction of Smallpox Vaccine*, 397.
90. *El Criterio Médico, Órgano Official de la Sociedad Hahnemanniana Matritense* (Madrid: Imprenta y Estereotipia de M. Rivadeneyra) 8 (1867): 143.
91. Govea, "Vacuna, su organización en Tamaulipas," 776–77.
92. AGEY, PE, Beneficencia, Box 308, Hospicios y Hospitales, Sanidad, Salubridad, September 7, 1897, Correspondence from the Director of the Consejo Superior de Salubridad to the Governor, no. 1095.
93. Ibid., Box 305, Hospitales, Correspondencia, Mérida, November 23, 1897, no. 1307.
94. There are also a few cases where the local jefe político begs for a cow, instead of children, to be sent so that the *linfa* can be properly produced. Ibid., Gobernación, Box 277, Correspondencia, Telegramas, Correspondencia Oficial, Asuntos de Gobierno, Mérida, 1892. See also earlier requests for *niños vacunados*, ibid., Box 101, Prefectura del Distrito de Mérida, 1855. Adam Warren found similar occurrences of propagation journeys to colonial Lima, Peru. Please see his dissertation, "Piety and Danger."
95. AGEY, PE, Beneficencia, Box 308, Hospicios y Hospitales, Sanidad, Salubridad, September 29, 1897, Correspondence no. 1176.
96. AGEY, PE, Varios Partidos/Municipios, Esteban Chan is listed in the Registro Civil for Motul, Box 304, December 1897 as having died at seven years of age from viruela. Considering that 1897 was a particularly harsh year of epidemic smallpox, it is interesting to note that Esteban's was the only death reported during the month of December for smallpox.
97. AGEY, PE, Beneficencia, Box 308, Hospicios y Hospitales, Sanidad, Salubridad, December 17, 1897.
98. The possibility that the unknown illnesses were in fact secondary infections contracted from tainted or spoiled shipments of smallpox vaccine can be seen in numerous Yucatecan town records. These "Unknown" deaths might also be linked to smallpox or smallpox-related deaths as a result of a shortfall in smallpox vaccine production. A decline in regional smallpox vaccine propagation may have prompted local officials to use out-of-date or tainted fluid, which may then have brought on secondary infections and even death. Similarly, if lancets were not sterilized or the vaccine itself were compromised, residents may have contracted hepatitis B. For more information, see Kiple, ed., *The Cambridge World History of Disease*, 795.
99. AGEY, PE, Gobernación, Box 254, 1889; AGEY, PE, Beneficencia, Box 304, Hospicios y Hospitales, Salubridad, Mérida, 1897.

100. Orvañanos, "Inaugural Address of the President," 710–11.
101. Colloredo-Mansfeld, "'Dirty Indians,'" 188.
102. NAWDC, Department of State (DOS), Consular Dispatches (CD), Mérida and Progreso, Record Group (RG) 59, Consul Edward Thompson to the Honorable U.S. Secretary of State, Progreso, December 20, 1900.
103. Chowning, *Wealth and Power in Provincial Mexico.* As testimony to how the Yucatán appeared to regional leaders within the Mexican republic, in 1850 the governor of Michoacán, Juan B. Ceballos, declared that "the keenest threat to the state's current calm was not the Indian population—which he believed was unlikely to follow the rebellious example of the 'casta primitiva' of the Sierra Gorda, the Yucatán, and the southern part of the state of Mexico" (230).
104. Alcereto, "Historia política," 346. As quoted in Wells and Joseph, *Summer of Discontent*, 45n123.
105. AGEY, PE, Box 330, Hacienda, Rentas, Contribuciones, Registro de la Propiedad, 1899. Also see Staples, "Policia y Buen Gobierno." Staples found that at midcentury a litany of regulations was implemented in Toluca, Mexico, prohibiting "both throwing garbage from the roof into the street and using the sidewalks for draining suet or curd" (120).
106. Tomes, *The Gospel of Germs*, 27.
107. Orvañanos, "President's Address," 6, presented at the Thirty-fifth Annual American Public Health Association Meeting, Atlantic City, NJ, September 30–October 3, 1907.
108. Estado de Yucatán, *Monografía*, 145.
109. Ibid., 91.
110. Ibid., 91–92.
111. Sowell, *The Tale of Healer*, 92.
112. Casares G. Cantón, ed., *Yucatán en el tiempo*, 2:162; also see Voekel, *Alone before God*, 222–23.
113. Ancona, *Colección de leyes*, 48.
114. As was the case earlier in Bolonchenticul, AGEY, PE, Gobernación, Box 95, Serie Petición del Vacunador de Bolonchenticul, 1853; ibid., Box 100, Secretaría de Estado y del Despacho de Gobernación, Mexico, 1855. Also observed by U.S. Consul Thompson later in 1900, NAWDC, DOS, CD, Mérida and Progreso, RG 59, Vol. 1, Correspondence no. 52 from Consul Thompson to Assistant Secretary of State, Progreso, November 30, 1900.
115. AGEY, PE, Gobernación, Box 85, Consejo del Estado, Mérida, Kanasin, 1851. The file contains over 150 pages of correspondence, mostly from the general directors of vaccine requesting that more vaccine was needed in the districts of Campeche, Hecelchakan, Hopelchen, Seybaplaya, and Isla del Carmen.
116. Between 1851 and 1857 approximately 80,000 inhabitants were lost due to the combined disasters of the Caste War, cholera, smallpox, yellow fever, and other diseases.
117. AGEY, PE, Beneficencia, Box 264, Salubridad, Sanidad, Hospicios, Hospitales, 1890.
118. Ibid., Box 304, Consejo Superior de Salubridad de Yucatán no. 1379, Mérida, December 4, 1897. Dr. Alfonso Peniche Rubio complains to the governor of the state that there is not enough assistance within the region to effectively end smallpox and stop its spread in the remote town of Cansahcab.

119. Ibid., Gobernación, Box 85, Consejo de Estado, Mérida, August 18, 1891. Campechanos complain that the rights of the members of the health board are not recognized, as they have to pay extra tariffs to receive goods from national and international ships.
120. During the 1890s Halachó was part of the partido of Maxcanú. It is located southwest of Mérida, bordering the state of Campeche.
121. Galaz, *Situación estadística de Yucatán*. In 1852 Halachó's population was 4,449 with ten haciendas, twelve ranchos, and 22,169 mecates of milpa (433); AGEY, PE, Beneficencia, Box 308, Hospicios y Hospitales, Sanidad, Salubridad, December 8, 1897.
122. AGEY, PE, Beneficencia, Box 308, Hospicios y Hospitales, Sanidad, Salubridad, Mérida, December 28, 1897.
123. Ibid., 1897.
124. Ibid., September 25, 1897. The Mayor of Halachó asks that a new vaccinator be sent because of the mistakes that Dr. Monsreal made. For examples of doctor-patient relations during smallpox epidemics, see Vaughan, *Curing Their Ills*, 43–44. According to Vaughan, the practice of hiding smallpox cases from the "smallpox police" was not unusual in colonial-era Africa.
125. AGEY, PE, Beneficencia, Box 308, Hospicios y Hospitales, Sanidad, Salubridad, December 22, 1897.
126. Ibid.
127. Ibid., 1897.
128. *Informes rendidos por los inspectores sanitarios de cuartel y los de los distritos al consejo superior de salubridad de 1898* (Mexico City: Imprenta del Gobierno, En El Ex-Arzobispado, 1899), 31.
129. Scott, *Domination and the Arts of Resistance*, 114.
130. Ibid., 20.
131. See correspondence from AGEC, 1119, Box 15, 1850. A new subvaccinator had yet to arrive since the previous one left his post. Also see ordinary session minutes from CAIHY, MC, Book 31, Mérida, 1853, 116 (reverse), November 25, 1853.
132. For more information on public "distrust" of state medicine, see Sowell, *The Tale of Healer*.
133. The same year that vaccination was made compulsory the Reglamento para la Forma de la Estadística del Estado de Yucatán was formed.
134. AGEY, PE, Box 304, Fomento, Estadísticas, *Boletín de Estadística*, no. 178, 1897. Halachó and Cansahcab are both considered henequen zone areas. Halachó is located near the present-day Campeche-Yucatán state line about forty-five miles southwest of Mérida. Canasahcab is located about forty miles to the east of Mérida.
135. AGEY, PE, Box 388, Milicia, 1900.
136. Ibid., Beneficencia, Box 264, Salubridad, Sanidad, Hospicios, Hospitales, 1890. Issued by the Secretaría de Estado y del Despacho de Gobernación, Circular.
137. Between 1893 and 1907, 256,000 persons were vaccinated in the Yucatán Peninsula. The first official census was conducted in 1895, thus population statistics for the peninsula before 1895 are somewhat erratic and unreliable. However, liberally speaking, if we can assume that the population statistics did not vary drastically during the 1893–1907 period, then it is reasonable to conclude that well over

three-quarters of the entire peninsula's population was vaccinated by the turn of the century.

138. AGEY, PE, Box 255, Población, Censos y Padrones, Registro Civil, Mérida, 1889.
139. A small margin of error may be attributed to the fact that the census did not separate out a category for smallpox survivors who would not have required vaccination.
140. AGEY, PE, Box 255, Población, Padrones Generales de los Habitantes, Sitilpech, 1889. Sitilpech is located about ten miles southeast of Mérida and twenty miles southwest of Motul.
141. AHAY, Municipios, Municipio de Espita, Yucatàn, Box 6, Vols. 30 and 33, 1898–1901. Many townships (*municipios*) like Espita were well aware of the mandatory vaccination policy through the circulation of announcements (bandos) and publication in *El Diario Oficial*. By 1901, it appears as though the vaccine was under control and no long tainted; previous to 1901, vaccination rates remained relatively low in Espita—local officials reasoned that it was related to rumors that the vaccine was tainted or bad.
142. Escalante, *Contribución al estudio*, 85.
143. Barbachano *La escuela de medicina*, 23.

Chapter 3

1. AGEY, Justicia, Tribunal Superior de Justicia Penal, Abuso de Autoridad, Citizens of Cacalchén against Don Esteban Herrera, October 24, 1854–March 1855.
2. Rosenberg, *The Cholera Years*, 113. Rosenberg also notes the particular threat free-roaming pigs posed to the public health of New York City during the 1849 cholera epidemic.
3. Wendt, ed., *A Treatise on Asiatic Cholera*, 20.
4. AGEY, Justicia, Tribunal Superior de Justicia Penal, Abuso de Autoridad, Citizens of Cacalchén against Don Esteban Herrera, October 24, 1854–March 1855.
5. French, "Imagining and the Cultural," 251. On economic liberalism in nineteenth-century Latin America, see Hale, *Mexican Liberalism in the Age of Mora*, 7; Gootenberg, "Beleaguered Liberals"; Platt, "Liberalism and Ethnocide."
6. McNamara, *A History of Asiatic Cholera*, 308–9; Pellarin, *Hygiéne des pays chauds*.
7. Watts, *Epidemics and History*, 194.
8. Voekel, "Piety and Public Space," 3. Pamela Voekel's work on the political and religious debates surrounding the burial of elites in late eighteenth-century Veracruz, Mexico, illustrates exactly how these Spanish traditions shaped modern Mexican burial practices.
9. For information on exchanges between the United States and Yucatán regarding cholera, see AAS, SFP, Box 38, Folder 3, January–April 1861 (1861: August to October); exchanges between Cuba and Yucatán are evident in *La Union Liberal*, Friday, March 28, 1856, 4–5, and in *Las Garantias Sociales* (Mérida), April 2, 1856, no. 80, 3.
10. For more information on the conceptualization of rebel Maya during the Caste War as "barbarians," see Gabbert, *Becoming Maya*, 53–55.

11. Kraut, *Silent Travelers*, 37.
12. Powers and Leiker, "Cholera among the Plains Indians," 320.
13. Rosenberg, *The Cholera Years*, 32.
14. For more information on Dr. John Snow's studies with cholera, see Snow, *Snow on Cholera*, 179.
15. Curtin, *Death by Migration*, 146.
16. For more information on Koch's study of cholera and the *Vibrio comma* bacillus, see Koch, *Essays of Robert Koch*, 171–86.
17. Holt, *Pestilential Foreign Invasion*, 6, at WRC, a division of the Historic New Orleans Collection: Kempre and Leila Williams Foundation, Rare Pamphlets, 669. H6, 1892.
18. *El Siglo XIX*, Thursday, June 6, 1850, no. 266, 2–3.
19. Requests on behalf of residents in small rural towns to dig new wells to ensure availability of drinking water during "dry times" were common; see AGEY, PE, Gobernación, Box 44, Vol. 1, Folder 4, 1841; ibid., Box 79, Comisión de Acopoio de Partidos, 1850.
20. The first global cholera pandemic occurred in the 1830s. For information on Mexico's first cholera pandemic, see Oliver Sánchez, *Un Verano Mortal;* Aguilar, *El Cólera*.
21. Estado de Yucatán, *Monografía*, 64.
22. Rosenberg, *The Cholera Years*, 75–78, 127. A compromise between older theories of contagion and burgeoning anticontagionist thought brought forth the school of contingent contagionists, who believed that cholera, while not inherently contagious, could become contagious provided it were to erupt among the right combination of environmental conditions. For opinions of contemporary observers, see the comparison between the danger zone for yellow fever and the more extensive one for cholera proposed by Dr. William Humboldt from work he conducted in a military hospital in Veracruz on behalf of the Mexican government in the Report of the Sanitary Commission of New Orleans on the epidemic yellow fever in 1854.
23. The backdrop for local struggles over cemetery control was the escalation of long-seated tensions between Liberal reformers and the Catholic Church. By the 1850s, many church and local officials had already experienced the horrors of the first cholera pandemic of the 1830s. Knowing that high mortality from such an epidemic led to an increase in burials, seasoned veterans of the first epidemic may have felt confident that they were better prepared for future episodes. Nonetheless, conflicts between church and state during the second cholera epidemic of the 1850s severely disrupted secular and clerical disease prevention efforts.
24. Cacalchén is located in the central henequen zone, east of Mérida, and directly east of Tixkokob. Cacalchén fell within the larger district confines of Motul. In 1851 the population of Cacalchén was estimated at 1,873; see Pérez Galaz, ed., "Situación estadística de Yucatán," "Jefatura Política de Motul," 501. According to an 1861 census report, Motul contained one city, twenty-six pueblos, 191 haciendas, and ninety-five ranchos and sitios (small farms). This number remained unchanged in the 1862 census report in which the number of haciendas decreased to twenty-five and the city was downgraded to a villa. Motul had an *ayuntamiento* with one president, eight *regidores*, and one *síndico;* a municipal junta with three representatives; and three jueces de paz. Each pueblo then had its

own designated number of municipal representatives and jueces de paz (usually no more than two or three for each pueblo). Herrera was one of the first jueces de paz for Cacalchén. See CAIHY, Section no. 37, Antonio G. Rejon, *Documentos justificativos de la memoria que el C. Antonio G. Rejon presentó a la legislatura de Yucatán como secretario general del gobierno del estado, en 8 de septiembre de 1862* (Mérida, Mexico: Imprenta de Jose Dolores Espinosa, 1862).

25. AGEY, Justicia, Tribunal Superior de Justicia Penal, Abuso de Autoridad, "Petición de los habitantes de Cacalchén para destituir de todo cargo público a don Esteban Herrera por abuso arbitrario en sus funciones," Cacalchén—Tixkokob—Motul—Izamal—Mérida, October 24, 1854–March 1855.
26. A capilla is a tiny church or chapel (usually a hacienda- or fajina-based church). Fajinas are the crops, lands, and property of the hacendado or capilla. The land comes entailed with an obligation from the townspeople, usually campesinos (farmers), to work a certain amount of time on the fajina or capilla.
27. AGEY, Justicia, Sección Tribunal Superior de Justicia Penal, Abuso de Autoridad, "Petición de los habitantes de Cacalchén para destituir de todo cargo público a don Esteban Herrera por abuso arbitrario en sus funciones," Cacalchén—Tixkokob—Motul—Izamal—Mérida, October 24, 1854–March 1855.
28. Rodriguez Losa, *Geografía política de Yucatán*, 2:95 and 123. There are no definitive population statistics or census records for the town of Cacalchén in 1853. However, the population estimate for Cacalchén in 1846 is 1,174 and for 1861, 1,962. If we calculate population growth between 1846 and 1861, we see an increase of 788 persons in Cacalchén over a fifteen-year period. Based on this growth rate, it is reasonable to estimate that, on average, the town of Cacalchén's population increased by approximately fifty-two persons per year. However, in consideration of the escalated death toll due to a combination of warfare and epidemic diseases, particularly smallpox and cholera, I have scaled the growth estimate per year down to forty-eight to compensate for increased mortality between 1847 and 1853. Given this projected growth rate, a population estimate for Cacalchén in 1853 can roughly be placed at 1,542. Cholera mortality estimates for 1853 are partially based on church records from the 1833 cholera epidemic. For instance, church records report 347 deaths from cholera in the pueblo of Motul in 1833, but there are no definitive mortality records for the town of Motul in 1853. Given the high number of cholera-related deaths in Motul in 1833, the death rate for the region may have been higher in 1853. However, the records of the church should be viewed with skepticism since they were recorded in 1849—some time after the 1833 cholera epidemic—and these records likely only reflect deaths in which there was enough time to obtain a priest for last sacraments. Records for specific districts, other than the city of Mérida, are scarce for the 1853 cholera epidemic. *El Regenerador* (1, no. 128, Monday, December 19, 1853) placed total deaths in Mérida from cholera at 2,629. A contemporary estimate places the total cholera-related deaths in the *parroquias* of Mérida in 1853 at more than 4,000; see Estado de Yucatán, *Monografía*, 64.
29. AGEY, Justicia, Tribunal Superior de Justicia Penal, Abuso de Autoridad, Citizens of Cacalchén against Don Esteban Herrera, October 24, 1854–March 1855. The article Herrera referred to is number 136 of the 1837 state legislative code.
30. Ibid.
31. Ibid.

32. CAIHY, MC, pamphlets. Numerous public health pamphlets were circulated following the crushing cholera epidemic of 1833. See, for example, "Medidas sanitarias adoptadas por el ayuntamiento de Mérida para el caso de que el cólera-morbus invada esta capital," by José Cristóbal Hernández, 12 pages, 1850; "Descubrimientos contra el cólera-morbus, interesantes al pueblo," Imprenta a cargo de Manuel Mimenza, 7 pages, 1850. Additionally, articles appeared daily in many Mérida and Campeche newspapers concerning new treatments from abroad, new public health regulations, and preventative disease theories. See *El Siglo XIX* for the months of May and June 1850, during which time several articles appeared in serial form concerning preventative measures against cholera with general advice to the public about hygiene, temperate behavior, and treatments. Also see AHSS, SP, Epidemias, Box 1, 23, July 12, 1850. Standard procedure for cemetery fumigation during the 1850 cholera pandemic is detailed in an *aviso* (advice column) by the Public Health Council of the Federal District, Mexico: "Hasta nueva orden y que se registraran las paredes y techos para reconocer si hay algunos endeduras las que si se encuentran se taparan inmediatamente haciendo al mismo tiempo fumigaciones tanto. . . . Convencido el consejo de la utilidad de las fumigaciones del cloro y los clorusos de cal y de sosa para destruir los miasmas orgánicos que muchos de ellos dan al ayre [*sic*] propiedades" (ibid.).
33. AGEY, Municipios, Motul, Yucatán, Vol. 1, Actas de Cabildo, 1833–50.
34. AHSS, SP, Epidemias Box 1, 1, June–August 1850; AGEY, Justicia, Tribunal Superior de Justicia Penal, Abuso de Autoridad, Citizens of Cacalchén against Esteban Herrera, October 24, 1854–March 1855.
35. Rugeley, *Yucatán's Maya Peasantry*, 77.
36. AGEY, Penal, Defunciones, 65, Box 161 F, April 30–May 25, 1888; ibid., Delitos contra la Salubridad Pública, 159, Box 16, January 24–Feburary 22, 1888; ibid., Infracción, 168, Box 130 B, May 26–June 20, 1881; ibid., Infracción de Leyes y Reglamentos sobre Inhumaciones, 85, Box 133, July 13–August 13, 1833.
37. Carey, *Our Elders Teach Us*, 123–24. Carey also notes cases of live burials during disease epidemics.
38. Scott, *Domination and the Arts of Resistance*.
39. Voekel, "Piety and Public Space," 3.
40. Staples, "La lucha por los muertos," 15.
41. Cooper, *Epidemic Disease in Mexico City*, 26.
42. Casares G. Cantón, ed., *Yucatán en el tiempo*, 2:161–62.
43. Staples, "La lucha por los muertos," 16.
44. Ibid.
45. Taylor, *Drinking, Homicide and Rebellion*, 134.
46. Voekel, "Piety and Public Space," 2–3.
47. Ibid., 2. Voekel explains that the Spanish buried their dead in temples as early as the eighth century.
48. Brading, *Church and State in Bourbon Mexico*, 144.
49. Tutino, *From Insurrection to Revolution in Mexico*.
50. Brading, *The First America*, 512.
51. Hale, *Mexican Liberalism in the Age of Mora*, 125.
52. Mora, *Obras sueltas*, 232.

53. The Ley Lerdo was passed by provisional president Ignacio Comonfort's secretary of treasury, Miguel Lerdo de Tejada, and was an outgrowth of the Revolution of Ayutla of 1855.
54. See Voekel, *Alone before God.*
55. Some literature on the interaction between bodies (collective and individual), space, and power includes Deleuze, "Klossowski or Bodies-Language"; and Deleuze and Foucault, "Intellectuals and Power." For a discussion of the colonial body in the Philippians, see Anderson, "Excremental Colonialism."
56. Cline, "Regionalism and Society in Yucatán," pt. 5, 608. Also cited in Dumond, *The Machete and the Cross*, 87n10.
57. Dumond, *The Machete and the Cross*, 87.
58. Bazant, "From Independence to the Liberal Republic," 32.
59. Katz, "The Liberal Republic," 50.
60. AHSS, SP, HP (Higiene Pública), IP (Inspección de Panteones), Box 1, 49, January 6, 1861, "Bando del gobernador del Distrito Federal del decreto de la secularización de cementerios en la República Mexicana (impreso)."
61. AGN, Group no. 120, Justicia Eclesiastica, Vol. 180 (old numbering system), 62–66.
62. Morrison, "The Life and Times of José Canúto Vela."
63. Casares G. Cantón, ed., *Yucatán en el tiempo*, 6:84–85.
64. Gijaba y Patrón, *Estudios comentario*, 1296.
65. On economic liberalism in nineteenth-century Latin America, see Hale, *Mexican Liberalism*, 7; Gootenberg, "Beleaguered Liberals," 3–18.
66. French, "Imagining and the Cultural History," 251; Lempérière, "¿Nación moderna o república barroca?"
67. Zapata, *El libro del Judío.*
68. See, for instance, *El Regenerador*, Friday, June 17, 1853, no. 54, 1: the secretary general of the national government stated that all public health regulations dictated "in the case of an epidemic are necessary and require immediate compliance."
69. *El Fénix*, September 25, 1849, no. 66, 1–2.
70. Rodríguez, *Iglesia y poder*, 33–35.
71. AHAY, Oficios, Vols. 30–35, 1848–56. There are several reports of priests dying of smallpox, cholera, or fever throughout these volumes. Also, for general information on population decline in Yucatán at midcentury, see Cook and Borah, *Essays in Population History*, 120–29.
72. AHAY, Oficios, 1855, Vol. 34.
73. Morrison, "The Life and Times of José Cantu Vela."
74. AGEY, PE, Gobernación, Box 44 (5), Vol. 1, 19, 1841.
75. Ibid.
76. Pérez Galaz, ed., "Situación estadística de Yucatán," 547–67. Folder no. 7, Partido del Carmen, Jefatura Política del Partido del Carmen: "Relación que hace el jefe político del expresado Partido sobre el estado actual de los diferentes ramos a que se contrae, formada en cumplimiento de la orden del superior Gobierno, fecha 18 de julio último." Many of Carmen's residents were not officially reincorporated into the Yucatecan state until President Santa Anna mandated the end of their segregation in 1853.
77. AHSS, SP, Epidemias, Box 1, 19, Mexico City, June 1, 1850, "Bando de las medidas preventivas que ha tenido a bien dictar el gobernador del distrito de acuerdo con

el Sr. Virario Capitular, venerable cuerpo de párrocos y Sres. Alcaldes de Cuartel, en la presente epidemia del cólera morbo" (Mexico City: Imprenta de Vicente G. Torres á cargo de Luis Vidaurri, 1850); ibid., 24, Mexico City, June 1, 1850. "Bando: Miguel Maria de Azcarate, coronel retirado y gobernador del Distrito Federal, á sus habitantes sabed"; AGN, Gobernación/Legajos, Legajo 2062, 1853, Circulares (medidas precauciones para epidemias), August–September 1853, public health circulars issued from Mexico City to various state capitals, including Mérida, Yucatán, on August 31, 1853.

78. Drake, ed., *The Western Journal of the Medical and Physical Sciences*, 335–36.
79. In this particular instance, the use of the term *pantheon* (*panteón*) refers to a special place for the entombment of famous or important dead persons; AHSS, SP, HP, IP, Box 1, 32, 1852.
80. Ibid.
81. Ibid.
82. Freidel, Schele, and Parker, *Maya Cosmos*, 283–85. For a contemporary view of burial rites, see Echeverría León, "Prácticas y costumbres funerarias," 41; Redfield, *A Village That Chose Progress*, 106.
83. Roys, *The Indian Background of Colonial Yucatán*, 28.
84. Cannon, "The Historical Dimension in Mortuary Expressions," 437.
85. Echeverría León, "Prácticas y costumbres funerarias," 55.
86. The four cardinal directions or points are a foundational element of ancient Maya religious ideology. The Maya also linked specific colors with the directions: red with the east, white with the north, black with the west, and yellow with the south. See Roys, *The Book of Chilam Balam*, 170.
87. Echeverría León, "Prácticas y costumbres funerarias," 47.
88. For an interesting study on conflicts of custom over burial rituals, see Larson, "Austronesian Mortuary Ritual in History."
89. AHSS, SP, HP, IP, Box 1, 36, August 9, 1855. Antonio de Bonilla, the superintendent of the municipal police of Mexico, wrote to the secretary of the Superior Health Council to report that in the Panteón de San Fernando they had complied with the preventative measures dictated by the governor of the district concerning the burial of cholera victims. Also see ibid., 39, September 1, 1855. Padre José Miguel Zurita, of the Iglesia Metropolitao, wrote to the Superior Health Council to inform them that the panteón under his charge had complied with the proper orders concerning those who had died of cholera. In his correspondence, the padre assured the council that he had familiarized the *mozo* (servant) of the panteón with the legislation passed the previous March. Zurita also explained that he, and no one else, was responsible for reorganization of the panteón and creation of specific nichos (nooks) in which the coléricos were buried "se arregló todo lo conserviente á poner en practica las órdenes superiores que dicen relacion á esta material." On the fourteenth of September the secretary of the council, D. José Vargas, responded to Zurita's letter by simply stating that he agreed it was his obligation to maintain the rules set forth by the council.
90. Ibid., 41, January 19, 1855.
91. Ibid.
92. *El Siglo XIX*, May 31, 1850, no. 261, "Las últimas disposiciones adoptadas por la autoridad, son referentes á los enterramientos," 3–4.
93. Carey, *Our Elders Teach Us*, 123.

94. TULALWGC, No. 2, Box 7, Folder no. 78 (in oversize Box no. 11, Folder no. 3), Catalog no. 1448, Mérida, Yucatán, September 18, 1853, Broadside, "Método curativo contra el cólera morbo, sin necesidad de medico ni botica"; AMC, Box 6, 285, Campeche, April 9, 1856, "Notificación sobre la construcción y limpieza de una capilla en el cementerio general." Also, see Rosenberg, *The Cholera Years*, 105.
95. AGEY, PE, Justicia, Box 96, Juzgado de Paz de Seybaplaya, August 8, 1853.
96. Reed, *The Caste War of Yucatán*, 153–54.
97. Estado de Yucatán, *Monografía*, 64.
98. AHAY, Oficios, 1854, Vol. 33.
99. For information on disease and burial in a highland Maya community, see Dunn, "A Cry at Daybreak." Dunn presents a case from 1789 in which a Maya woman sat up all night near her child's grave in an effort to observe a Maya ritual that required a twenty-four-hour pre-interment time. We know about this case because it violated a rule laid down by a group of Spanish doctors who had been sent to the community and had ordered all bodies of those who died of typhus to be buried almost immediately.
100. AHAY, Oficios, 1854, Vol. 33.
101. AHAY, Book de Licencias de Exhumaciones de Restos Año 1888; Licencias de Exhumaciones de Restos 1897–1902.
102. AHAY, Oficios, 1854, Vol. 33.
103. The city of New Orleans also required death certificates to be issued by a physician during the height of the 1853 yellow fever epidemic. See, E. D. Fenner, M.D., *History of the Epidemic Yellow Fever, at New Orleans, LA. in 1853*, 43, WRC, Rare books and Manuscript Collection, 211.L9 F3.
104. CAIHY, pamphlet by Dr. F. Pedrera, "Método profiláctico y curativo del cólera morbo," 31 (Mérida, Mexico: Imprenta de *La Revista de Mérida*, 1892), vol. 1, no. 2, 14. Also see *El Siglo XIX*, May 31 and April 21, 1850, no. 261, 3–4.
105. AHSS, SP, HP, IP, Box 1, 45, February 1857.
106. Roediger, "And Die in Dixie." Roediger's study on African American funeral rituals in the American South reverses the 1914 findings of H. M. Henry that blacks were allowed to attend funerals and gather in groups of more than seven because of the white community's prevailing belief that they posed no harm in such instances due to their overwhelming commitment to "superstitions." Rather, Roediger contends that "Henry's argument might, in fact, be reversed since there is evidence that lawmakers specifically sought out funerals as special occasions for repression" (164).
107. Poc-Boc and Pomuch are north of the city of Campeche, on the coast, just south of today's Yucatán-Campeche state line in the state of Campeche.
108. Drake, ed., *The Western Journal of the Medical and Physical Sciences*, 322–23.
109. Similar conditions were found in New York City during the second cholera pandemic; see Rosenberg, *The Cholera Years*, 113.
110. ABH, Record Group (R) 39, Records Inwards (RI), 1852, 424–25.
111. Ibid., R 99, House of Assembly, RI, 1867–70, 171–74, February 8, 1868.
112. AHSS, SP, HP, IP, Box 1, 49, "El C. Justino Fernandex, bando del gobernador interino del Distrito de Mexico, á sus habitantes," passed into law by C. Melchor Ocampo—minister of government—on behalf of President Benito Juárez on

July 31, 1859, and signed by Justino Fernandez and Secretary Rafael Dondé, January 6, 1861.

113. Ibid.

114. Voekel, "Piety and Public Space." Voekel found that during the late colonial period in Veracruz, it was common practice to not charge a set fee, but rather require a "customary donation" in order to obtain a burial spot (3).

115. AGEY, PE, Gobernación, Box 134, Inhumación Fuera de Cementerios, Mérida, March 5, 1863.

116. Reed, *The Caste War of Yucatán*, 152.

117. "Juzgado Primero de Paz," *El Regenerador*, November 7, 1853, vol. 3, no. 110, 2–3.

Chapter 4

1. *El Siglo XIX* (Mérida), Saturday, August 4, 1849, no. 4, 1–2. Correspondence is dated June 8, 1849, from Miguel Barbachano to Francisco Martinez de Arredondo, Secretary General and the Minister of State and Chief of Interior and Exterior Relations.
2. Quintal Martín, *Correspondencia de la Guerra de Castas*, 19. Letter from Miguel Barbachano to Jacinto Pat, Tekax, March 1, 1848.
3. Martínez Alomía, *Historiadores de Yucatán*, 137.
4. The following works represent only a sampling from a vast body of work on nineteenth-century civilizing campaigns or missions that were central to this study: Larson, *Trials of Nation Making*, 57–59; Wells and Joseph, *Summer of Discontent;* Alonso, *Thread of Blood*, 50 and 98; Jacobson, *Whiteness of a Different Color*.
5. Reed, *The Caste War of Yucatán*, 153.
6. Anderson, "Disease, Race, and Empire"; Anderson, "Immunities of Empire"; Curtin, *Death by Migration*.
7. ABH, MC-396, from the Jubilee Library of Capt. M. S. Metzgen, MBE, Book 1841–49. Superintendents, Lieutenant Governors and Governor 1841–84, 139; 1849, January 5, 1849, R 22b, Superintendent to Commandant to Bacalar.
8. ABH, R 32(a), Letters Outwards (LO), 1849–50, 1–195. Letter no. 186, Belize, November 30, 1850. Letter to John Young, Chair of the Board of Health, from George Barkely.
9. Rugeley, "The Maya Elites," 477.
10. Ortega, "Revolts and Peasant Mobilizations in Yucatán," 295.
11. See, for example, *El Siglo XIX*, Friday, May 31, 1850, no. 261, 1; *El Regenerador* (Mérida), Friday, December 9, 1853, no. 124, 3.
12. Quote is from *La Union*, Tuesday, February 22, 1848, no. 24, 4; ibid., Saturday, February 19, 1848, no. 23, 4; ibid., Tuesday, April 4, 1848, no. 36, 4; AGEY, PE, Gobernación, Box 101, Tesoreria Municipal de Seybaplaya, 1855.
13. Classic treatments of the Caste War remain Reed, *The Caste War of Yucatán;* and Navarro, *Raza y tierra*. In large part, these studies are based on the works of Baqueiro, *Ensayo histórico*. *Ensayo histórico* was first published in 1865 and then again in 1871–79; O'Reilly, *Los indios de Yucatán*. For more recent contributions on the subject of the Caste War, see Joseph, *Rediscovering the Past at Mexico's Periphery* and Rugeley, *Yucatan's Maya Peasantry*.

14. Rugeley, *Yucatán's Maya Peasantry*, 107.
15. See Eric Van Young's comments on millenarian movements in nineteenth- and early twentieth-century Mexico in "The New Cultural History Comes to Old Mexico," 213. Also see Vanderwood, *The Power of God against the Guns of Government.*
16. Remmers, "Henequen, the Caste War," 312. This population figure is for 1850, and the percentage is from the population figure for 1846.
17. Bazant, "From Independence to the Liberal Republic," 25.
18. Morrison, "The Life and Times of José Canúto Vela"; Rugeley, "The Maya Elites"; Rugeley, *Yucatán's Maya Peasantry.*
19. Baqueiro, *Ensayo histórico;* O'Reilly, *Los indios de Yucatán;* Ancona, *Historia de Yucatán;* Solís, *Historia de Yucatán.*
20. Morrison, "The Life and Times of José Canúto Vela," 2–3; Rugeley, *Yucatán's Maya Peasantry.* Rugeley contends, "Between 1800 and 1847, taxes generated more incentive and spilled more ink than all other peasant grievances combined. It is impossible to overestimate the importance of this long-ignored issue in generating insurrectionary tension" (xv).
21. Menéndez, *Historia del infame;* Remmers, "Henequen, the Caste War," 454.
22. FMUNAM, Legajo 121, 1, 1–75, 35–52, covering cholera at 1850. CAIHY, Pamphlets, X-1855, no. 46, "Método curativo contra el cólera morbo."
23. TULALWGC, No. 2, Box 7, Folder no. 78 (in oversize Box no. 11, Folder no. 3), Catalog no. 1448, Mérida, Yucatán, September 18, 1853, Broadside by Igancio Vado, "Método curativo contra el cólera morbo, sin necesidad de medico ni botica."
24. Casares G. Cantón, ed., *Yucatán en el tiempo*, 4:113.
25. TULALWGC, No. 2 (1015 pieces: manuscripts, autographs, broadsides, newspapers, periodicals, and printed items), Box 7, Folder no. 78 (in oversize Box no. 11, Folder no. 3), Catalog no. 1448, Mérida, Yucatán, September 18, 1853, Broadside, "Método curativo contra el cólera morbo."
26. For a complete understanding of the differences between contagionists, contingent contagionists, anticontagionists, and animalcular and atmospheric theories of disease, see Rosenberg, *The Cholera Years*, 75–78.
27. Pío Pérez, *Diccionario de la lengua maya*, xv.
28. AGEC, Box 11, 820, Acuerdo para augmentar los vocales que forman la Junta de Sanidad para evitar la propagación de la epidemia del cólera, 1849.
29. Stillé, *Cholera*, 82.
30. Ray, *Cholera*, 103–4.
31. Several historians of public health and medicine have examined state-building and changes in international relations through the lens of cholera epidemics: Rosenberg, *The Cholera Years;* Kudlick, *Cholera in Post-Revolutionary Paris;* Evans, *Death in Hamburg.* The following is only a partial representation of published and unpublished works dealing specifically with cholera: Chambers, *The Conquest of Cholera;* Durey, *The Return of the Plague;* Longmate, *King Cholera;* Pelling, *Cholera, Fever and English Medicine;* Morris, *Cholera 1832;* van Heyningen and Seal, *Cholera;* Oliver Sánchez, *Un verano mortal;* Cuenya and others, *El cólera de 1833.*
32. Pío Pérez, *Diccionario de la lengua maya.* Pío Pérez served as mayor of Mérida from 1848 to 1853; he also served as the jefe político for Peto in the 1840s. Juan

Pérez married Nicolasa Peón, cementing a relationship with the powerful Peón family; see Casares G. Cantón, *Yucatán en el tiempo*, 5:122.

33. CAIHY, Pamphlets, Book 31, 103, Verso del September 17, 1853, Sesión Ordinaria, "Colera morbus." Grandin traces key shifts in Guatemala's early national politics through the cholera epidemic of the 1830s in *The Blood of Guatemala*. In particular, see chapter 3, "A Pestilent Nationalism: The 1837 Cholera Epidemic Reconsidered," 82–98; also see Palmer and Jiménez, *Educando a Costa Rica*.
34. A lazaretto is a hospital for the poor and diseased. Lazarettos are commonly used as quarantine stations for those with particularly horrible and infectious conditions: "The term is derived from Lazarus (Luke 16), the beggar full of sores who was laid at the rich man's gate but who achieved ultimate salvation in Abraham's bosom" (Walton, Beeson, and Scott, eds., *The Oxford Companion to Medicine*, 1:668).
35. CAIHY, Pamphlets, Book 31, 105, Verso del September 18, 1853, Sesión Ordinaria, "Colera en Valladolid."
36. Casares G. Cantón, ed., *Yucatán en el tiempo*, 5:143.
37. García y García, *Historia de la Guerra de Castas*, 27.
38. Wells, "Forgotten Chapter of Yucatán's Past," 211n38.
39. AHAY, Box Defunción Cólera Morbuz, 1833–53.
40. Ibid., Oficios, 1854, Vol. 54, República Mejicana, Parroquia de Ichmul, Partido de Peto, Distrito de Tekax, Departamento de Yucatán, September 26, 1854, letter from Pedro Badillo.
41. AGEY, PE, Gobernación, Box 101, Tesoreria Municipal de Seybaplaya, 1855; ibid., Iglesia, Box 97, Gobernación del Obispado de Yucatán, Mérida, 1853.
42. During Guatemala's first bout with epidemic cholera in 1831, health committees took to the streets, pruning trees, banning liquor sales, and encouraging the formation of community assistance and sanitation watch groups (Grandin, *The Blood of Guatemala*, 89); Asturias, *Historia de la medicina*, 169. According to Asturias, the Commission on Health in Guatemala was founded in 1837 specifically to fight cholera. For more information on intrusive cholera preventatives, see Evans, *Death in Hamburg;* Kudlick, *Cholera in Post-Revolutionary Paris*.
43. AGEY, PE, Iglesia, Box 97, Parroquia de Tekantó, 1853.
44. *El Siglo XIX* (Mérida), Friday August 3, 1849, no. 3, 1. Correspondence is dated June 12, 1849, from Miguel Barbachano to Francisco Martinez de Aredondo, Secretary General and His Excellency the Minister of State and Chief of Interior and Exterior Relations.
45. On the northern margins of the Mexican republic, see Alonso, *Thread of Blood;* Radding, *Wandering Peoples;* Hu-DeHart, *Yaqui Resistance and Survival*.
46. *El Siglo XIX* (Mérida), Saturday, August 4, 1849, no. 4, 1–2. Correspondence is dated June 8, 1849, from Miguel Barbachano to Francisco Martinez de Arredondo, Secretary General and His Excellency the Minister of State and Chief of Interior and Exterior Relations.
47. Ibid.
48. Ibid.
49. AGEY, Judicial, Box 06-B, 02 Departamento Judicial de Tekax, Serie 20 Juzgado de 1st Instancia de Tekax, 1882, Asunto 029 Designación de Curador/Depositario de Bienes, Promoventes May, Pablo, Observaciones Menor Chable, Maria Soledad. The legal age of adulthood was sixteen.

50. The mother, Agipata May, died before her husband at the age of forty-five from dysentery.
51. Civil code 1525, as listed in Pérez, *Colección de leyes.*
52. We should note that as was common among many Maya citizens at this time, neither Pablo May nor any of the village elders could write, so they had their sworn statements taken down by an official scribe, accompanied by the appropriate seals of verification and authenticity.
53. *El Grano de Arena* (Campeche), July 2, 1852, no. 62. Citing a report from New Orleans in Veracruz's newspaper *El Eco del Comercio*, public health experts declared that children seemed to be particularly vulnerable to the disease and constituted a high percentage of the fatalities: "It is not in our spirit to turn around and spread alarm in our town, therefore in this instance to improve the situation," they argued, "we have decided that we should call attention to our authorities so that in time they can adopt certain methods to prevent the malady, in the Health Commission of New Orleans has declared, of 342 dead between the 11 and the 28 of this past May, 188 were dead from cholera. [They have concluded that] it seems as though children have a fatal predilection to this terrible plague" (4).
54. AGEY, PE, Iglesia, Box 97, Parroquia de Tekantó, 1853, Letter from Jose Manuel Torres, February 12, 1853, to the Sr. Secretary General D. Cresencio José Pirrelo.
55. Blum, *Domestic Economies*, xxxiii. *El Siglo XIX* (Mérida), Saturday, August 4, 1849, no. 4, 1–2. Correspondence is dated June 8, 1849, from Miguel Barbachano to Francisco Martinez de Arredondo, Secretary General and His Excellency the Minister of State, Chief of Interior and Exterior Relations.
56. Wells, *Yucatán's Gilded Age*, 106.
57. Pérez, *Colección de leyes*, 353. Decreto de 23 de Mayo de 1850, "Permitiendo la libre importación de maíz." Also see AGEC, 1850, Box 13, 983, "Notificaciones de las medidas aplicadas por el ayuntamiento de Campeche por la escasez de maíz" (Correspondence regarding what measures can be implemented in order to address the shortage of grains for internal consumption).
58. Pérez, *Colección de leyes*, 344. Orden de 12 de Abril, "Que los jefes políticos envien hidalgos para cosechar las milpas de los sublevados" (The jefes políticos send hidalgos to harvest the milpas of the rebels).
59. Cook and Borah, *Essays in Population History*, 2:115.
60. Menéndez, *Historia del infame*; Remmers, "Henequen, the Caste War," 454.
61. Evans, *Death in Hamburg*. Evans investigates circumstances that led up to the 1888 cholera outbreak in the city of Hamburg and seeks to understand the political and social dimensions of the city's experience with cholera. In choosing Hamburg, Evans creates a paradigm for understanding how regional separatism is articulated in public health practices and disease prevention.
62. AGEY, PE, Gobernación, Box 98, Prefectura del Distrito de Valladolid, Sucilá, Valladolid and Mérida, 1854.
63. Baqueiro, *Ensayo histórico*, 2:37.
64. AGEY, PE, Gobernación, Box 98, Prefectura del Distrito de Valladolid, Sucilá, Valladolid and Mérida, 1854.
65. Ibid., Prefectura del Distrito de Valladolid, October 28, 1854, Letter to the Sr. Prefecto de Valladolid from the citizens of Sucilá.
66. Ibid., Prefectura del Distrito de Valladolid, Governor Vega to the Prefectura of the District of Valladolid, November 4, 1854.

67. CAIHY, Rejon, Documentos Justificativos, Section no. 37.
68. Gibson, *Spanish Tradition in America.*
69. AHAY, Box Defunción Cólera Morbus, 1833–53, January 11, 1853. Mortality records are sporadic at best for the peninsula during the height of the Caste War. From October to December 1852, 1,008 people died from cholera in Umán and the satellite pueblos of Bolon and Samahil.
70. Reed, *The Caste War of Yucatán*, 71.
71. ANEY, Vol. Escrituras of 1852, Book no. 12, Section 1, Mérida, Yucatán, May 22, 1852, 154.
72. TULALWGC, No. 2 (1015 pieces: manuscripts, autographs, broadsides, newspapers, periodicals, and printed items), Box 7, Folder no. 78 (in oversize Box no. 11, Folder no. 3), Catalog no. 1448, Mérida, Yucatán, September 18, 1853, Broadside, "Método curativo contra el cólera morbo," signed by Ignacio Vado.
73. Ibid.
74. Rosenberg, *The Cholera Years*, 75–78.
75. Quoted in Watts, "Cholera Politics in Britain in 1879," 295.
76. For more information on Dr. John Snow's studies with cholera, see Snow, *Snow on Cholera*, 179.
77. Snow, *On the Mode of Communication of Cholera*, 162. For more information on Robert Koch's work on cholera and other diseases, see Carter, *Essays of Robert Koch*, 171–86.
78. *Public Health Reports and Papers*, 351.
79. For a complete understanding of the differences between contagionists, contingent contagionists, noncontagionists, and animalcular and atmospheric theories of disease, see Rosenberg, *The Cholera Years*, 75–78.
80. *El Fénix*, "Variedades: Consejos al pueblo," Monday, May 20, 1850, no. 113, 3 (advice from Dr. Quin of Europe regarding homeopathic methods of prevention and treatment for cholera). Dr. Quin's advice appears throughout the latter half of the nineteenth century in almost all Yucatecan and Mexican periodicals.
81. FMUNAM, Legajo 121, 1, 1–75, 35–52, covering cholera at 1850. CAIHY, Pamphlets, X-1855, No. 46, "Método curativo contra el cólera morbo." TULALWGC, No. 2, Box 7, Folder no. 78 (in oversize Box no. 11, Folder no. 3), Catalog no. 1448, Mérida, Yucatán, September 18, 1853, Broadside by Igancio Vado, "Método curativo contra el cólera morbo, sin necesidad de medico ni botica."
82. CAIHY, Pamphlets, 7, 01, *Cura homeopática del cólera, por Fredrico Foster Quin, M.D. Médico ordinario de S.M. Leopolde, rey de los belgas, miembro del instituto real de Lóndres, de la real sociedad de medicina de Edimburgo, de la academia de medicina y del instituto real de Nápoles, de la sociedad homeopática de Leipsick & c.*, trans. from French into Spanish by Safiago Savage, doctor of medicine at Harvard University (Mérida, Mexico: Nazario Novelo, 1850). *El Siglo XIX*, Monday, June 3 1850, no. 263; ibid., "Continua de la memoria del Dr. F. F. Quin," Tuesday, June 4, 1850, no. 264, 1–3; ibid., "La memoria del Dr. F. F. Quin" (continued), Wednesday, June 5, 1850, no. 265, 2–3; ibid., "La memoria del Dr. F. F. Quin," Thursday, June 6, 1850, no. 266.
83. Cook, "The Management of Cholera." Cook traces the historical record of rehydration treatment for cholera patients.
84. See the table of treatments proposed by nineteenth-century American doctors in Carpenter's "The Treatment of Cholera," 4.

85. *Azumbre*, the term utilized in the documents, indicates a quantity of measurement equivalent to twenty-one liters.
86. CAIHY, Dr. Canú, *Remedios preservativos y curativos contra el cólera morbus*, Joaquín Castillo Peraza, ed., (8 pages) Mérida, Yucatán, ca. 1833.
87. CAIHY, Manuscripts, 1890, Francisco Xavier Ramirez, *Ramillete de flores de la medicina para que los pobres se puedan curar sin ocupar otra persona. Escrito por el hermano Francisco Xavier Ramirez, natural de Murcia. Varios remedios fáciles para todos los males que naturalmente se padecen; dichos remedios los ha recogido de varios autores médicos y de la práctica que tiene en esta providencia de Yucatán, y de otras partes de América y Europa* (Mérida, Mexico: Imprenta de Florentino M. González, 1890). See the appendix "El folklorismo," February 3, 1785, 128–32.
88. Morales Pereira, "Clínica interna," 38.
89. Laudanum usually contained a mixture of about 45 percent alcohol with 45.6 grains of opium per fluid ounce.
90. Morales Pereira, "Clínica interna," 39.
91. Kudlick, *Cholera in Post-Revolutionary Paris*. Kudlick argues that *instructions populaires*, published during nineteenth-century cholera outbreaks in Paris, shed light on how an emerging bourgeoisie used medical advice to construct their own image of the disease and the government (105).
92. Homeopathy is a system of medicine founded by Samuel "Hahnemann" of Germany in the late seventeenth and early eighteenth centuries. The general theory dictates that administering small doses of substances that in large doses will invoke a true occurrence of the disease can cure disease, in other words, treating like with like. Hydrotherapy is known as the "water cure" and was originated by Vincenz Preissnitz in Germany in the early 1800s. The idea is to use water both internally and externally to treat maladies and disease (Walton, Beeson, and Scott, eds., *The Oxford Companion to Medicine*, 1:549 and 570).
93. *El Siglo XIX*, "Havana, April 21 Homeopathy and Cholera," Saturday, May 25, 1850, no. 256; ibid., "La homeopatía y el cólera," Monday, June 3, 1850, no. 263, 1–3.
94. Morales Pereira, "Clínica interna," 452–53.
95. Crandon-Malamud, *From the Fat of Our Souls*; Palmer and Jimenez, *Educando a Costa Rica*.
96. Probably the most popular, or widely read, of the nineteenth-century travel writers was John Lloyd Stephens, a British adventurer-archaeologist, who authored a travel series including *Incidents of Travel in Yucatán*, published in 1843. Mr. Stephens's traveling companion, Frederick Catherwood, was among the first to use the daguerreotype to produce glass-collodion plate photo-etchings of Maya ruins. Stephens and Catherwood's depictions of indigenous peoples were among the first to be published throughout the Western Hemisphere. See Stephens, *Incidents of Travel in Yucatán*. For a complete listing of Augustus Le Plongeon's publications, see Desmond and Messenger, *A Dream of Maya*, 137–39.
97. *La Redacción* (Mérida), July 19, 1850, no. 9, 4.
98. Ibid., August 7, 1850, no. 17, 2. Reported from Veracruz June 29, 1850, in *El Arco de Iris*.
99. Also spelled "xkantumbub"; see Zapata, *El Libro del Judio*, 113, and Sierra and Calero Quintana, *Registro Yucateco*, 172, but Sierra and Calero Quintana spell it "xkantumbu."
100. García y García, *Historia de la Guerra de Castas*, 130.

101. Daly and DuPont, "The Controversial and Short-Lived Early Use," 1317–18.
102. AHSS, SP, EM, Box 4, 8, 1922.
103. AGN, Gobernación/Legajos, Legajo 2062, 1853, Circulares (Medidas Precautorias para Epidemias). This collection of confirmations from state leaders contains brief statements that they have received the information on preventative methods for the epidemic of fevers that had appeared in the state of Guerrero as well as the possible cholera that had appeared in Puebla and Tehuacan. Among the first to confirm receipt of the circular were the areas of Toluca, Talxcala, the Distrito Federal, Puebla, Veracruz, Querétaro, Oaxaca, Guanajuato, Michoacán, Aguascalientes, San Luis Potosí, Guadalajara, Tamaulipas, Durango, Saltillo, and Colima—all of whom responded between August 4 and August 15. Among the last to confirm receipt were those on the northern and southern peripheries such as Chihuahua, Sonora, Tabasco, San Cristobal, and Mérida, who did not receive the information until the latter half of the month or early in September.
104. See, for instance, Turin, *Instrucción sobre el cólera-morbo.*
105. CAIHY, Rejón, Documentos Justificativos, Section no. 37.
106. Laudanum is a liquid medicine in an opium base, usually a combination of opium and alcohol.
107. Baldwin, *Contagion and the State*, 192.
108. *Scientific American: The Advocate of Industry and Journal of Scientific, Mechanical, and other Improvements* (New York, 1846–69); *The Lancet: A Journal of British and Foreign Medical and Chemical Science, Criticism, Literature and News* (1823–).
109. AGEY, PE, Gobernación, Box 100, Republica Mexicana Comandancia Principal del Marina del Departamento del Norte en Su Capital, December 10, 1855.
110. Heller, *Alone in Mexico*, 152–53. Heller also had to await the arrival of "the sanitation boat" while anchored outside of Campeche harbor in 1846. According to Heller, "They demanded the necessary papers. . . . After two hours I was taken ashore, presented before the port captain and the *jefe político*, and questioned."
111. AGEY, PE, Gobernación, Box 100, Republica Mexicana Comandancia Principal del Marina del Departamento del Norte en Su Capital, December 10, 1855.
112. AGEC, 893, Box 12, 1850, Notificaciones de las precauciones por la epidemia del cólera morbo; ibid., Box 10, 587, 1885, Acuerdo de la Junta de Sanidad del Estado, relativo a las precauciones que se tomarán contra la epidemia de la viruela negra y del cólera; *El Siglo XIX*, Thursday, June 27, 1850, no. 284, 1; AHSS, SP, Epidemias, Box 1, 47, November 1867.
113. Grandin, *The Blood of Guatemala*, 89. Grandin also found that medical professionals who attempted to combat cholera during Guatemala's 1837 epidemic derived much of their knowledge from experiences with smallpox epidemics. Additionally, Grandin found that Paris-based physicians significantly influenced cholera treatments used in Guatemala. Indeed, the noncontagionist position was quite popular among French medical professionals throughout the first worldwide cholera pandemic of the 1830s and hence came to influence sanitary methods implemented in Guatemala.
114. Estado de Yucatán, *Monografía*, 63–64.
115. *El Siglo XIX* (Mérida), "Campeche May 15—El Cólera," May 20, 1850, no. 251, 3.
116. ABH, R 36, LI, 1850–51, 1–133, 78, December 6, 1850, Letter to His Excellency Colonel Hemcourt from John Young, Chairman of the Board of Health.

117. WRC, Rare Pamphlet, RA, 74, H1, L6, *Report of the Joint Committee, Public Health. Majority Report* (New Orleans: Printed by Emile la Sere, State Printer, 1854), 5, 20.
118. Ibid., 5–25.
119. Donald F. Stevens discusses how "immoral and excessive" sexual behavior was also thought to contribute to the onset of cholera during the 1833 epidemic in Mexico City; see Stevens, "Eating, Drinking, and Being Married," 78.
120. WRC, RP, RA, 74, H1, L6. *Report of the Joint Committee*, 5–25.
121. ABH, R 36, 78, LI, November 30, 1850, Chairman of the Board of Health, Dr. Young, to His Excellency Colonel Hemcourt; ibid., R 32, 186, LO, December 7, 1850, John Fancourt to Dr. Young.
122. AGEC, Box 12, 935, 1850–52, Solicitud de la información de la noticia de que en Campeche se ha desarrollado la epidemia del cólera morbo.
123. Ibid., Box, 11, 850, 1849, Se notificó al H. Ayuntamiento del Carmen y la Junta de Sanidad la disposición superior relativa a suspender la observación de los buques a la Habana.
124. For example, see ibid., Box 13, 968, 1850, May 1, 1850, Letter from Jose del Rosario Gil to the Jefatura Política Subalterna del Carmen. Gil states that cholera remained in the capital of Tabasco without contaminating other areas.
125. AHAY, Oficios, Vol. 54, Parroquia de Tekantó, September 24, 1854, Letter from José Torres to El Excelentísimo y Altísimo Sr. Obispo; ibid., Parroquia de Calotmul, September 18, 1854, Letter from Vicente Marín to El Excelentísimo y Altísimo Sr. Obispo; and ibid., Parroquia de Sotuta, September 6, 1854.
126. "Plain Advice to All during the Visitation of the Cholera," 356.
127. AHSS, SP, Epidemia, Box 1, 30, May 17, 1850, Letter from Jose M. Reyes to the Consejo de Salubridad in Mexico City.
128. Ibid., 34, May 1850, "Acta de reconocimiento de un cadáver de una mujer que murió de cólera," de Mariano Guerra.
129. Ibid., 36, April 1850, "Acta de reconocimiento de un enfermo de cólera," Ingresado al Hospital de San Andrés, Rendida por el Practicante Menor, Felipe Castillo, al Secretario del Consejo de Dres. Erazo y Reyes.
130. AGEC, Box 12, 943, March 12, 1850, Notificación de los presupuestos para la construcción de dos carros para la limpieza pública.
131. AGEY, PE, Gobernación, Box 101, Tesoreria Municipal de Seybaplaya, Seybaplaya, 1855, Letter from José Cadenas the Sr. Subprefecto de Seybaplaya to the Prefectura del Distrito de Campeche en el Departamento de Yucatán, October 4, 1854.
132. See, for example, requests for funds in the 245-page file, AGEY, PE, Gobernación, Serie Disposición y Decretos en Repuesta a Exposiciones y Solicitudes 1849–53, Mérida, Yucatán.
133. Ibid., Secretaría General de Gobierno, Prefectura de Distrito de Campeche, 1854.
134. AGN, Gobernación, Sin Sección, 20, Box 365, 1849, Decretos y Leys, Relativo al cobro y préstamo del ayuntamiento, por la epidemia de cólera morbus; AHSS, SP, Epidemias, Box 1, 24, June 1, 1850; ibid., 25, September 2, 1850, Bandos de la epidemia de cólera.
135. AHSS, SP, Epidemias, Box 1, 31, May 1850, Surgencia del consejo sobre varias medidas preventivas a ejecutar, para preservar a los alumnos de los colegios de la epidemia de cólera que amenaza a la capital.
136. CAIHY, Pamphlets, Folder 7, No. 11, José Cristóbal Hernández, *Medidas sanitarias adoptadas por el ayuntamiento de Mérida para el caso de que el cólera-morbus*

invada esta capital (Mérida, Mexico: Manuel Mimenza, 1850). Also see Manuel Mimenza (printer), *Descubrimientos contra el Cólera-Morbus, interesantes al pueblo* (Yucatán: Manuel Mimenza, 1850), 7 pages.

137. García y García, *Historia de la Guerra de Castas*, 7; Cook and Borah, *Essays in Population History*, 2:178.
138. Estado de Yucatán, *Monografía*, 81.
139. Remmers, "Henequen, the Caste War," 330–31.
140. Ibid., 395.
141. Dumond, *The Machete and the Cross*. Dumond argues that the region had been under federal control for so long that there were probably no other alternatives (397).

Chapter 5

1. AGEY, PE, Gobernación, Box 254, 1889.
2. Ibid., JSS (Junta Superior de Sanidad), Copiador de Oficios, Book 1, June 1, 1891–January 16, 1894.
3. Ibid.; ibid., Book 2, February 9, 1894–March 26, 1895; ibid., Book 3, April 8, 1895–August 4, 1897.
4. See Evans, *Bound in Twine*, chapter 1.
5. Estado de Yucatán, *Monografía*, 101, 105. Between 1900 and 1910, Yucatán's population increased 0.96 percent and between 1910 and 1920, 0.40 percent.
6. Wedeen, "Seeing Like a Citizen." While Wedeen's example is modern Yemen, her remarks apply to many modernizing state situations, including modern Yucatán.
7. Joseph, "The United States, Feuding Elites," 177.
8. Remmers, "Henequen, the Caste War," 779.
9. Knight, *The Mexican Revolution*, 1:80.
10. Wells, *Yucatan's Gilded Age*; Evans, *Bound in Twine*.
11. Hart, *Revolutionary Mexico*, 161, 177–86.
12. Gordon, *The Great Arizona Orphan Abduction*, 49. For more on Mexican land tenure, see the classic, Tannenbaum, *The Mexican Agrarian Revolution*.
13. Casares G. Cantón, *Yucatán en el tiempo*, 3:249.
14. For more information on competition between cordage companies and the McCormick Harvesting Machine Company, see Wells, *Yucatán's Gilded Age*, 40–41.
15. Ober, *Travels in Mexico*, 83.
16. AGEY, "Entradas y salidas del Hospital O'Horan," Vol. 1, 1906; Vol. 1, 1907; Vol. 1, 1916; Vols. 1–2, 1917; Vol. 1, 1923; Vol. 1, 1925. These volumes contain information beyond their ascribed title. For instance, the 1906 volume contains material beginning in 1891 and ending in 1907, while the 1907 volume extends into the summer of 1909. There are numerous entries in these volumes detailing skin irritations, rashes, and fractured and broken limbs among *jornaleros* and *trabajadores*. I am indebted to Elías Teyer Carmona at the AGEY for releasing these uncataloged volumes to me and to Cinthia Vanessa Fernández Vergara for taking the time to help compile the information contained within these extensive volumes.

17. *Monthly Bulletin of the International Bureau of the American Republics, International Union of American Republics* (Washington Government Printing Office) 20 (April–June 1905): 420.
18. Ortega, "La hacienda henequenera," 152.
19. Evans, *Bound in Twine*, 4; Joseph, "From Caste War to Class War," 121. Withington sold Cyrus McCormick the rights to his mechanical binder in 1872.
20. Winberry, "Development of the Mexican Railroad System," 118. Moreover, it was not until 1951 that a rail system connected the peninsula to the rest of the nation.
21. Yoder, "Globalization and the Evolving Port Landscape," 48.
22. The construction of railroads began in 1881, telegraph and telephone wires between 1870 and 1883, and Yucatán's Government Palace was constructed between 1883 and 1892. Maximilian had granted the land for the railroads in the 1860s. For more on railroad development in Porfirian Yucatán, see Wells, "All in the Family."
23. Winberry, "Development of the Mexican Railroad System," 118.
24. Echeverría, *¡Nos llevó el tren!*, 24.
25. Abel, *Health, Hygiene, and Sanitation in Latin America*, 13.
26. Echeverría, *¡Nos llevó el tren!*, 142.
27. Wells and Joseph, *Summer of Discontent*, 177.
28. Ibid., 179.
29. Turner, *Barbarous Mexico*, 8. Careful consideration should be given to the context in which Turner's reports on Porfirian Mexico took place. The bulk of Turner's reporting was collected during two trips to Mexico in 1908 and 1909. Turner was clearly a product of the American Progressive era, in which sensationalistic yellow journalism prospered and muckraking reporters abounded. Wells and Joseph note that Turner's exposé that was serialized in *American Magazine* "provided the basis for a 'black legend' that many still accept for Porfirian Yucatán. Significantly, *campesinos* still often refer to the pre-Revolutionary period as 'the time of slavery'" (*Summer of Discontent*, 317n47).
30. Turner, *Barbarous Mexico*, 8.
31. Ibid., 16.
32. AGEY, PE, Gobernación, Box 259, Fomento, Industria y Comercio, Industría, Telegrafos, Colonización y Estadísticas de Producción, 1890. Hacienda Uelilá was owned by a Peón in 1890, Peón de Peón Lorieto, Uelilá, Buenavista y Ponthón. Also see Dumond and Dumond, eds., *Demography and Parish Affairs*, 379.
33. Wells and Joseph, *Summer of Discontent*, 179. The citizens of Hunucmá managed to hold off the advances of railroad construction until the close of the nineteenth century. There is even a case of a mysterious disappearance of a railroad surveyor from Southeastern Railway Company in 1900 from the area.
34. Ibid., 180.
35. Similar cycles of crop decline, famine, drought, and disease also affected Indians of Mexico's northern periphery during Spanish colonial rule and the early national period; see Gutiérrez, *When Jesus Came*, 130.
36. Rodriguez Losa, *Geografía política de Yucatán*, 2:170–71.
37. AGEY, PE, Gobernación, Box 224, Series Correspondencia, Asuntos de Gobierno Leyes y Decretos, Circulares, Mérida, 1883. On social banditry in Mexico, see Vanderwood, *The Power of God*, 139; Joseph, "On the Trail of Latin American Bandits."

38. Wells and Joseph, *Summer of Discontent*, see map on page 178; and see Echeverría, *¡Nos llevó el tren!*, 16–17.
39. Rodriguez Losa, *Geografía política de Yucatán*, 2:216–18. The population for Hunucmá and its surrounding pueblos was approximately 18,902 in 1895. In 1900 the population of the partido was estimated at 9,508. A drop by almost half of the partido's population in a five-year period merits pause. In 1837 Hunucmá was absorbed into the district of Mérida, but less than ten years later in 1849, new divisions for the state were implemented and Hunucmá was incorporated into the partido of Mérida as a pueblo.
40. *Boletín de Higiene: Revista mensual, medicina: Cirugía y farmacia. Órgano del consejo superior de salubridad del estado de Yucatán* (Mérida) 17 (third year, September 15, 1897): 129.
41. Rodriguez Losa, *Geografía política de Yucatán*, 3:230. In 1900 other pueblos, villas, and ports were listed as part of the partido of Hunucmá. They were Bolón, Hunucmá (villa), Kinchil, Smahil, Sisal (port), and, incorporated into the partido of Hunucmá in 1872, Tetiz, Ucú, and Umán (villa). It is likely that Hunucmá, although a territorial component of the partido of Mérida after 1849, still operated as its own partido with its own villas and pueblos, as indicated in the 1900 census report. The death toll reported in 1897 from the mystery illness in Hunucmá probably included the aforementioned villas and pueblos.
42. Although population statistics are not available for the year 1897, they are for 1895 and 1900, and a clear decline in population is evident over this five-year period (Rodriguez Losa, *Geografía política de Yucatán*, 3:230).
43. Joseph, "The United States, Feuding Elites," 191.
44. *La Revista de Mérida*, January 25, 1871, 3.
45. Wells and Joseph, *Summer of Discontent*, 160.
46. *El Siglo XIX*, Wednesday, August 14, 1850, no. 20. Information received from Campeche August 9, 1850.
47. Cook and Borah, *Essays in Population History*, 178.
48. AGEY, PE, Gobernación, Box 224, Correspondencia Oficial, Asuntos de Gobierno, Leyes y Decretos, Circulares, Mérida, 1883.
49. As governor of Yucatán, Olegario Molina provided more funds for the medical school in order to create special studies in laboratory science and a school of nursing. See Casares G. Cantón, *Yucatán en el tiempo*, 4:229. Also see Chowning, *Wealth and Power in Provincial Mexico*. Chowning found that at midcentury Michoachán's liberal elites "sought to cast themselves . . . as champions of the people. Juan B. Ceballos took great pride in recounting the roads that had been improved, and the bridges, jails, cemeteries, aqueducts and fountains that had been constructed during his administration" (231).
50. Tenenbaum, "Streetwise History," 143. Construction on the Paseo de la Reforma began after 1900 (Agostoni, *Monuments of Progress*).
51. Wells and Joseph, *Summer of Discontent*, 64.
52. Pérez de Sarmiento, *Historia de una elección*, 70–76.
53. Wells and Joseph, *Summer of Discontent*, 64, 133. Construction on the Paseo de Montejo began in 1902.
54. AGEY, PE, Box 360, Beneficencia, Salubridad, Sanidad, 1900, 1901, 1902.
55. Wells and Joseph, *Summer of Discontent*, 89.
56. Casares G. Cantón, *Yucatán en el tiempo*, 4:229.

57. See, for instance, Robertson, *A Visit to Mexico*; Desmond and Messenger, *A Dream of Maya*; Le Plongeon, *Here and There in Yucatan*.
58. Beezley, *Judas at the Jockey Club*, 67; Robertson, *A Visit to Mexico*, 152–53; Salisbury, "Letter from Augustus Le Plongeon," 66.
59. NAWDC, DOS, CD Mérida and Progreso, RG 59, Consul Edward Thompson to the Honorable U.S. Secretary of State, Progreso, December 20, 1900.
60. Staples, "Policía y buen gobierno." Staples found that at midcentury a litany of regulations were implemented in Toluca, Mexico, prohibiting "both throwing garbage from the roof into the street and using the sidewalks for draining suet or curd" (120).
61. AGEY, PE, Beneficencia, Box 304, Hospicios y Hospitales, Salubridad, Mérida 1897.
62. Ibid., Box 146-C, 3, Penal, Infanticidio (the following case against Pech, Manuela Mul, and Veronica Cauich for infanticide and violation of Civil Register law regarding the interment of cadavers), Valladolid-Mérida, August 18, 1885–March 10, 1886.
63. Ibid., Box 304, Hospicios, Hospitales, Salubridad, Mérida, 1897. Especially see Consejo de Salubridad de Yucatán, Correspondence no. 1378, regarding cemetery fumigations, corpse deposits, and roaming animals in the cemeteries.
64. Agostoni, "Discurso médico," 5.
65. AGEY, Poder Judicial (PJ), Archivo Histórico, 02, Departamento Judicial de Tekax, 20 Juzgado de 1st instancia de Tekax, 1891, case no. 013129, 077 Diligencia: de Infracción de Leyes de Inhumación-Exhumación, Promovente: Mendoza Ireneo—Demandado: Uc Marcelina.
66. Ibid., 02 Departamento Judicial de Tekax, 20, Juzgado de 1st Instancia de Tekax, 1905, case no. 013645, 077 Diligencia/Causa por Infracción de Leyes Inhumación-Exhumación, Oficialia del Registro Civil-Tekax, Demandado, Cano Jose Concepcion.
67. Ibid., JSS, Copiador de Oficios, Book 1, June 6, 1891–January 16, 1894; ibid., Book 2, February 9, 1894–March 26; ibid., Book 3, April 8, 1895–August 4, 1897.
68. Pérez, *Colección de leyes*.
69. AGEY, PE, Box 254, Gobernación, 1889.
70. Ibid.
71. Ibid., Justicia, Tribunal Superior de Justicia, Penal, Abuso de Autoridad, Petición de los Habitantes de Cacalchén para Destituir de Todo Cargo Público a Don Esteban Herrera por Abuso Arbitrario en sus Funciones, October 24, 1854–March 1855, Cacalchen—Tixcocob—Motul—Izamal—Mérida; ibid., PE, Gobernación, Box 254, 1889; ibid., JSS, Copiador de Oficios (asunto), March 3, 1920–May 31, 1920, Mérida, Vol. 86. This listing of sources across a wide range of dates illustrates the pervasive and enduring problem animals posed to sanitation. Yet, despite the regular litany of complaints lodged against animals as harbingers of disease, their control was not specifically addressed until the passing of the 1891 public health regulations.
72. On the links between patriotic thinking, civilizing missions, and public health campaigns, see Kashani-Sabet, "Hallmarks of Humanism."
73. AGEY, PE, Box 254, Gobernación, 1889.

74. Public health officials similarly sought to clean the streets as a means to control filth and promote sanitation in Los Angeles; see Cruz, "Urbanización y modernidad en el Porfiriato."
75. Parker, "Civilizing the City of Kings." Parker also argues that nineteenth-century intellectuals in Lima saw public health and hygiene as a "powerful rationale for urban reform, and advances of the Balta years had been justified in the fight against yellow fever, typhoid, and other contagious diseases" (158).
76. Estado de Yucatán, *Monografía*, 83–85.
77. Casares G. Cantón, *Yucatán en el tiempo*, 2:72.
78. Ibid., 2:130.
79. "Deaths in the Profession Abroad," *British Medical Journal* 1, no. 2423 (1907): 1402; Casares G. Cantón, *Yucatán en el tiempo*, 5:113.
80. Wells and Joseph, *Summer of Discontent*, 105; "Mexican Railroad Merger: Amalgamated Corporation of Yucatan Roads has a Capital of 30,000,0000," *New York Times*, September 28, 1902, 1.
81. Wells, "All in the Family," 190.
82. Barbachano, *La escuela de medicina de Mérida*, 91; Santos Fernández, "Una visita a Mérida (Yucatán)," 79.
83. Ramos and others, *El Indio*, 209.
84. Ibid., 231. Apache raids on March 8, 1890. On Rancho Batepito, fires were set to dye-wood forests and "Indians employed on ranches that cut the wood are disgusted with the work," May 14, 1890 (253); schools are relocated to avoid "becoming victims of the fury of the savages, as has happened before," June 25, 1890 (267).
85. On the northern frontiers, see Alonso, *Thread of Blood*; Radding, *Wandering Peoples*; Hu-DeHart, *Yaqui Resistance and Survival*.
86. Vanderwood, *The Power of God*, 152–53.
87. Ibid., 147–48; AGEY, PE, Gobernación, Box 277, Official Correspondence, Telegrams, and Various Government Subjects, Mérida, 1892.
88. Wells and Joseph, *Summer of Discontent*, 45.
89. Farriss, *Maya Society under Colonial Rule*.
90. Katz, "The Liberal Republic and the Porfiriato," 101.
91. Dumond, *The Machete and the Cross*, 395.
92. Wells, *Yucatán's Gilded Age*, 105.
93. Menéndez, *Quintana Roo*, 47.
94. Dumond, *The Machete and the Cross*, 127.
95. Menendez, *Historia del infame*.
96. Richard, *Nueva frontera mexicana*, 70.
97. Dumond, *The Machete and the Cross*, 186.
98. Konrad, "Capitalism on the Tropical-Forest Frontier," 146, table 6.1.
99. Wells, *Yucatán's Gilded Age*, 107–8.
100. Konrad, "Capitalism on the Tropical-Forest Frontier," 157.
101. Wells, *Yucatán's Gilded Age*, 107–8.
102. Turner, *Barbarous Mexico*, 41. Turner is unclear as to whether the victims that the old man spoke of died from exhaustion or some type of illness. Turner indicated that malaria did strike during the transport of Yaquis to Yucatán. With the cautions outlined in note 29, however, I use Turner here to provide valuable social

background and insights into what was likely to have been a brutally oppressive experience for the Yaqui and Mayo Indians of Sonora and the Maya of Yucatán.

103. Hu-DeHart, *Yaqui Resistance and Survival*, 181. According to Hu-DeHart, "The exact number of deported Yaquis has never been officially tabulated. Izábel claimed that he had sent some two thousand out of the state by 1907. Many more were deported in 1908, which saw the peak of deportations. Unlike the earlier period, this time few women and children were spared the terrible fate." Hu-DeHart further contends, "As the final solution to the Yaqui crisis, deportation illustrates some of the contradictions that arose out the limits of Porfirian growth. In the more general sense, Mexico did not experience the kind of industrialization that could have absorbed its displaced, dispossessed rural populations, such as the Yaquis, into a modern work force" (198).
104. Wells and Joseph, *Summer of Discontent*, 131.
105. "Better Drainage for Mexico," *New York Times*, April 14, 1893, 5.
106. Wells and Joseph, *Summer of Discontent*, 131.
107. Ibid.
108. Starr, *In Indian Mexico*, 299.
109. Watts, "Yellow Fever Immunities," 958.
110. Carrillo, "Economía, política y salud pública," 75.
111. See Soluri, *Banana Cultures*.
112. Abel, *Health, Hygiene, and Sanitation*, 24–25. The use of quinine to prevent malaria began in the 1830s primarily among European military troops stationed in the West Indies. Americans also began to use mosquito nets in Cuba and Panama, which gave them a decided advantage over mosquito-vector diseases such as malaria. See Curtin, *Death by Migration*, 136.
113. Curtin, *Death by Migration*. Curtain found that "Beriberi . . . became increasingly common in the second half of the nineteenth century" (77). Krauss, *Inside Central America*, 252.
114. See, for example, Le Plongeon, *Here and There in Yucatán*; Norman, *Rambles in Yucatán*; Stephens, *Incidents of Travel in Yucatán*. Shortly after his return from Panama, Stephens succumbed to malaria in New York City on October 13, 1852. "He was simply worn out, battered by malaria and internal ailments, aggravated from years in the tropics. . . . Quinine had been discovered to lessen malarial fevers, and although he consumed large doses of the bitter drug, it was too late to have any effect" (Sutton and Sutton, *Among the Maya Ruins*, 191).
115. AGEY, PE, Beneficencia, Box 559, Hospitales, Salubridad, Mérida, 1907.
116. By the 1880s, experiments with mosquitoes (initiated by Cuban scientist Carlos Finlay, Jesse Lazear, and later Ronald Ross, Patrick Manson, and Walter Reed) revealed that the transmission of malaria occurred through an insect agent. In spite of the research conducted by these scientists, physicians still considered all forms of febrile disease to be one and the same. Contemporaries of Dr. Finlay argued that, in particular, malaria was difficult to connect to an origination point "because of the various types of fever that may be produced by a single kind of parasite and the varying degrees of severity in different individual cases, however, it seems a hopeless task to trace to its place of origin any one of the three kinds of malaria" (Shattuck, *The Peninsula of Yucatán*, 356). At the time of the publication, Dr. Shattuck was assistant professor of tropical medicine at Harvard University

Medical School. The study was conducted in collaboration with thirteen other professionals. Also see Nash, *Inescapable Ecologies*, 106–7.

117. AGEY, PE, Beneficencia, Box 559, Hospitales, Salubridad, Mérida, 1907.
118. NAWDC, DOS, CD Mérida and Progreso, RG no. 59, Vol. 1, Correspondence no. 52 from Consul Thompson to Assistant Secretary of State, Progreso, November 30, 1900.
119. Ibid.
120. Ibid.
121. Ibid., Unnumbered Correspondence from Consul Thompson to Assistant Secretary of State, Progreso, July 8, 1900.
122. Martínez-Fernández, "Don't Die Here," 26n5. The quote about the Canary Islands and Havana comes from NAWDC, DOS, CD, RG 59, United States Consuls in Havana, William H. Roberston to William L. Marcy, July 27, 1854; Ballou, *Due South*, 141; Marero, *Cuba*, 14, 67.
123. Martínez-Fernández, "Don't Die Here," 26n4, 26n6.
124. Zumárraga, "Vomito prieto."
125. AGEY, Entradas y Salidas del Hospital O'Horan, Vol. 1, 1906–7.
126. Cisneros Cámara, *Segunda colección de leyes*, 244.
127. AGEY, PE, Beneficencia, Box 360, Salubridad, Sanidad, Mérida, September 8, 1900; 1901 and 1902.
128. Ibid., Beneficencia, Box 394, Salubridad, Hospitales, Mérida, 1903.
129. Richard, *Nueva frontera mexicana*, 62.
130. NAWDC, DOS, CD, Mérida and Progreso, RG 59, Vol. 6, Letter from Henry Goldthwaite in Mobil, Alabama, to the Surgeon General of the U.S. Marine Hospital Service, October 17, 1901.
131. Estado de Yucatán, *Monografía*, 64.
132. "Informe que el agente sanitario extraordinario en Yucatán rinde al Consejo S. Salubridad de México acerca de los casos de fiebre amarilla observados en la ciudad de Mérida," *Boletín del Consejo Superior de Salubridad* 4, no. 3 (September 30, 1898): 83.
133. Santos Fernández, "Una visita a Mérida (Yucatán)," 80–81. Dr. Fernández was the first Cuban doctor to practice ophthalmology on the island.
134. Carrillo, "Economía, política y salud pública," 76.
135. *Código Sanitario del Estado de Yucatán*. Reglamento del Artículo 222 del Código Sanitario para el Régimen de la Prostitución Reglamento para la Comprobación de la Tuberculosis en las Vacas de Ordeña el Sacrifico de Las Que Resulten Enfermas y Aplicación que se Dará á los Despojos de Éstas. Reglamento para el Régimen de Servicio Antirrábico, Índice Cronológico de las Leyes Que sobre la Sanidad en Sus Diversos Ramos se han Dictado en Yucatán, desde 1810 hasta 1909.
136. Casares G. Cantón, *Yucatán en el tiempo*, 3:35.
137. Tabulations of yellow fever cases were usually recorded in the *Boletín Sanitario*. See, for instance, AGEY, PE, Beneficencia, Box 599, Hospitales, Salubridad, Correspondencia, 1908.

Chapter 6

1. On October 19, 1915, the United States and six Latin American nations extended official recognition to the Carranza government. One month later Carrancista forces overpowered revolutionary leader Pancho Villa in the battle of Agua Prieta.
2. Casares G. Cantón, *Yucatán en el tiempo*, 1:427–28.
3. For more on language of the "liberation decree" and historical memory associated with the decree, see Eiss, "Redemption's Archive."
4. Joseph, *Revolution from Without*, 7.
5. Eiss, "Redemption's Archive," 116–17.
6. Gonzales, *The Mexican Revolution*, 168.
7. Joseph, *Revolution from Without*, 176.
8. RAC, RFA, Record Group (RG) 1.1 (Projects), Series 323 (Mexico) J (Public Health Demonstrations), Box 19, Folder 156, 1928–30, Letter from Dr. Russell to Dr. Carr, December 29, 1928.
9. For a typical U.S. business view, see the chapter "The Rape of the Yucatán" in Thompson's *Trading with Mexico*. He writes that "Alvarado, in his 'conquest' of Yucatán, frankly spread terror throughout the peninsula" (177). Characteristically, Thompson defends debt peonage as actually good for the Indians, who were "able to have some of the good things of life" by getting advances and "spent gaily, careless of the future" (179).
10. NLBLAC, Rare Books and Manuscripts (RBM), García Genero Collection (GGC), Folder A (a–c, 1486).
11. On the use of the term *age of slavery*, see Menéndez, *Historia del infame*.
12. Knight, *The Mexican Revolution*, 1:88; Turner, *Barbarous Mexico;* Reed, *Insurgent Mexico*.
13. Joseph, *Revolution from Without*, 126.
14. Fallaw, *Cárdenas Compromised*, 10.
15. Turner's *Barbarous Mexico* and Reed's *Insurgent Mexico* "stand out as principal examples of U.S. yellow journalist–styled coverage of Mexico during the revolution. . . . " For a contemporary overview of U.S. media coverage of the Mexican Revolution and revolutionary-era propaganda, see Anderson, "'What's to Be Done with 'Em?'"; Smith, "Carrancista Propaganda"; Wells, "Family Elites in a Boom-and-Bust Economy."
16. NLBLAC, RBM, GGC, "Papeles varios sobre la revolución" (c–d, 1486). The language Alvarado invoked during his speech of 1915 is consistent with Mexico's national Constitutionalist Party discourse headed by revolutionary president Venustiano Carranza. See "Call to Arms," March 4, 1913, broadside.
17. Knight, *The Mexican Revolution*, 2:238; Higuera, *Actuación revolucionaria del General Salvador Alvarado* (located at NLBLAC), 44, excerpt from Alvarado's public speech made in February of 1915.
18. For more on the connection between Carranza and Alvarado, see Alvarado's *La traición de Carranza*. Also see Joseph, *Revolution from Without*, 6–10. In 1917 Felipe Carrillo Puerto ascended to the presidency of the Socialist Party of Yucatán, and in the winter of 1918, he served as interim governor of the state of Yucatán. By the time the 1919 elections arrived, a coup had disrupted the process of gubernatorial succession, and local officials detained Carrillo Puerto, forcing him to leave Yucatán. In 1920 the publication of the *Plan de Agua Prieta* facilitated Carrillo

Puerto's return to Yucatán and emboldened the activities of the Socialist Party. In 1921 the Second Socialist Party Congress met in Izamal, Yucatán, and changed the name of the party from Partido Socialista del Sureste to Partido Socialista de Yucatán (Socialist Party of Yucatán). Between 1918 and 1922 the governor's chair of Yucatán changed hands a total of ten times, with many governors serving only brief terms.

19. Joseph, *Revolution from Without*, 101 and 234.
20. Higuera, *Actuación revolucionaria del General Salvador Alvarado*, 44, excerpt from Alvarado's public speech made in February of 1915.
21. Alvarado, *The Agrarian Law of Yucatán;* and Eiss, "Redemption's Archive," 118.
22. Alvarado, *The Agrarian Law of Yucatán*, 3.
23. Ibid., *The Fundamental Problem of Mexico*, 7.
24. Evans, *Bound in Twine*, 165.
25. Alvarado's Five Sisters Plan referred to agrarian, property, tax, labor, and municipal laws. See Valadés, "Salvador Alvarado," 429.
26. AGEY, PE, Gobernación, Box 564, Departamento de Trabajo, Leyes, Quejas, Memoriales, Peticiones, Correspondencia, Elecciones, Reglamentos, Gobernador Salvador Allende, 1917.
27. Casares G. Cantón, *Yucatán en el tiempo*, 6:108. A declaration of smallpox eradication for the peninsula came in 1919 and for the Mexican nation in 1951. For more about the entrance of smallpox and yellow fever with Alvarado's troops, see Escalante, *Historia de la medicina en Yucatán*.
28. AGEY, PE, Gobernación, Box 478, Beneficencia Pública, Sanidad, 1915. Annual salaries for state-appointed medics varied largely depending on whether or not they still attended medical school or had obtained license to practice medicine. Standard salaries ranged from 35 pesos per month for a vacunador (vaccinator)—trained only in the vaccination technique—to 150 pesos per month for the secretary of the Superior Health Council. For more information regarding salaries of medical professionals and technicians, see AGEY, PE, Gobernación, Box 478, Beneficencia Pública, Sanidad, 1915.
29. Casares G. Cantón, *Yucatán en el tiempo*, 1:198–99.
30. NLBLAC, RBM, GGC, "Papeles varios sobre la revolución" (c–d, 1486); and Higuera, *Actuación revolucionaria del General Salvador Alvarado*, 67.
31. King, "Security, Disease, Commerce," 765.
32. AGEY, PE, JSS, Mérida, 1920, Vol. 87, January 7, 1920–July 31, 1920: a three-page report dated July 27, 1920, explaining the transition in 1917 from the Junta Superior de Salud to the Dirección General de Salubridad e Higiene.
33. Alvarado, *Cartilla revolucionaria* (located at NLBLAC, RBM, GGC).
34. Knight, *The Mexican Revolution*, 2:423.
35. Alvarado, *Cartilla revolucionaria*.
36. Joseph, *Revolution from Without*, 101.
37. AGEY, PE, JSS, September 4, 1917–October 31, 1917, Book 69, Copiador de Oficios.
38. Ibid., Registro General de Entradas de Enfermos, January 1, 1917–August 31, 1920.
39. Ibid., PE, Gobernación, Box 740, 1921; ibid., Box 757, 1922. Also see Fallaw, "Dry Law, Wet Politics."
40. Fallaw, "Dry Law, Wet Politics," 45–46.
41. AGEY, PE, Gobernación, Box 740, 1921; ibid., Box 757, 1922; ibid., Box 770, 1923.

42. Ibid., Box 740; also see Bliss, *Compromised Positions*.
43. AGEY, PE, Gobernación, Box 748, Informes, Memoriales, Solicitudes, Quejas, 1921.
44. Cueto, "Sanitation from Above," 4.
45. RAC, RFA, RG 1.1 (Projects), IHB/D, Series 3, Box 13, Series 323 A (Mexico) (Medical Sciences), 1920, 1922, 1925, Folder 93. In particular, see correspondence between Rockefeller Foundation president Dr. George E. Vincent and Mr. A. A. Moll regarding the importance of hygiene instruction in Mexico. Moll was the Spanish editor for the *Journal of the American Medical Association* between 1920 and 1922.
46. Katz, *The Secret War in Mexico*, 195–99.
47. Sandos, "Pancho Villa and American Security."
48. Deverell, *Whitewashed Adobe*, 201–5.
49. Molina, *Fit to Be Citizens?*, 60–61.
50. Crosby, *America's Forgotten Pandemic*.
51. Birn, *Marriage of Convenience*, 46.
52. RAC, RFA, Rockefeller Archive Center (RFC), RG 12.5, Box 38—Diaries, T. C. Lyster, Major, Medical Corps, U.S. Army, Diplomatic Notes, 1916 and 1919–21.
53. Ibid.
54. Noguchi, "*Leptospira icteroides* and Yellow Fever." *Leptospira icteroides* is a spiral organism transferred human to human via the stegomyia mosquito. In 1918 the Rockefeller Foundation sponsored a trip to Guayaquil, Ecuador, so that IHB doctors, including Dr. Noguchi, could study yellow fever in an endemic region. In Guayaquil, Dr. Noguchi conducted experiments with guinea pigs, and later puppies, by inoculating the animals with yellow fever cultures extracted from human victims. Dr. Noguchi observed similarities in the outward manifestations of the disease in the guinea pigs to those expressed in humans such as skin lesions, jaundice, and hemorrhaging of blood into the lungs and stomach (recognized in humans as the "black vomit" victims emit in the acute stages of infection). Based on these initial findings, Dr. Noguchi continued to explore, in other regions, the immunological relationship between *Leptospira icteroides* as an instigator of yellow fever and the development of a vaccine and curative serum.
55. Bliss, *Compromised Positions*.
56. Among other places, the Rockefeller Foundation conducted public health work in China and Russia in the 1920s and 1930s. For more information on the Rockefeller Foundation in China, see Thomson, *While China Faced West*, 122–50; and Ma, "The Rockefeller Foundation." On Rockefeller Foundation work in Russia, see Solomon, "Knowing the 'Local.'"
57. RAC, RFA, RG 12.5, Box 38—Diaries, T. C. Lyster, Major, Medical Corps, U.S. Army, Diplomatic Notes, 1916 and 1919–21.
58. RAC, RFA, RG 5, Series 1.2, Various Private Sector/IHD Correspondence: Typhus—1916, Box, 29, Folder 461. The RFA's Dr. Rose reported that after a conference with Señor Cabrera of Mexico—the head of the Mexican delegation on the American and Mexican joint commission—on October 23, 1916, the two discussed the possibility of the IHB coming to Mexico to aid in the control of typhus fever. Rose stated that the IHB would need a public statement from Mexico that ensured the country's cooperation, emphasizing that the program would not be connected politically and that the work would not be exploited by the press.

Also see ibid., RG 1.1 (Projects) IHB, Series 3, Box 13, Series 323 A (Mexico) (Medical Sciences), 1920, 1922, 1925, Folder 93, Letter to James R. Sheffield from George Vincent, May 5, 1925.

59. Birn, *Marriage of Convenience*, 3.
60. Duffy, *The Sanitarians*.
61. Smith, "The United States and the Mexican Revolution," 186. Ryan's work in Mexico and Washington contributed to the formation of the Bucareli Conference and Treaty in the spring of 1923. The Bucareli Treaty stipulated that the contentious Article 27 of the Mexican Constitution of 1917, prohibiting foreign ownership of land and subsoil rights in Mexico, would not be applied retroactively. Thus, subsoil rights purchased before 1917 were not subject to seizure. For more on the Bucareli Conference and Treaty see Hart, *Revolutionary Mexico*, 343.
62. RAC, RFA, RG 1.1 (Projects), IHB/D, Series 3, Box 13, Series 323 A (Mexico) (Medical Sciences), Folder 93, 1920, 1922, 1925, Letter from General J. A. Ryan to President of the Rockefeller Foundation, George E. Vincent, December 1, 1922.
63. The title "International Health Board" endured until 1927 when the Rockefeller Foundation changed the title to "International Health Division." As Anne-Emanuelle Birn points out in her study of the Rockefeller Foundation in Mexico, the terms *International Health Board, International Health Division*, and *Rockefeller Foundation* are used "interchangeably, rarely distinguishing one entity from the other" by both Rockefeller Foundation men and their Mexican counterparts. As Birn indicates in her work, in order to remain "true to the language of the original sources, we may not always be able to avoid the overlapping use of institutional names," and I have adopted a similar strategy in distinguishing between the International Health Board and International Health Division. Since the majority of this work falls before 1927, *International Health Board* is more commonly used. After 1927, I use *International Health Division;* however, like Birn, if a Rockefeller Foundation doctor refers to the International Health Board after 1927 or simply uses the term *RFA* for the International Health Board or IHB, I give privilege to the original document by employing the language embedded in the sources (Birn, *Marriage of Convenience*, 11).
64. See *Annual Report of the Surgeon General of the Public Health Service of the United States, 1915* (Washington, D.C.: Government Printing Office, 1915), 124.
65. Knight, *The Mexican Revolution*, 2:423.
66. RAC, RFA, RG 1.1 (Projects), IHB/D, Series 323 A (Mexico) (Medical Sciences), Box 13, 1920, 1922, 1925, Folder 93, Letter from Mr. Moll to Dr. George E. Vincent, President, the Rockefeller Foundation, February 2, 1920.
67. For more information on Hideyo Noguchi and his work, see Eckstein, *Noguchi;* D'Amelio and Banbery, *Taller than Bandai Mountain;* and Plesset, *Noguchi and His Patrons*.
68. Cueto, "Sanitation from Above," 5.
69. When boiled and then cooled, the gel-like substance swelled and settled around a culture, thus preserving it. The gelatinous substance is considered resistant to most bacteria and therefore was commonly used as a basis of solid bacterial culture media or used as a gel diffusion.
70. RAC, RFA, RG 5 (Correspondence), Series 1.2, Sub-series 323, Box 96, Folder 1129, Letter to Pruneda from Noguchi regarding yellow fever vaccine development, November 23, 1920.

71. Ibid., IHB/D, Series 1.2, Sub-series 323 (Mexico), Box 96, Folder 1129, 1920; for a corollary situation involving Noguchi's vaccine in Bolivia, see Zulawski, *Unequal Cures*.
72. Noguchi's vaccine was ineffective in combating yellow fever, but Max Theiler and his associates formulated an effective yellow fever vaccine in 1937. See Cueto, "Sanitation from Above," 6n21.
73. RAC, RFA, RG 5, IHB/D, Series 1.2, Sub-series 323 (Mexico), Box 96, Folder 1129, 1920. For information on smallpox vaccination campaigns in Yucatán see *Las Garantías Sociales* (Mérida), Friday, July 11, 1856, no. 123; AHAY, Municipios, Municipio de Espita, Yucatán, Box 6, Vol. 30 and 33, 1898–1901. Many municipalities like Espita were well aware of the mandatory vaccination policy through the circulation of bandos and publication in *El Diario Oficial*. Before 1901, vaccination rates remained relatively low in Espita—local officials reasoned that it was related to rumors that the vaccine was tainted or bad.
74. Delaporte, *The History of Yellow Fever*, 23–24.
75. RAC, RFA, RG 12.1, Box 38—Diaries, "Rockefeller Yellow Fever Commission in Mexico," January 1920 and May 1921; also see Birn, *Marriage of Convenience*, 51.
76. AGEY, PE, JSS, Mérida, 1920, Vol. 87: January 7, 1920–July 31, 1920, see "Reglamento interior de la Junta Superior de Sanidad."
77. RAC, RFA, RG 5, IHB, Series 2, Box 33, Series 323 (Mexico), Folder 194, 1922.
78. Peard, *Race, Place, and Medicine*.
79. Manzanilla Domínguez, *Los enemigos del Indio;* Licéaga, *Algunas considerciones*.
80. AGEY, PE, Gobernación, Box 564, Departamento de Trabajo, Leyes, Quejas, Memoriales, Peticiones, Correspondencia, Elecciones, Reglamentos, 1917, Gobernador Salvador Allende; ibid., Box 740, 1921.
81. Ibid., Box 740, 1921.
82. Ibid., Box 748, 1922.
83. *Código sanitario del estado de Yucatán* (Mérida: Imprenta de la "Escuela Correccional de Artes y Oficios," 1911), 37–38.
84. See, for instance, cases brought by the state against those allegedly practicing witchcraft and those impersonating medical doctors, AGEY, Gobernación, Box 753-Bis, Beneficencia y Salud, Correspondencia, 1922.
85. Carrillo, "The New Yucatán," 138, 141.
86. AGEY, PE, Gobernación, Box 747 and 748, 1921–23. Numerous complaints were filed with state military and the state government regarding a lack of trust or "*desconfianza*" that had developed between residents of urban and rural areas and newly imported teachers, doctors, and military garrisons.
87. Ibid., Box 753-Bis, Beneficencia y Sanidad, Serie Correspondencia (Sanidad), Mérida, 1922.
88. Ibid., Box 747 and 748, Gobernación, 1921–23.
89. Fallaw, *Cárdenas Compromised*, 61.
90. AGEY, PE, Gobernación, Box 748, Informes, Memoriales, Solicitudes, Quejas, 1921.
91. Casares G. Cantón, *Yucatán en el tiempo*, 3:35; Solorzano, "The Rockefeller Foundation in Revolutionary Mexico," 52–71.
92. AGEY, PE, Beneficencia, Box 679, Sanidad, Salubridad, Mérida, 1919.
93. Ibid., JSS, Vol. 93, Mérida, October 31, 1920–September 9, 1921.
94. Ibid., Vol. 94, Mérida, December 31, 1921–March 11, 1921.

95. RAC, RFA, RG 5, Series 2, Sub-series 323, Box 33, Folder 194, "Log of Yellow Fever Inspection Trip to Mexico, 1924," Dr. M. E. Connor.
96. Ibid., RG 12.1, Box 38—Diaries, "Journal of T.C. Lyster, Colonel Medical Corps, U.S. Army (Retired), Representing the Rockefeller Yellow Fever Commission in Mexico, 1920," 11.
97. Ibid., RG 1.1 (Projects), IHB/D, Series 323 (Mexico), Box 17, Folder 139, Russell to Warren, September 13, 1924.
98. "Rockefeller Foundation Leads World Fight on Disease," *Science News-Letter* 8, no. 272 (June 26, 1926): 2–3.
99. RAC, RFA, RG 1.1 (Projects), Series 323, Box 13, Folder 95, 21, Medical Education in Mexico 1923—2nd half.
100. Ibid., 35, Medical Education in Mexico 1923—2nd half.
101. Ibid., RG 12.1, Box 53, (Diaries, Officer's Logs), F. Russell 1925–26, Vol. 2 of 4, Interview with M. E. Connor, Saturday, April 17, 1926, 311. Dr. Connor packed his bags in 1926 and left Mexico for El Salvador, a nation he posited was likely to be the endemic center for yellow fever proliferation.
102. AHSS, SP, Epidemias, Box 40, Mexico City, 1924; RAC, RFA, RG 5, Series 3, Series 323, Box 148, Folder 1758, Report of Yellow Fever Control in Mérida, May 1923.
103. AHSS, SP, Epidemias, Box 40, Mexico City, 1924.
104. *Informes rendidos por el C. Gral. Plutarco Elias Calles*, 102. Contains a report from the National Department of Public Health declaring that no cases of yellow fever had appeared since 1922.
105. For more on the PSS's reforms in Yucatán, see Fallaw, *Cárdenas Compromised*, 17 and 109.
106. AGEY, PE, Gobernación, Box 740, 1921.
107. Ruz Menéndez, *Liga acción social.*
108. RAC, RFA, RG 12.1 (Diaries, Officer's Logs), F. Russell 1922–24, Vol. 1 of 4, Box 53, Interviews from Thursday April 4, 1924, with Dr. M. E. Connor, 137.
109. See, for instance, Joseph, *Revolution from Without;* Sánchez Novelo, *La rebelión delahuertista en Yucatán;* Fallaw, "Felipe Carrillo Puerto."
110. Betancourt Pérez, *El asesinato de Carrillo Puerto*. Betancourt views Carrillo Puerto as a self-made martyr persecuted and ultimately executed by the henequeneros of Yucatán.
111. Fallaw, *Cardenas Compromised*, 61; Betancourt Pérez, *El asesinato de Carrillo Puerto;* Cardona, *Oda roja a la memoria*.
112. Ethel Nelson, letter to the editor, "Revolution in Yucatán: Two Views of the System Introduced by Carrillo and Swept Away by Followers of de la Huerta," *New York Times*, January 20, 1924, special features section.
113. Casares G. Cantón, *Yucatán en el tiempo*, 3:425; Fallaw, "Dry Law, Wet Politics," 53; and Estado de Yucatán, *Monografía*, 148–49. Between 1922 and 1923 Carrillo Puerto's administration distributed 438,866 hectares of land to 22,525 peasants (see Spenser, "Workers Against Socialism?," 234).
114. AGEY, Libros de la JSS, Book 108, 1924 (first trimester), Oficio 118.
115. Evans, *Bound in Twine*, 199.
116. RAC, RFA, RG 1.1, Series 323 J (Mexico), Box 19, Folder 156, Yellow Fever Chronology, MX Expenditures—1929.

117. Ibid. (Projects), IHB/D, Series 323 (Mexico), Box 17, Folder 140, Dr. Carr to Dr. Ferrell, September 30, 1929; ibid., Series 323 J (Mexico), Box 19, Carr and Ferrell discuss new project budgets for 1931.
118. "Control of Yellow Fever," *New York Times*, March 5, 1922, 84.
119. "Rockefeller Foundation Leads World Fight on Disease," *Science News-Letter* 8, no. 272 (June 26, 1926): 2–3.
120. "Rockefeller Help to World Reviewed," *New York Times*, November 10, 1929, 14.
121. AGEY, PE, Beneficencia, Box 700, Hospitales, 1920.
122. Ibid., Libros Históricos, JSS, Copiador de Oficios, Books 111–42, Years 1925–30. See, in particular, Book 113, January 8, 1926–February 26, 1926, Document 53.
123. AGEY, Libros Históricos, JSS, Copiador de Oficios, Books 108–18, Years 1924–26; ibid., Books 90–136, Years 1920–30. Collectively, these administrative records of the JSS detail page after page of fines implemented for failure to comply with mandatory gynecological exams for prostitutes, fees imposed for failure to comply, apprehension of prostitutes, and exams conducted. Equal efforts are concentrated on fees imposed on owners of allegedly rabid dogs, the observation of and extermination of allegedly rabid dogs, and the administration of antirabies treatments to humans bitten by dogs; Solorzano, *Fiebre dorada o fiebre amarilla?*
124. *Informe rendido por el gobernador*, 29–32; *Informe rendido por el gobernador constitucional de Yucatán*, 31.
125. Cueto, "The Rockefeller Foundation's Medical Policy," 229.
126. *Informe rendido por el gobernador constitucional de Yucatán*, 47–50.

Conclusion

1. Anderson, *Colonial Pathologies*, 8.
2. Birn and Solórzano, "Public Health Policy Paradoxes," 1198.
3. AGEY, PE, Gobernación, Box 101, Prefectura del Distrito de Mérida, April 24, 1855.
4. AGEC, Box 13, 968, 1850, "Notificaciones de las precauciones por la propagación del cólera en la Habana y San Juan Bautista."
5. *El Siglo XIX*, June 3, 1850, no. 263; ibid., "Continua de la memoria del Dr. F. F. Quin," June 4, 1850, no. 264, 1–3; ibid., "La memoria del Dr. F. F. Quin" (continued), Wednesday, June 5, 1850, no. 265, 2–3; ibid., "La memoria del Dr. F. F. Quin," Thursday, June 6, 1850, no. 266.
6. AAS, SFP, Box 38, Folder 6 (March–May), April 8, 1862.
7. Stephens, *Incidents of Travel*, 1:61–64.
8. Shattuck, *The Peninsula of Yucatán*.
9. Ibid., 25.
10. Ibid., 62.
11. Ibid., 389, table 65.
12. Ibid., 427.
13. Allen W. Lloyd, "Lloyd Mexico Economic Report January-2002," July 20, 2002, www.mexconnect.com/MEX/lloyds/llydec00102.html#quintana_roo_tourism (accessed January 8, 2010).
14. Hostettler, "New Inequalities."

15. Ardren, "Conversations"; Savage, "Ecological Disturbance"; Stronza, "Anthropology of Tourism"; www.tourbymexico.com/tours/about.htm (accessed January 8, 2010).
16. Crist and Paganini, "Pyramids, Derricks and Mule Teams in the Yucatán Peninsula."
17. Tibbetts, "Toxic Tides."
18. Tenenbaum, "Trampling Paradise"; Diego Cevallos, "Environment: Health Is Victim of Climate Change, Scientists Say," *Inter Press Service* (Mérida), December 2, 2008.
19. "Mexico Expected to Reach Millennium Development Goals before 2015," *Xinhua General News*, September 25, 2008.
20. Cueto, *Cold War, Deadly Fever*, 145–46.
21. Although there is an abundant literature focusing on environmental consequences of DDT and chemical spraying on the environment and on human populations, one of the most famous and timeless studies is *Silent Spring* by Rachel Carson. Also see Wright, *The Death of Ramón González;* Fenster and others, "Association of In Utero Organochlorine Pesticide Exposure," 598; Salazar-García and Gallardo-Díaz, "Reproductive Effects of Occupational DDT Exposure."
22. Cueto, *Cold War, Deadly Fevers*, 41; Spielman and D'Antonio, *Mosquito*, 150.
23. Spielman and D'Antonio, *Mosquito*, 174.
24. Roberts, "DDT Risk Assessments."
25. Loroño-Pino and others, "Introduction of the American/Asian Genotype"; Kendall and others, "Urbanization, Dengue, and the Health Transition."
26. "Mexico, Venezuela Implement Counter-dengue Measures," *Xinhua General News Service*, August 29, 2007.
27. Danis-Lozano and others, "Risk Factors for *Plasmodium vivax*," 466.
28. See, for instance, a recent study linking rates of breast cancer in adult women to DDT exposure at a young age: Cohn and others, "DDT and Breast Cancer in Young Women."
29. Servicios de Salud de Yucatán, Hospital General Dr. Augustín O'Horan, horan.yucatan.gob.mx/wp/2009/01/en-breve-entrara-en-funcionamiento-ampliacion-del-area-de-urgencias-del-hospital-escuela-o'horan/%20-%20more-168 (accessed January 8, 2010).
30. Camara Milan, "El Dr. Hideyo Noguchi en Yucatán." According to the World Health Organization, yellow fever vaccine is safe and highly effective and offers protective immunity to 95 percent of those infected. See www.who.int/mediacentre/factsheets/fs100/en/index.html (accessed January 8, 2010).
31. "Ambassador Garza Travels to Mérida, Yucatán Inaugurates Exhibition of Modern Sculpture," *US Fed News*, April 15, 2005. Ambassador Garza donated microscopes to the Hospital General Dr. Agustin O'Horan while in Mérida for the sculpture exhibit. The donation was part of a seventeen-million-dollar cooperative program between the United States and Mexico to prevent and treat tuberculosis throughout Mexico.
32. "Denuncian medicos mayas malos tratos de funcionarios," *Milenio* (Progreso), February 4, 2009, 20.
33. "Más apoyo a las culturas populares," *Diario de Yucatán*, January 27, 2009.

Afterword

1. "Mérida: La contigencia sanitaria," *Diario de Yucatán*, September 18, 2009; Carrie Kahn, "Why So Many Swine Flu Deaths in Mexico?," National Public Radio, May 7, 2009, www.npr.org/templates/story/story.php?storyId=103887262 (accessed July 23, 2010).
2. La Secretaría de Salud de México, "Situación actual de la epidemia," February 17, 2010, portal.salud.gob.mx/sites/descargas/pdf/influenza/situacion_actual_epidemia_170210.pdf (accessed July 23, 2010).
3. Barry, *The Great Influenza*, 452.
4. Centers for Disease Control and Prevention, "Questions & Answers 2009 H1N1 Flu ('Swine Flu') and You," December 19, 2009, www.cdc.gov/H1N1flu/qa.htm (accessed July 23, 2010).
5. See www.who.int/csr/don/2010_07_23a/en/index.html (accessed July 23, 2010).
6. Saúl Ortega, "Cronología de influenza," *El Diaro NTR Zacatecas, Periodismo Crítico*, May 4, 2009, ntrzacatecas.com/secciones/salud/2009/05/04/cronologia-de-la-influenza-2 (accessed July 23, 2010).
7. Gostin, "Influenza."
8. Laurie Garrett, "The Path of a Pandemic," *Newsweek*, May 2, 2009, www.newsweek.com/id/195692 (accessed July 23, 2010).
9. Gostin, "Influenza," 2376.
10. "Hoteleros de Cancún retan a turistas," *El Universal*, May 12, 2009, www.eluniversal.com.mx/notas/597597.html (accessed July 23, 2010); Gostin, "Influenza," 2377.
11. Gostin, "Influenza," 2378.
12. Chris Buckley, "China niega disciminación a mexicanos por influenza," *International Business*, May 4, 2009, www.ibtimes.com.mx/articles/20090504/china-influenza-discriminacion-mexicanos.htm (accessed July 23, 2010); "No existe discriminación contra mexicanos en China: Alfonso Araujo," *La Jornada Michoacán*, May 6, 2009.
13. Gostin, "Influenza," 2377; "The Butcher's Bill: Flu and the Global Economy," *Economist*, May 2, 2009.
14. Cecilia González, "Desata polémica discriminación a mexicanos en Argentina," SDP noticias.com, May 6, 2009, sdpnoticias.com/sdp/contenido/2009/05/06/392427 (accessed July 23, 2010).
15. "Israel Renames Unkosher Swine Flu," BBC News, April 27, 2009, news.bbc.co.uk/2/hi/8021301.stm (accessed July 23, 2010).
16. Marc Brodsky, "'Swine Flu' Name Won't Be Changed in Israel," *JTA* (The Global News Service of the Jewish People), April 29, 2009, jta.org/news/article/2009/04/29/1004758/swine-flu-name-wont-be-changed-in-israel (accessed July 23, 2010).
17. Brodsky, "'Swine Flu.'"
18. Ángeles Cruz Martínez, "El virus a/H1N1 es amenazador y caprichoso, advierte la OMS," *La Jornada*, July 3, 2009.
19. See www.dgepi.salud.gob.mx/pandemia/PS%20materiales/PANDEMIA%20DE%20INFLUENZA%20AMIS.pdf (accessed July 23, 2010).
20. Kahn, "Why So Many Swine Flu Deaths?"

21. This population statistic qualifies Mexico City's metropolitan area as the third largest in the world and the largest in the Americas. See Instituto Nacional de Estadística y Geografía, "Población total," table 19.5.
22. Davis, *Planet of Slums*, 133.
23. E. Vega and others, "Fine and Coarse Particulate Matter"; Zeger, and others, "Mortality in the Medicare Population."
24. José Miguel González Rivero, "Sin miedo a la influenza H1N1 miles de feligreses en los centros de religión del estado," *Diario de Yucatán*, July 20, 2009.
25. "H1N1: What You Need to Know," Public Radio International, October 1, 2009, www.pri.org/health/h1n1-what-you-need-to-know1646.html (accessed July 23, 2010).
26. "La vacuna antiinfluenza aplicada en México es segura: Sector salud," *La Jornada en Línea*, December 17, 2009, boletinnoticioso.wordpress.com/2009/12/17/boletin-noticioso-17–12–09 (accessed July 23, 2010).
27. Gostin, "Influenza," 2378.
28. "Ministros rechazan barreras a carne de cerdo," Informador.com.mx, December 27, 2009, www.informador.com.mx/mexico/2009/101144/1/ministros-rechazan-barreras-a-carne-de-cerdo.htm (accessed July 23, 2010).
29. "Mérida: La contigencia sanitaria."
30. Ana María Aragonés, "Reflexiones en el contexto de la influenza," *La Jornada*, May 11, 2009, www.jornada.unam.mx/2009/05/11/index.php?section=opinion&article=022a2pol (accessed July 23, 2010); Saulo Padilla and Cathryn Clinton, "Reflection: Fears Concerning the H1N1 Virus Have Led to Discrimination," *Mennonite*, May 19, 2009, www.themennonite.org/issues/12–10/articles/Reflection_Fears_concerning_the_H1N1_virus_have_led_to_discrimination (accessed July 23, 2010).

BIBLIOGRAPHY

Archives and Manuscript Collections

AAS	American Antiquarian Society (Worcester, Massachusetts)
ABH	Archives of British Honduras (Belmopán)
AGEC	Archivo General del Estado de Campeche (Campeche)
AGEY	Archivo General del Estado de Yucatán (Mérida)
AGN	Archivo General de la Nación (Mexico City)
AHAY	Archivo Histórico de Archidiócesis de Yucatán (Mérida)
AHFM-UNAM	Archivo Histórico del Facultad de Medicina, Universidad Nacional Autónoma de México (Mexico City)
AHSS	Archivo Histórico de la Secretaría de Salud (Mexico City)
AMC	Archivo Municipal de Campeche (Campeche)
ANEY	Archivo Notorial del Estado de Yucatán (Mérida)
BCCA	Biblioteca Crecencillo Carrillo y Ancona (Mérida)
CAIHY	Centro de Apoyo de Investigaciones Históricos de Yucatán (Mérida)
COC	Casa de Oswaldo Cruz (Rio de Janeiro)
CONDUMEX	Centro de Estudios de Historia de México Archivo Histórico (Mexico City)*
FMUNAM	Facultad Medicina del Universidad Nacional Autónoma de México (Mexico City)
NAWDC	United States National Archives (Washington, D.C.)
NLBLAC	Nettie Lee Benson Latin American Collection at the University of Texas, Rare Books and Manuscripts, García Genero Collection (Austin)
RAC	Rockefeller Archive Center (Sleepy Hollow, New York)

* Since the publication of this book, CONDUMEX has changed its name to the Centro de Estudios de Historia de México Carso (CEHM).

RFA	Rockefeller Family Archives (Sleepy Hollow, New York)
SFP	Salisbury Family Papers (Worcester, Massachusetts)
TULALWGC	Tulane University, Latin American Library, William Gates Collection (New Orleans, Louisiana)
VEMC	Mexican Viceregal and Ecclesiastical Collection at Tulane University Latin American Library (New Orleans, Louisiana)
WRC	Williams Research Center, a Division of the Historic New Orleans Collection (Kempre and Leila Williams Foundation)

Newspapers and Periodicals

Boletín de Higiene
El Álbum Yucateco
El Amigo del País
El Chisgarabis
El Eco del Comercio
El Eco del Oriente
El Estudiante de Medicina
El Fénix
El Folklorismo
El Gallo
El Grano de Arena
El Hijo de la Patria
El Museo Yucateco
El Regenerador
El Siglo XIX: Boletín Oficial del Gobierno de Yucatán
La Aurora Mérida
La Caridad
La Emulación
La Ley de Amor
La Pelota, Campeche
La Razón del Pueblo
La Redacción
La Reforma
La Revista de Mérida
La Revista Yucateca
Las Garantías Sociales
Las Mejoras Materiales
La Unión
La Unión Liberal
La Voz de la Revolución
Mosaico
New York Times
Periódicos Peninsulares

Published Primary Sources

Ancona, Eligio. *Colección de leyes, decretos, ordenes y demás disposiciones de tendencia general, expedidas por el poder legislativo del estado de Yucatan desde 1851 hasta la presente época. Formada con autorización del gobierno.* Vol. 6. Mérida, Mexico: Tipografía del Gil Canto, 1887.

———. *Historia de Yucatán desde la época más remota hasta nuestros días.* 4 vols. Mérida, Mexico: Heredia Arguelles, 1878.

Alvarado, Salvador. *The Agrarian Law of Yucatan (1915).* Mérida, Mexico: 1915.

———. *Cartilla revolucionaria para los agentes de propaganda de la causa constitucionalista.* Mérida, Mexico: 1915.

———. "The Fundamental Problem of Mexico." Lecture given in New York City, March 1920. San Antonio, TX: 1920.

———. *Gobierno constitucionalista reglamento de la inspección médica de las escuelas del estado decreto, no. 411.* Mérida, Mexico: Imp. Y Linot, "La Voz de la Revolución," 1916.

———. *La traición de Carranza.* New York: s.n., 1920.

Annual Report of the Surgeon General of the Public Health Service of the United States, 1915. Washington, D.C.: Government Printing Office, 1915.

Asturias, Francisco. *Historia de la medicina en Guatemala.* Guatemala: Impreso en la Tipografía Nacional, 1902.

Aznar Barbachano y Juan Carbó, Tomás. *Memoria sobre la conveniencia, utilidad y necesidad de erigir constitucionalmente en estado de la confederación mexicana el antiguo distrito de Campeche: Constituido de hecho en estado libre y soberano desde mayo de 1848, por virtud de los convenios de división territorial que celebró con el estado de Yucatán, de que era parte.* Mexico City: Imprenta de Ignacio Cumplido, 1861.

Ballou, Maturin M. *Due South: Or Cuba Past and Present.* New York: Negro Universities Press, 1891. Reprint, New York: Negro Universities Press, 1969.

Baqueiro, Serapio. *Ensayo histórico sobre las revoluciones de Yucatán desde el año de 1840 hasta 1864.* Edited by Salvador Rodríguez Losa. 5 vols. Mérida, Mexico: Ediciones de la Universidad Autónoma de Yucatán, 1990.

———. *Renseña geográfica, histórica y estadística del estado de Yucatán desde los primitivos tiempos de la península.* Mexico City: Imprenda de Franciso Diaz de Leon, 1881.

Cardona, Rafael. *Oda roja a la memoria de Felipe Carrillo Puerto, gobernador de Yucatán, fusilado recientemente por las fuerzas reaccionarias de Adolfo de la Huerta, y cuyo lema era una promesa de redención para América: Tierra y libertad.* México City: Talleres Sánchez & de Guise, 1924.

Carrillo, Felipe. "The New Yucatán: A Message to All Americans from the Martyred Maya Leader." *Survey Index* 102 (April–September 1924): 138–42.

Cisneros Cámara, Antonio. *Segunda colección de leyes, decretos y órdenes y demás disposiciones de tendencia general expedidos por los poderes legislativo y ejecutivo del estado de Yucatán—Año 1902.* Vol. 1. Mérida, Mexico: Imprenta de "El Eco del Comercio," 1904.

Código sanitario del estado de Yucatán. Mérida: Imprenta de la "Escuela Correccional de Artes y Oficios," 1911.

Creelman, James. "President Díaz: Hero of the Americas." *Pearson's Magazine* 19, no. 3 (March 1908): 231–77.

Drake, Daniel, MD, ed. *Western Journal of the Medical and Physical Sciences*. Vol. 7. Cincinnati: E. Deming, 1834.

Escalante, Alvaro Avila. *Contribución al estudio de la historia de la medicina yucatán*. Leido en las sesiones del Comité en Mérida de la Asociación Medica Mexicana, March 12 and October 15. Mérida, Mexico: Imprenta y Rayado Universal, 1925.

———. *Historia de la medicina en Yucatán*. Mérida, Mexico: Imprenta y Rayado Universal, 1926.

Espinosa Rendon, José D., and Crescencio Carrillo Ancona, eds. *El repertorio pintoresco: Ó miscelánea instructiva y amena consagrada a la religión, la historia del país, la filosofía, la industria y las bellas letras*. Mérida, Mexico: Imprenta de José D. Espinosa, 1863.

Estado de Yucatán. *Estadística de Yucatán. Publicase por acuerdo de la R. Sociedad de Geografía y Estadística*. 1853. Copy located at AGEY, Mérida, Mexico.

———. *Recuerdo de la primera visita del Sr. Presidente de la República Mexicana, General don Porfirio Díaz*. 1906. Copy located at the Getty Research Institute, Los Angeles.

García y García, Apolinar. *Historia de la Guerra de Castas de Yucatán, sirviéndole de prólogo una reseña de los usos, costumbres é inclinaciones peculiares de los indígenas*. Mérida, Mexico: Tipografía de Manuel Aldana Rivas, 1865.

Govea, Carlos. "Vacuna, su organización en Tamaulipas." In Memorias del *Transactions of the Second Pan-American Medical Congress*, 771–85. Held in Mexico City, November 16–19, 1896. Mexico City: Hoeck y Compania Impresores y Editores, 1898.

Hibbard, David R. *A Treatise on Cow-Pox in Which the Existence of Small-Pox, or Variloid in a New York Form, Subsequent to Vaccination, Is Shown to Arise from Some Imperfection in Its Performance, and Not the Result of Inefficacy on the Part of the Vaccine to Shield the System Entirely from These Diseases*. New York: Harper & Brothers, 1835.

Higuera, Ernesto, ed. *Actuación revolucionaria del General Salvador Alvarado en Yucatán*. Mexico City: Costa-Amic, 1965.

Holt, Joseph. *Pestilential Foreign Invasion as a Question of States' Rights and the Constitution: The Failure of the Maritime States Demands a Common Defense; An Address Delivered before the Tri-State Medical Society of Georgia, Alabama and Tennessee, at Chattanooga, October 26, 1892*. New Orleans, LA: L. Graham & Son, 1892.

Humboldt, William. "Extract from a Communication Addressed to the Sanitary Commission." In Report of the Sanitary Commission of New Orleans on the Epidemic Yellow Fever of 1853, 127–34. New Orleans, LA: City Council of New Orleans, 1854.

Huntington, Ellsworth. *The Climactic Factor as Illustrated in Arid America 1914*. Publication 192. Washington, D.C.: Carnegie Institution of Washington, 1914.

Informe rendido por el gobernador constitucional de Yucatán, C. Dr. Alvaro Torre Diaz, ante la XX legislatura del estado, el 1st de enero de 1929. Mérida, Mexico: Talleres Tipográficos del Gobierno del Estado, 1929.

Informe rendido por el gobernador constitucional interino de Yucatán Jose M. Iturralde Traconis ante la H. XXVIII legislatura del estado el 1st de enero de 1925. Edición oficial. Mérida, Mexico: Talleres Tipográficos del Gobierno 58 con 61, 1925.

Informes rendidos por el C. Gral. Plutarco Elias Calles, presidente constitucional de los Estado Unidos Mexicano ante H. congreso de la unión los días 1st de Septiembre de 1925 y 1st de

Septiembre de 1926 y contestación de los CC. presidentes del citado. Congreso. Mexico City: Talleres Gráficos de la Nación, "Diario Oficial," 1925.

Knox, Thomas W. *The Boy Travelers in Mexico: Adventures of Two Youths in a Journey to Northern and Central Mexico, Campechey, and Yucatán, with a Description of the Republics of Central America and the Nicaragua Canal.* New York: Harper and Brothers, 1890.

Landa, Fray Diego de. *Relación de las cosas de Yucatán.* Mexico City: Consejo Nacional para la Cultura y las Artes, 1994.

———. *Yucatan Before and After the Conquest.* Translated by William Gates. New York: Dover, 1978.

Le Plongeon, Alice D. *Here and There in Yucatan: Miscellanies.* New York: John W. Lovell, 1889.

Licéaga, Eduardo. *Algunas consideraciones acerca de la hygiene social en México.* México City: Tipográficas Vda. De F. Diaz de Leon, Sucs., 1911.

———. "A Century of Arm to Arm Vaccination in Mexico." *Indiana Medical Journal* 21, no. 1 (1902): 290–94.

Martínez Alomía, Gustavo. *Historiadores de Yucatán: Apuntes biográficos y bibliográficos de los historiadores de esta península desde su descubrimiento hasta fines del siglo XIX.* Campeche: Tipografía "El Fénix," 1906.

Mason, Gregory. "A Socialist Despot in Yucatan." *New Outlook* 114 (September–December 1916): 655–65.

———. *South of Yesterday.* New York: H. Holt, 1940.

———, and Herbert Joseph Spinden. *Silver Cities of Yucatán.* New York: G. P. Putnam's Sons, 1927.

McNamara N. C., FCU (surgeon to the Westminster Hospital). *A History of Asiatic Cholera.* London: Macmillan, 1876.

Menéndez, Carlos R. *Historia del infame y vergonzosos comercio de indios vendidos a los esclavistas de Cuba por los políticos yucatecos, desde 1848 hasta 1861; Justificación de la revolución indígena de 1847; Documentos irrefutables que lo comprueban.* Mérida, Mexico: Talleres Gráficos de "La Revista de Yucatán," 1923.

Morales Pereira, Samuel. "Clínica interna: Algunas reflexiones y recopilación de opiniones sobre el cólera morbo." *Gaceta Médica, Periódico de la Academia de Medicina de Méjico* 21, no. 2 (January 15, 1886): 34–39.

Noguchi, Hideyo. "*Leptospira icteroides* and Yellow Fever." *Proceedings of the National Academy of Sciences USA* 6 (1920): 110–11.

Norman, B. M. *Rambles in Yucatan: Including a Visit to the Remarkable Ruins of Chi-chen, Kabah, Zayi, Uxmal & C.* New York: J&H Langley, 1844.

Ober, Frederick A. *Travels in Mexico and Life among the Mexicans.* Boston: Estes and Lauriat, 1884.

O'Reilly, Justo Sierra. *Los indios de Yucatán: Consideraciones sobre el origen, causas y tendencias de la sublevación de los indígenas, sus probables resultados y su posible remedio.* Vol. 1. Mérida, Mexico: Universidad Autónoma de Yucatán, 1994.

Orvañanos, Domingo. "President's Address." *Public Health Papers and Reports* 33, pt. 1. Columbus, OH: Press of Fred J. Heer, 1908.

———. "Inaugural Address of the President of the Section of Hygiene and Demography." In *Transactions of the Second Pan-American Medical Congress*, 710–13. Held in Mexico City, November 16–19, 1896. Mexico City: Hoeck y Compania Impresores y Editores, 1898.

Pellarin, Augustin. *Hygiéne des pays chauds. Contagion du cholera démontrée par l'épidémie de la Guadeloupe, conditions hygiéniques de l'émigration dans les pays chauds et de la colonization de ces pays*. Paris: J. B. Bailliére, 1872.

Pérez, Alonso Aznar, compiler. *Colección de leyes, decretos y ordenes ó acuerdos de tendencia general: Que comprende todas las disposiciones legislativas, desde 1 de enero de 1846, hasta fin de diciembre de 1850*. 3 vols. Mérida, Mexico: Rafael Pedrera, 1851.

———, compiler. "Law of December 11, 1849." In *Colección de leyes, decretos y ordenes ó acuerdos de tendencia general del poder legislativo del estado libre y soberano de Yucatan, 1832–[1850]*, 303–4. Vol. 3. Mérida, Mexico: Rafael Pedrera, 1851.

———, compiler. "Medidas para la conservación y propagación del fluido vacuno." In *Colección de leyes, decretos y ordenes ó acuerdos de tendencia general: Que comprende todas las disposiciones legislativas, desde 1 de enero de 1846, hasta fin de diciembre de 1850*, vol. 3, edited by Rafael Pedrera, 47. Mérida, Mexico: Rafael Pedrera, 1851.

Pérez Galaz, Juan de Dios, ed. "Situación estadística de Yucatán en 1851." Boletín del Archivo General de la Nación (Mexico) ser. 1, vol. 19, no. 3 (1948–49).

Pío Pérez, Juan. *Diccionario de la lengua maya*. Mérida, Mexico: Imprenta Literaria de Juan F. Molina Solís, 1866–77.

"Plain Advice to All during the Visitation of the Cholera." *Medical Times and Gazette: A Journal of Medical Science, Literature, Criticism, and News* 7 (October 1, 1853): 355–56.

Priestley, Herbert Ingram. *José de Gálvez, Visitor-General of New Spain (1765–1771)*. Berkeley: University of California Press, 1916.

Public Health Reports and Papers (presented at the Meetings of the American Public Health Association, 1873). Vol. 1. New York: Hurd and Houghton, 1875.

Ray, D. N. *Cholera and Its Preventive and Curative Treatment*. New York: A. L. Chatterton, 1884.

Reclus, Elisée. *The Earth and Its Inhabitants*. Vol. 2: *North America: Mexico, Central America, West Indies*. New York: D. Appleton, 1893.

Regil, José Maria. *Estadística de Yucatán*. Vol. 3. Mexico City: Publicase por acuerdo de la R. Sociedad de Geografía y Estadística, 1853.

Rejón, Antonio G. *Documentos justificativos*. Mérida, Mexico: Imprenta de Jose Dolores Espinosa, 1862.

Robertson, William Parish. *A Visit to Mexico, the West India Islands, Yucatan and the United States*. London: Simpkin, Marshall, 1859.

Ruz Menéndez, Rodolfo. *Liga acción social*. Mérida, Mexico: Empresa Editora Yucateca, S.A., 1913.

Salisbury, Stephen, Jr. "Letter from Augustus Le Plongeon to the President of the Mexican Republic, Señor Don Sebastian Lerdo de Tejada, Mérida, January 27, 1876." In *The Mayas, the Sources of Their History: Dr. Le Plongeon in Yucatan, His Account of Discoveries*, 93–103. Worchester, MA: Press of Charles Hamilton, 1877.

———. *The Mayas, the Sources of Their History: Dr. Le Plongeon in Yucatan, His Account of Discoveries*. Worchester, MA: Press of Charles Hamilton, 1877.

Santero, D. Francisco Javier. *Elementos de higiene privada y pública*. Vol. 2. Madrid: El Cosmos Editorial, 1885.

Santos Fernández, Dr. Juan. "Una visita a Mérida (Yucatán)." *Anales de la Academia de Ciencias Médicas Físicas y Naturales de la Habana, Revista Cientifica* 39 (June 22, 1902): 72–82.

Sierra, Justo, and Vicente Calero Quintana. *Registro yucateco: Periódico literario redactado por una sociedad de amigos*. Vol. 1. Mérida, Mexico: Imprenta de Castillo y Companía, 1845.

Snow, John. *On the Mode of Communication of Cholera*. 2nd ed. London: J. Churchill, 1855.

Solís, Juan Francisco Molina. *Historia de Yucatán desde la independencia de España, hasta la época actual*. Mérida, Mexico: Talleres Gráficos de *La Revista de Yucatán*, 1921.

Spinden, Herbert Joseph. *Ancient Civilizations of Mexico and Central America*. 3rd ed. American Museum of Natural History, Handbook 3. New York: American Museum of Natural History, 1928. First published 1917.

———. *The Reduction of Maya Dates*. Cambridge, MA: Peabody Museum, 1924.

Starr, Fredrick. *In Indian Mexico: A Narrative of Travel and Labor*. Chicago: Forbes, 1908.

Stillé, Alfred. *Cholera: Its Origin, History, Causation, Symptoms, Lesions, Prevention and Treatment*. Philadelphia: Lea Brothers, 1885.

Thompson, Wallace. *Trading with Mexico*. New York: Dodd, Mead, 1921.

Trachtenberg, Alexander, ed. *The American Labor Year Book, 1917–1918*. New York: Rand School of Social Science, 1918.

Turin, L. A. Calvi de. *Instrucción sobre el cólera-morbo asiático, y método curativo que le conviene*. Translated by El Conde de la Cortina. Mexico City: Impreso de F. Escalante y C., 1854.

United States, Department of State, Consular Reports: Commerce, Manufactures, etc. Vol. 71, no. 271. Washington, D.C.: Government Printing Office, 1903.

Villasenor, Roberto. *El separatismo en Yucatán: Novela histórico política mexicana*. Mexico City: Andres Botas, 1916.

Wendt, Edmund Charles, ed. *A Treatise on Asiatic Cholera*. Prepared with John Charles Peters, Ely McCellan, John B. Mailton, and George Miller Sternberg. New York: William Wood, 1885.

Zumárraga, Eduardo Arceo. "Vómito prieto, Tesis presentada á la Facultad de Medicina, Cirugía y Framácia de Yucatán, para obtener el grado de doctor en medicina y cirugía." Medical thesis. Mérida, Mexico: Imprenta Cecilio Leal, 1909–10.

Secondary Sources

Abel, Christopher. *Health, Hygiene, and Sanitation in Latin America c. 1870 to c. 1950*. London: Institute of Latin American Studies, University of London, 1996.

Adamo, Sam. "The Sick and the Dead: Epidemic and Contagious Disease in Rio de Janeiro, Brazil." In *Cities of Hope: People, Protests, and Progress in Urbanizing Latin America, 1870–1930*, edited by Ronn Pineo and James A. Baer, 218–39. Boulder, CO: Westview, 1998.

Adams, Walter Randolph, and John P. Hawkins. *Health Care in Maya Guatemala: Confronting Medical Pluralism in a Developing Country*. Norman: University of Oklahoma Press, 2007.

Adas, Michael. *Machines as the Measure of Men: Science, Technology, and Ideologies of Western Dominance*. Ithaca, NY: Cornell University Press, 1989.

Agostoni, Claudia. "Discurso médico, cultura higiénica y la mujer en la ciudad de México al cambio de siglo (XIX–XX)." *Mexican Studies/Estudios Mexicanos* 18, no. 1 (Winter 2002): 1–22.

———. *Monuments of Progress: Modernization and Public Health in Mexico City, 1876–1910*. Calgary, Alberta: University of Calgary Press, 2003.

Aguilar, Rafael Valdez. *El cólera: Enfermedad de la pobreza*. Culiacán, Mexico: Universidad Autónoma de Sinaloa, 1993.

Alcereto, Albino. "Historia política desde del descubrimiento Europeo hasta 1920." In *Enciclopedia yucatanense*, vol. 3, edited by Carlos A. Echánove Trujillo, 5–388. México City: Gobierno de Yucatán, 1944–47.

Alchon, S. A. *Native Society and Disease in Colonial Ecuador*. New York: Cambridge University Press, 1991.

Alonso, Ana Maria. *Thread of Blood: Colonialism, Revolution, and Gender on Mexico's Northern Frontier*. Tucson: University of Arizona Press, 1995.

Anderson, Benedict. *Imagined Communities: Reflections on the Origin and Spread of Nationalism*. New York: Verso, 1983.

Anderson, Mark C. "'What's to Be Done with 'Em?' Images of Mexican Cultural Backwardness, Racial Limitations, and Moral Decrepitude in the United States Press, 1913–1915." *Mexican Studies/Estudios Mexicanos* 14, no. 1 (1998): 23–70.

Anderson, Warwick. *Colonial Pathologies: American Tropical Medicine, Race, and Hygiene in the Philippines*. Durham, NC: Duke University Press, 2006.

———. "Disease, Race, and Empire." *Bulletin of the History of Medicine* 70, no. 1 (1996): 62–67.

———. "Excremental Colonialism: Public Health and the Poetics of Pollution." *Critical Inquiry* 21, no. 3 (Spring 1995): 640–69.

———. "Immunities of Empire: Race, Disease, and the New Tropical Medicine, 1900–1920." *Bulletin of the History of Medicine* 70, no. 1 (Spring 1996): 94–118.

———. *Tropical Pathologies: American Tropical Medicine, Race, and Hygiene in the Philippines*. Durham, NC: Duke University Press, 2006.

Aparecida de S. Lopes, María. "Revolución y ganadería en el norte de México." *Historia Mexicana* 57, no. 3 (January–March 2008): 863–900.

Ardren, Traci. "Conversations about the Production of Archaeological Knowledge and Community Museums at Chunchucmil and Kochol, Yucatán, México." *World Archaeology* 34, no. 2 (October 2002): 379–400.

Arnold, David, ed. *Imperial Medicine and Indigenous Societies*. New York: St. Martin's, 1988.

———. "Smallpox and Colonial Medicine in Nineteenth-Century India." In *Imperial Medicine and Indigenous Societies*, edited by David Arnold, 45–65. New York: St. Martin's, 1988.

Arrom, Silva Marina. *Containing the Poor: The Mexico City Poor House, 1774–1871*. Durham, NC: Duke University Press, 2000.

Baklanoff, Eric N., and Edward Moseley, eds. *Yucatán in an Era of Globalization*. Tuscaloosa: University of Alabama Press, 2008.

Baldwin, Peter. *Contagion and the State in Europe, 1830–1930*. New York: Cambridge University Press, 1999.

Barbachano, M. C. Arturo Erosa. *La escuela de medicina de Mérida, Yucatán*. Mérida, Mexico: Universidad Autónoma de Yucatán, 1997.

———. "La salud pública en Yucatán durante el siglo XIX." *Cuadernos de la Facúltad de Medicina* 13 (1992).

Barrera Vasquez, Alfredo, ed. *El libro del Judío: Su ubicación en la tradición botánica y en la medicina tradicional yucatanense*. Jalapa, Mexico: Instituto Nacional de Investigaciones sobre Recursos Bióticos, 1983.

Barry, John M. *The Great Influenza: The Epic Story of the Deadliest Pandemic in History*. New York: Penguin, 2004.

Bazant, Jan. "From Independence to the Liberal Republic, 1821–1867." In *Mexico since Independence*, edited by Leslie Bethell, 1–48. Cambridge: Cambridge University Press, 1991.

Beezley, William H. *Judas at the Jockey Club and Other Episodes of Porfirian Mexico*. Lincoln: University of Nebraska Press, 1987.

———, and Linda A. Curcio-Nagy, eds. *Latin American Popular Culture: An Introduction*. Wilmington, DE: Scholarly Resources, 2000.

———, and Judith Ewell, eds. *The Human Tradition in Latin America: The Nineteenth Century*. Wilmington, DE: Scholarly Resources, 1989.

———, Cheryl English Martin, and William E. French, eds. *Rituals of Rule, Rituals of Resistance: Public Celebrations and Popular Culture in Mexico*. Wilmington, DE: Scholarly Resources, 1994.

Bellingeri, Marco. "Del peonaje al salario: El caso de San Antonio Tochatlaco de 1880 a 1920." *Revista Mexicana de Ciencias Políticas y Sociales* 24, no. 91 (1978): 121–35.

Betancourt Pérez, Antonio. *El asesinato de Carrillo Puerto: Refutación de las tesis sustentadas por el escritor don Roque Armando Sosa Ferreyro en su libro "El crimen del miedo."* Mérida, Mexico: Imprenta Zamora, 1974.

Bethell, Leslie, ed. *Mexico since Independence*. New York: Cambridge University Press, 1991.

Bhaba, Homi K. *The Location of Culture*. New York: Routledge, 1994.

Birn, Anne-Emanuelle. *Marriage of Convenience: Rockefeller International Health and Revolutionary Mexico*. Rochester, NY: University of Rochester Press, 2006.

———, and Armando Solórzano. "Public Health Policy Paradoxes: Science and Politics in the Rockefeller Foundation's Hookworm Campaign in Mexico in the 1920s." *Social Science and Medicine* 49 (1999): 1198–1213.

Blichfeldt, E. H. *A Mexican Journey*. New York: Thomas Y. Crowell, 1912.

Bliss, Katherine Elaine. *Compromised Positions: Prostitution, Public Health, and Gender Politics in Revolutionary Mexico City*. University Park: Pennsylvania State University Press, 2002.

Blum, Ann Shelby. "Children without Parents: Law, Charity, and Social Practice, Mexico City, 1867–1940." PhD diss., University of California–Berkeley, 1998.

———. *Domestic Economies: Family, Work, and Welfare in Mexico City, 1884–1943*. Lincoln: University of Nebraska Press, 2009.

Boone, Elizabeth Hill, and Walter D. Mignolo, eds. *Writing without Words: Alternative Literacies in Mesoamerica and the Andes*. Durham: University of North Carolina Press, 1994.

Brading, David Anthony. *Church and State in Bourbon Mexico*. New York: Cambridge University Press, 2002.

———. *The First America: The Spanish Monarch, Creole Patriots, and the Liberal State, 1492–1867.* New York: Cambridge University Press, 1991.

Brannon, Jeffery, and Gilbert Joseph. *Labor and Capital in Modern Yucatán: Essays in Regional and Political Economy.* Tuscaloosa: University of Alabama Press, 2002.

———. Review of *Land, Labor, and Capital*, by Thomas Benjamin. *Hispanic American Historical Review* 72, no. 4 (November 1992): 630–32.

Bricker, Victoria. *Indian Christ, Indian King: The Historical Substrate of Maya Myth and Ritual.* Austin: University of Texas Press, 1981.

Briggs, Asa. "Cholera and Society in the 19th Century." *Past and Present* 19 (1961): 76–96.

Brown, JoAnne. *Matters of Life and Death: Political Hygiene and Historical Memory in the U.S., 1805–1915.* Baltimore, MD: Johns Hopkins University Press, 1998.

Brunk, Samuel, and Ben Fallaw, eds. *Heroes and Hero Cults in Latin America.* Austin: University of Texas Press, 2006.

Burns, Allen F. *An Epoch of Miracles: Oral Literature of the Yucatec Maya.* Austin: University of Texas Press, 1983.

Camara Milan, Pedro. "El Dr. Hideyo Noguchi en Yucatan." *Revista Biomédica* 11, no. 3 (2000): 207–12.

Cannon, Aubrey. "The Historical Dimension in Mortuary Expressions of Status and Sentiment." *Current Anthropology* 30, no. 4 (August–October 1989): 437–58.

Capozzola, Christopher. "The Only Badge Needed Is Your Patriotic Fervor: Vigilance, Coercions, and the Law in World War I America." *Journal of American History* 88, no. 4 (March 2002): 1354–82.

Carey, David, Jr. *Our Elders Teach Us: Maya-Kaqchikel Historical Perspectives Xkib'ij Kan Qate' Qatata'.* Tuscaloosa: University of Alabama Press, 2001.

Carey, James C. *The Mexican Revolution in Yucatán, 1915–1924.* Boulder, CO: Westview, 1984.

Carpenter, Charles C. J. "The Treatment of Cholera: Clinical Science at the Bedside." *Journal of Infectious Diseases* 166, no. 1 (July 1992): 2–14.

Carrillo, Ana María. "Economía, política y salud pública en el México porfiriano (1876–1910)." *História, Ciencias, Saúde—Manguinhos* 9 (Supplement 2002): 67–87.

Carson, Rachel. *Silent Spring.* 40th anniversary ed. With essays by Edward O. Wilson and Linda Lear. New York: Houghton Mifflin, 2002. First published 1962.

Casares G. Cantón, Raúl E., ed. *Yucatán en el tiempo: Enciclopedia alfabética.* 6 vols. Mérida, Mexico: Inversiones Cares, S.A. de C.V. Col. México, 1998–2001.

Castañeda, Quetzil E. *In the Museum of the Maya: Touring Chichén Itzá.* Minneapolis: University of Minnesota Press, 1996.

Chambers, J. S. *The Conquest of Cholera: America's Greatest Scourge.* New York: Macmillan, 1938.

Chen, C. C. *Medicine in Rural China: A Personal Account.* Berkeley: University of California Press, 1989.

Chowning, Margaret. *Wealth and Power in Provincial Mexico: Michoacán from the Late Colony to the Revolution.* Stanford, CA: Stanford University Press, 1999.

Clendinnen, Inga. *Ambivalent Conquests: Maya and Spaniard in Yucatán, 1517–1570.* New York: Cambridge University Press, 1987.

Cline, Howard F. "Civil Congregations of the Indians in New Spain, 1598–1606." *Hispanic American History Review* 29 (1949): 349–69.

———. "Regionalism and Society in Yucatán, 1825–1847: A Study of 'Progressivism' and the Origins of the Caste War." PhD diss., Harvard University, 1947.

———. "Remarks on a Selected Bibliography." In *The Maya of East Central Quintana Roo* by Alfonso Villa Rojas. Washington, D.C.: Carnegie Institute, 1944.

———. *The United States and Mexico.* Cambridge, MA: Harvard University Press, 1965.

Coatsworth, John. "Indispensible Railroads in a Backwards Economy: The Case of Mexico." *Journal of Economic History* 39, no. 4 (December 1979): 939–60.

Cohn, Barbara A., Mary S. Wolff, Piera M. Cirillo, and Robert I. Sholtz. "DDT and Breast Cancer in Young Women: New Data on the Significance of Age at Exposure." *Environmental Health Perspectives* 115, no. 10 (October 2007): 1406–14.

Colloredo-Mansfeld, Rudi. "'Dirty Indians,' Radical Indígenas, and the Political Economy of Social Difference in Modern Ecuador." *Bulletin of Latin American Research* 17, no. 2 (1998): 185–205.

Conklin, Alice L. "Colonialism and Human Rights, a Contradiction in Terms? The Case of France and West Africa, 1895–1914." *American Historical Review* 103, no. 2 (1998): 419–42.

Conrad, Geoffrey W., and Arthur A. Demarest. *Religion and Empire: The Dynamics of Aztec and Inca Expansionism.* New York: Cambridge University Press, 1984.

Cook, David Noble. *Born to Die: Disease and New World Conquest, 1492–1650.* Cambridge: Cambridge University Press, 1998.

———, and W. George Lovell, eds. *Secret Judgments of God: Old World Disease in Spanish Colonial America.* The Civilization of the American Indian Series. Norman: University of Oklahoma Press, 1992.

Cook, G. C. "The Management of Cholera: The Vital Role of Rehydration." In *Cholera and the Ecology of* Vibrio cholerae, edited by B. S. Drasar and Bruce D. Forrest, 54–67. London: Chapman and Hall, 1996.

Cook, Sherburne F., and Woodrow Borah. *Essays in Population History: Mexico and the Caribbean.* Vol. 2. Berkeley: University of California Press, 1974.

Cooper, Donald B. *Epidemic Disease in Mexico City, 1761–1813: An Administrative, Social, and Medical Study.* Austin: University of Texas Press, 1965.

Cosminsky, Sheila. "Alimento and Fresco: Nutritional Concepts and Their Implications for Health Care." *Human Organization* 36, no. 2 (1977): 203–7.

Crandon-Malamud, Libbet. *From the Fat of Our Souls: Social Change, Political Process, and Medical Pluralism in Bolivia.* Berkeley: University of California Press, 1991.

Crist, Raymond E., and Louis A. Paganini. "Pyramids, Derricks and Mule Teams in the Yucatán Peninsula: A Second Effort in 2,500 Years to Develop a Jungle and Forest Area." *American Journal of Economics and Sociology* 39, no. 3 (July 1980): 217–26.

Crosby, Alfred W. *America's Forgotten Pandemic: The Influenza of 1918.* 2nd ed. Austin: University of Texas Press, 2003.

———. *The Columbian Exchange: Biological and Cultural Consequences of 1492.* Westport, CT: Greenwood, 1972.

Cruz, Carlos Contreras. "Urbanización y modernidad en el Porfiriato. El caso de la ciudad de Puebla." In *Limpiar y obedecer. La basura, el agua y la muerte en la puebla de Los Angeles, 1650–*

1925, edited by Rosalva Loreto L. and Francisco J. Cervantes B. Puebla, 187–219. Puebla, Mexico: Centro de Estudios Mexicanos y Centroamericanos, Universidad de Puebla, 1994.

Cuenya, Miguel, Elsa Malvido, Concepcion Lugo O., Ana Maria Carrillo, and Lilia Oliver Sánchez. *El cólera de 1833. Una nueva patología en México: Causas y efectos*. Mexico City: Instituto Nacional de Antropología e Historia, 1992.

Cueto, Marcos. *Cold War, Deadly Fever: Malaria Eradication in Mexico, 1955–1975*. Baltimore, MD: Johns Hopkins University Press, 2007.

———, ed. *Missionaries of Science: The Rockefeller Foundation and Latin America*. Bloomington: Indiana University Press, 1994.

———. "The Rockefeller Foundation's Medical Policy and Scientific Research in Latin America: The Case of Physiology." In *Missionaries of Science: The Rockefeller Foundation and Latin America*, edited by Marcos Cueto, 126–48. Bloomington: Indiana University Press, 1994.

———. "Sanitation from Above: Yellow Fever and Foreign Intervention in Peru, 1919–1922." *Hispanic American Historical Review* 72, no. 1 (February 1992): 1–22.

Curtin, Philip D. *Death by Migration: Europe's Encounter with the Tropical World in the Nineteenth Century*. New York: Cambridge University Press, 1989.

Daly, Walter J., and Herbert L. DuPont. "The Controversial and Short-Lived Early Use of Rehydration Therapy for Cholera." *Clinical Infectious Diseases* 47 (2008): 1315–19.

D'Amelio, Dan, and Fred Banbery. *Taller than Bandai Mountain; The Story of Hideyo Noguchi*. New York: Viking, 1968.

Danis-Lozano, R., M. H. Rodriguez, L. Gonzalez-Ceron, and M. Hernandez-Avila. "Risk Factors for *Plasmodium vivax* Infection in the Lacandon Forest, Southern Mexico." *Epidemiology and Infection* 122, no. 3 (June 1999): 461–69.

Davis, Mike. *Planet of Slums*. New York: Verso, 2006.

De Bevoise, Ken. "The Compromised Host: The Epidemiological Context of the Philippine-American War." PhD diss., University of Oregon, 1986.

Debré, Patrice. *Louis Pasteur*. Translated by Elborg Forster. Baltimore, MD: Johns Hopkins University Press, 2000.

De Kruif, Paul. *The Microbe Hunters: The Classic Book on the Major Discoveries of the Microscopic World*. Orlando, FL: Harcourt, 1996. First published 1926.

Delaporte, François. *The History of Yellow Fever: An Essay on the Birth of Tropical Medicine*. Cambridge, MA: MIT Press, 1991.

del Castillo, Francisco Fernandez. *Los viajes de don Francisco Xavier de Balmis: Notas para la expedición vacunal de España y Filipinas (1803–1806)*. Mexico City: Sociedad Médica Hispano Mexicana, 1985.

Deleuze, Gilles. "Klossowski or Bodies-Language." In *The Logic of Sense*. Translated by Mark Lester with Charles Stivale. Edited by Constantin V. Boundas. New York: Columbia University Press, 1990.

———, and Michel Foucault. "Intellectuals and Power." In *Language, Counter-Memory, Practice: Selected Essays and Interviews by Michel Foucault*, edited by D. F. Bouchard, 205–17. Ithaca, NY: Cornell University Press, 1977.

Desmond, Lawrence Gustave, and Phyllis Mauch Messenger. *A Dream of Maya: Augustos and Alice Le Plongeon in Nineteenth-Century Yucatan*. Albuquerque: University of New Mexico Press, 1988.

Deverell, William. *Whitewashed Adobe: The Rise of Los Angeles and the Remaking of Its Mexican Past*. Berkeley: University of California Press, 2005.

Díaz y de Ovando, Clementina. *El Doctor Manuel Carmona y Valle y la fiebre amarilla: Son noticia periodista (1881–1886)*. Mexico City: Universidad Nacional Autónoma de México, 1993.

Díaz Zermeño, Héctor. *Cancerbero del traidor Victoriano Huerta ó military leal? Aureliano Blanquet (1848–1919)*. México City: Universidad Nacional Autónoma de México, 2004.

Douglas, Mary. *Purity and Danger: An Analysis of the Concepts of Pollution and Taboo*. Boston: Ark Paperbacks, 1985.

Drake, Paul W., ed. *Money Doctors, Foreign Debts, and Economic Reforms in Latin America from 1890s to the Present*. Wilmington, DE: Scholarly Resources, 1994.

Dudgeon, J. A. "Development of Smallpox Vaccine in England in the Eighteenth and Nineteenth Centuries." *British Medical Journal* 1, no. 5342 (May 1963): 1367–72.

Duffin, Jacalyn. *History of Medicine: A Scandalously Short Introduction*. Toronto, Ontario: University of Toronto Press, 1999.

Duffy, John. *The Sanitarians: A History of American Public Health*. Chicago: University of Illinois Press, 1990.

Dumond, Carol Steichen, and Don E. Dumond, eds. *Demography and Parish Affairs in Yucatán 1797–1897: Documents from the Archivo de la Mitra Emeritense Selected by Joaquín de Arrigunaga Peón*. University of Oregon Anthropological Papers 27. Eugene, OR: Department of Anthropology, University of Oregon, 1982.

Dumond, Don E. *The Machete and the Cross: Campesino Rebellion in Yucatán*. Lincoln: University of Nebraska Press, 1997.

Dunn, Alvis E. "A Cry at Daybreak: Death, Disease, and Defense of Community in a Highland Ixil-Mayan Village." *Ethnohistory* 42, no. 4 (1995): 595–604.

Durey, Michael. *The Return of the Plague: British Society and the Cholera, 1831–1832*. Dublin: Gill and Macmillan, 1979.

Echeverría, Pedro V. *¡Nos llevó el tren!: Los ferrocarrileros de Yucatán*. Mérida, Mexico: Facultad de Arquitectura Universidad Autónoma de Yucatán, 1999.

Echeverría León, Emilia Esther. "Prácticas y costumbres funerarias en Mani, Yucatán." Tesis de licenciado, Universidad de Yucatán Escuela de Ciencias Antropológicas, 1984.

Eckstein, Gustav. *Noguchi*. New York: Harper & Brothers, 1931.

Eiss, Paul K. "Redemption's Archive: Remembering the Future in a Revolutionary Past." *Comparative Studies in Society and History* 44, no. 1 (January 2002): 106–36.

Estado de Yucatán, ed. *Monografía sobre la salud pública de Yucatán 50 aniversario de la creación de la secretaría de salud*. Mérida, Mexico: Impreso en los Talleres Gráficos del Sudeste, S.A. de C.V., 1993.

Evans, Richard. *Death in Hamburg: Society and Politics in the Cholera Years, 1830–1910*. New York: Oxford University Press, 1987.

Evans, Sterling. *Bound in Twine: The History and Ecology of the Henequen-Wheat Complex for Mexico and the American and Canadian Plains, 1880–1950*. College Station: University of Texas A&M Press, 2007.

Fallaw, Ben. *Cárdenas Compromised: The Failure of Reform in Postrevolutionary Yucatán*. Durham, NC: Duke University Press, 2001.

———. "Dry Law, Wet Politics: Drinking and Prohibition in Post-revolutionary Yucatán, 1915–1935." *Latin American Research Review* 37, no. 2 (2002): 37–64.

———. "Felipe Carrillo Puerto of Revolutionary-Era Yucatán, Mexico: Popular Leader, Caesar, or Martyr?" In *Heroes and Hero Cults in Latin America*, edited by Samuel Brunk and Ben Fallaw, 128–48. Austin: University of Texas Press, 2006.

———. "The Life and Deaths of Felipa Poot: Women, Fiction, and Cardenismo in Postrevolutionary Mexico." *Hispanic American Historical Review* 82, no. 4 (November 2002): 645–83.

Farriss, Nancy. *Maya Society under Colonial Rule: The Collective Enterprise of Survival.* Princeton, NJ: Princeton University Press, 1984.

Fenn, Elizabeth A. "Biological Warfare in Eighteenth-Century North America: Beyond Jeffery Amherst." *Journal of American History* 86, no. 4 (2000): 1552–80.

Fenster, Laura, Brenda Eskenazi, Meredith Anderson, Asa Bradman, Kim Harley, Hedy Hernandez, Alan Hubbard, and Bana B. Barr. "Association of In Utero Organochlorine Pesticide Exposure and Fetal Growth and Length of Gestation in an Agricultural Population." *Environmental Health Perspectives* 114, no. 4 (April 2006): 597–602.

Florescano, Enrique, and Elsa Malvido, eds. *Ensayos sobre la historia de las epidemias en México.* 2 vols. Mexico City: Instituto Mexicano del Seguro Social, 1982.

Freidel, David, and Linda Schele. *A Forest of Kings: The Untold Story of the Ancient Maya.* New York: William Morrow, 1990.

———, and Joy Parker. *Maya Cosmos: Three Thousand Years on the Shaman's Path.* New York: William Morrow, 1993.

French, William E. "Imagining and the Cultural History of Nineteenth-Century Mexico." In "Mexico's New Cultural History: Una Lucha Libra," special issue, *Hispanic American Historical Review* 79, no. 2 (May 1999): 249–67.

Gabbert, Wolfgang. *Becoming Maya: Ethnicity and Social Inequality in Yucatán since 1500.* Tucson: University of Arizona Press, 2004.

Gann, Thomas William Francis. *Ancient Cities and Modern Tribes: Exploration and Adventure in Maya Lands.* New York: Scribner's Sons, 1926.

García Quintanilla, Alejandra. "Reshaping the Social Body: Hunger among the Yucatec—Maya at the Turn of the Century." Paper presented at "Rethinking the Post-Colonial Encounter: Transitional Perspectives on the United States' Presence in Latin America," Yale University, October 18–21, 1995.

Gibson, Charles. *Spanish Tradition in America.* Columbia: University of South Carolina Press, 1968.

Gijaba y Patrón, Antonio. *Estudios comentario a las revoluciones sociales de México.* Mexico City: Tradición, SA, 1973.

Gómez-Pompa, Arturo. *The Lowland Maya Area: Three Millennia at the Human-Wildland Interface.* Binghamton, NY: Food Products, 2003.

Gonzales, Michael J. *The Mexican Revolution, 1910–1940.* Albuquerque: University of New Mexico Press, 2002.

Gootenberg, Paul. "Beleaguered Liberals: The Failed Generation of Free Traders in Peru." In *Guiding the Invisible Hand: Economic Liberalism and the State in Latin American History*, edited by Joseph L. Love and Nils Jacobsen, 63–97. Westport, CT: Praeger, 1988.

Gordon, Linda. *The Great Arizona Orphan Abduction*. Cambridge, MA: Harvard University Press, 1999.

Gorn, Elliot J. "Black Magic: Folk Beliefs of the Slave Community." In *Science and Medicine in the Old South*, edited by Ronald Numbers and Todd L. Savitt, 295–326. Baton Rouge: Louisiana State University Press, 1989.

Gostin, Lawrence O. "Influenza A (H1N1) and Pandemic Preparedness under the Rule of International Law." *JAMA* 301 (2009): 2376–78.

Grandin, Greg. *The Blood of Guatemala: A History of Race and Nation*. Durham, NC: Duke University Press, 2000.

Gutiérrez, Ramón A. *When Jesus Came, the Corn Mothers Went Away: Marriage, Sexuality, and Power in New Mexico, 1500–1846*. Stanford, CA: Stanford University Press, 1991.

Hale, Charles A. *Mexican Liberalism in the Age of Mora, 1821–1853*. New Haven, CT: Yale University Press, 1968.

Harris, Cole. "Voices of Disaster: Smallpox around the Strait of Georgia in 1782." *Ethnohistory* 41, no. 4 (Fall 1994): 591–626.

Harrison, Mark. "The Tender Frame of Man: Disease, Climate, and Racial Difference in India and the West Indies, 1760–1860." *Bulletin of the History of Medicine* 70, no. 1 (1996): 68–93.

Hart, John Mason. *Revolutionary Mexico: The Coming and Process of the Mexican Revolution*. Berkeley: University of California Press, 1987.

Hawkins, John P. *Health Care in Maya Guatemala: Confronting Medical Pluralism in a Developing Country*. Norman: University of Oklahoma Press, 2007.

Headrick, Daniel R. "The Tools of Imperialism: Technology and the Expansion of European Colonial Empires in the Nineteenth Century." *Journal of Modern History* 51, no. 2 (1979): 231–63.

Heller, Karl Bartholomäus. *Alone in Mexico: The Astonishing Travels of Karl Heller, 1845–1848*. Translated and edited by Terry Rugeley. Tuscaloosa: University of Alabama Press, 2007.

Henderson, Peter V. N. *In the Absence of Don Porfirio: Francisco León de la Barra and the Mexican Revolution*. Wilmington, DE: Scholarly Resources, 2000.

Herring, D. Ann. "'There Were Young People and Old People and Babies Dying Every Week': The 1918–1919 Influenza Pandemic at Norway House." *Ethnohistory* 41, no. 1 (Winter 1993): 73–105.

Hopkins, Donald R. *Princes and Peasants: Smallpox in History*. Chicago: University of Chicago Press, 1983.

Hostettler, Ueli. "New Inequalities: Changing Maya Economy and Social Life in Central Quintana Roo, Mexico." In *Anthropological Perspectives on Economic Development and Integration*, edited by Norbert Dannhaeuser and Cynthia Werner, 25–59. Research in Economic Anthropology Series 22. Oxford: Elsevier, 2003.

Hübbe, Ricardo Molina. *Las hambres de Yucatan*. Mexico City: Editorial Orientaciones, 1941.

Hu-DeHart, Evelyn. *Yaqui Resistance and Survival: The Struggle for Land and Autonomy, 1821–1910*. Madison: University of Wisconsin Press, 1984.

Hudson, Robert P. *Disease and Its Control: The Shaping of Modern Thought*. Westport, CT: Greenwood, 1983.

Instituto Nacional de Estadística y Geografía. "Población total por principales ciudades 2010 y 2015." In *Agenda estadística de los Estados Unidos Mexicanos*, table 19.5. Mexico City: INEGI, 2009. Electronic document, www.inegi.org.mx/prod_contenidos/espanol/bvinegi/productos/integracion/pais/agenda/2009/Agenda_2009.pdf (accessed July 10, 2010).

Jacobson, Matthew Frye. *Barbarian Virtues: The United States Encounters Foreign Peoples at Home and Abroad, 1876–1917*. New York: Hill and Wang, 2000.

———. *Whiteness of a Different Color: European Immigrants and the Alchemy of Race*. Boston: Harvard University Press, 1998.

Jannetta, Ann. *The Vaccinators: Smallpox, Medical Knowledge, and the "Opening" of Japan*. Palo Alto, CA: Stanford University Press, 2007.

Jiménez, Iván Molina, and Steven Palmer. *La voluntad radiante: Cultura impresa, magia y medicina en Costa Rica, 1897–1932*. San José, Costa Rica: Editorial Porvenir, Plumsock Mesoamerican Studies, 1996.

Joseph, Gilbert M. "From Caste War to Class War: The Historiography of Modern Yucatán (c. 1750–1940)." *Hispanic American Historical Review* 65, no. 1 (February 1985): 111–34.

———. "Mexico's 'Popular Revolution': Mobilization and Myth in Yucatán, 1910–1940." *Latin American Perspectives* 4, no. 3 (Summer 1979): 46–65.

———. "On the Trail of Latin American Bandits: A Reexamination of Peasant Resistance." *Latin American Research Review* 25, no. 3 (1990): 7–53.

———. *Rediscovering the Past at Mexico's Periphery: Essays on the History of Modern Yucatan*. Tuscaloosa: University of Alabama Press, 1986.

———. "Rethinking Mexican Revolutionary Mobilization: Yucatán's Seasons of Upheaval, 1909–1915." In *Everyday Forms of State Formation: Revolution and the Negotiation of Rule in Modern Mexico*, edited by Joseph Nugent and Daniel Nugent, 135–69. Durham, NC: Duke University Press, 1994.

———. *Revolution from Without: Yucatán, Mexico, and the United States, 1880–1924*. Durham, NC: Duke University Press, 1988.

———. "The United States, Feuding Elites, and Rural Revolt in Yucatán, 1836–1915." In *Rural Revolt in Mexico: U.S. Intervention and the Domain of Subaltern Politics*, edited by Daniel Nugent, 173–206. Durham, NC: Duke University Press, 1998.

———, and Daniel Nugent, eds. *Everyday Forms of State Formation: Revolution and the Negotiation of Rule in Modern Mexico*. Durham, NC: Duke University Press, 1994.

Kashani-Sabet, Firoozeh. "Hallmarks of Humanism: Hygiene and Love of Homeland in Qujar Iran." *American Historical Review* 105, no. 4 (October 2000): 1171–1203.

Katz, Friedrich. "The Liberal Republic and the Porfiriato, 1867–1910." In *Mexico since Independence*, edited by Leslie Bethell, 49–124. Cambridge: Cambridge University Press, 1991.

———, ed. *Riot, Rebellion, and Revolution: Rural Social Conflict in Mexico*. Princeton, NJ: Princeton University Press, 1988.

———. *The Secret War in Mexico: Europe, the United States, and the Mexican Revolution*. Chicago: University of Chicago Press, 1981.

Keeney, Elizabeth Barnaby. "Unless Powerful Sick: Domestic Medicine in the Old South." In *Science and Medicine in the Old South*, edited by Ronald Numbers and Todd L. Savitt, 276–94. Baton Rouge: Louisiana State University Press, 1989.

Kendall, Carl, Patricia Hudelson, Elli Leontsini, Peter Winch, Linda Lloyd, and Fernando

Cruz. "Urbanization, Dengue, and the Health Transition: Anthropological Contributions to International Health." In "Contemporary Issues of Anthropology in International Health," special issue, *Medical Anthropology Quarterly* 5, no. 3 (September 1991): 257–68.

King, Linda. *Roots of Identity: Language and Literacy in Mexico.* Stanford, CA: Stanford University Press, 1994.

King, Nicholas B. "Security, Disease, Commerce: Ideologies of Postcolonial Global Health." *Social Studies of Science* 32, no. 5/6 (October–December 2002): 763–89.

Kiple, Kenneth F., ed. *The Cambridge World History of Human Disease.* New York: Cambridge University Press, 1993.

Knaut, Andrew Louis. "Disease and the Late Colonial Public Health Initiative in the Atlantic Ports of New Spain." PhD diss., Duke University, 1994.

Knight, Alan. *The Mexican Revolution.* Vol. 1: *Porfirians, Liberals and Peasants.* Lincoln: University of Nebraska Press, 1986.

———. *The Mexican Revolution.* Vol. 2: *Counter-revolution and Reconstruction.* Lincoln: University of Nebraska Press, 1986.

———. "The Peculiarities of Mexican History: Mexico Compared to Latin America, 1821–1992." In "The Colonial and Post Colonial Experience: Five Centuries of Spanish and Portuguese America," quincentenary supplement, *Journal of Latin American Studies* 24 (1992): 99–144.

Koch, Robert. *Essays of Robert Koch.* Translated by K. Codell Carter. Contributions in Medical Studies 20. New York: Greenwood, 1987.

Konrad, Herman W. "Capitalism on the Tropical-Forest Frontier: Quintana Roo, 1880s to 1930." In *Land, Labor and Capital in Modern Yucatán: Essays in Regional and Political Economy*, edited by Jeffrey Brannon and Gilbert Joseph, 143–78. Tuscaloosa: University of Alabama Press, 2002.

Koplow, David. *Smallpox: The Fight to Eradicate a Global Scourge.* Berkley: University of California Press, 2003.

Koth, Karl B. *Waking the Dictator: Veracruz, the Struggle for Federalism, and the Mexican Revolution, 1870–1927.* Calgary, Alberta: University of Calgary Press, 2002.

Krauss, Clifford. *Inside Central America: Its People, Politics and History.* New York: Summit Books, 1991.

Kraut, Alan M. *Silent Travelers: Germs, Genes, and the "Immigrant Menace."* Baltimore, MD: Johns Hopkins University Press, 1994.

Kudlick, Catherine J. *Cholera in Post-Revolutionary Paris: A Cultural History.* Berkeley: University of California Press, 1996.

Kunitz, S. J. *Disease and Social Diversity: The European Impact on the Health of Non-Europeans.* New York: Oxford University Press, 1994.

LaFeber, Walter. *The American Age: U.S. Foreign Policy at Home and Abroad.* Vol. 1. 2nd ed. New York: W. W. Norton, 1996.

Larson, Brooke. *Trials of Nation Making: Liberalism, Race, and Ethnicity in the Andes, 1810–1910.* New York: Cambridge University Press, 2004.

———, and Olivia Harris, eds. *Ethnicity, Markets, and Migration in the Andes: At the Crossroads of History and Anthropology.* Durham, NC: Duke University Press, 1995.

Larson, Pier M. "Austronesian Mortuary Ritual in History: Transformations of Secondary

Burial (Famadihana) in Highland Madagascar." *Ethnohistory* 48, no. 1–2 (Winter/Spring 2001): 123–55.

Leavitt, Judith Walker, and Ronald Numbers, eds. *Sickness and Health in America.* Madison: University of Wisconsin Press, 1985.

Lempérière, Annick. "Nación moderna o república barroca? México, 1823–1857." In *Imaginar la nación*, edited by Fraçois-Xavier Guerra and Mónica Quijada, 135–77. Münster, Germany: Lit, 1994.

Lincove, David A. "Radical Publishing to 'Reach the Million Masses': Alexander L. Trachtenberg and International Publishers, 1906–1966." *Left History* 10, no. 1 (Fall/Winter 2004): 85–40.

Lindenbaum, Shirley, and Margaret Lock, eds. *Knowledge, Power, and Practice: The Anthropology of Medicine and Everyday Life.* Berkeley: University of California Press, 1993.

Lipp, Frank J. *The Mixe of Oaxaca: Religion, Ritual, and Healing.* Austin: University of Texas Press, 1991.

Lira, Andrés. "Justo Sierra: La historia como entendimiento responsable." In *Historiadores de México en el siglo XX*, edited by Enrique Florescano and Ricardo Pérez Montfort, 22–40. Colección Obras de Historia Series. Mexico City: Fondo de Cultura Económica, 1995.

Lockhart, James. *We People Here: Nahuatl Accounts of the Conquest of Mexico.* Berkeley: University of California Press, 1992.

Logan, Michael H. "Humoral Medicine in Guatemala and Peasant Acceptance of Modern Medicine." *Human Organization* 32, no. 4 (1973): 385–95.

Longmate, Norman. *King Cholera: The Biography of a Disease.* London: Hamish Hamilton, 1966.

Lord, Rebecca A. "Vaccinating the Body Politic: The Campaign against Smallpox during the United States Military Occupation of the Dominican Republic, 1916–1924." Paper presented at the XXII Annual Latin American Studies Association Conference, Miami, March 16–18, 2000.

Loreto, Rosalva L., and Francisco J. Cervantes B., eds. *Limpiar y obedecer: La basura, el agua y la muerte en la Puebla de Los Angeles (1650–1925).* Puebla, Mexico: Centro de Estudios Mexicanos y Centroamericanos, Universidad de Puebla, 1994.

Loroño-Pino, María A., José A. Farfán-Ale, Alicia L. Zapata-Peraza, et al. "Introduction of the American/Asian Genotype of Genotype of Dengue 2 Virus into the Yucatán State of Mexico." *American Society of Tropical Medicine and Hygiene* 71, no. 4 (2004): 485–92.

Love, Joseph L., and Nils Jacobsen, eds. *Guiding the Invisible Hand: Economic Liberalism and the State in Latin American History.* Westport, CT: Praeger, 1988.

Ma, Quisha. "The Rockefeller Foundation and Modern Medical Education in China, 1915–1951." PhD diss., Case Western Reserve University, 1995.

Macpherson, Kerrie L. *A Wilderness of Marshes: The Origins of Public Health in Shanghai, 1843–1893.* New York: Oxford University Press, 1987.

Mallon, Florencia E. "Peasants and State Formation in Nineteenth-Century Mexico: Morelos, 1848–1858." *Political Power and Social Theory* 7 (1988): 1–54.

Manzanilla Domínguez, Anastasio. *Los enemigos del indio.* Mexico City: s.n., 1929.

Manzano, Juan Ramón Bastarrachea, and William Brito Sansores, eds. *The diccionario maya: Maya-Español/Español-Maya.* 3rd ed. Mexico City: Editorial Porrúa, 1995.

Marero, Levi. *Cuba: Economía y sociedad.* Madrid: Editorial Playor, 1988.

Martinez, Oscar J. *Troublesome Border.* Tucson: University of Arizona Press, 1988.

Martínez-Fernández, Luis. "Don't Die Here: The Death and Burial of Protestants in the Hispanic Caribbean, 1840–1885." *Americas* 49, no. 1 (July 1992): 23–47.

Mayer, Brantz. *Mexico: Lo que fué y lo que es.* Mexico City: Fondo de Cultura Económica, 1953.

McCaa, Robert. "Revisioning Smallpox in Mexico Tenochtitlán, 1520–1950: What Difference Did Charity, Quarantine, Inoculation and Vaccination Make?" In *Vivere in Citta/Living in the City: 14th–20th Centuries. Poverty, Charity and the City,* vol. 4, edited by Eugenio Sonnino, 455–88. Rome: Casa Editrice Universitá La Sapienza, 2004.

McKneill, William H. *Plagues and Peoples.* New York: Anchor Books, 1977.

McLynn, Frank. *Villa and Zapata: A History of the Mexican Revolution.* New York: Carrol & Graf, 2000.

Meade, Teresa A. *"Civilizing" Rio: Reform and Resistance in a Brazilian City, 1889–1930.* University Park: Pennsylvania State University Press, 1997.

Menéndez, Gabriel Antonio. *Quintana Roo: Una interrogación nacional.* México City: Partido Nacional Revolucionario, 1936.

Miller, Jeffery H. "The Princeton Codex of the Book of Chilam Balam of Nah." *Princeton University Library Chronicle* 53, no. 3 (1992): 287–96.

Molina, Natalia. *Fit to Be Citizens? Public Health and Race in Los Angeles, 1879–1939.* Berkeley: University of California Press, 2006.

Montellano, Bernard R. Ortiz de. *Aztec Medicine, Health and Nutrition.* New Brunswick, NJ: Rutgers University Press, 1990.

Morris, R. J. *Cholera 1832: The Social Response to an Epidemic.* New York: Holmes and Meier, 1976.

Morrison, Lynda Sanderford. "The Life and Times of José Cantu Vela: Yucatecan Priest and Patriot (1802–1859)." PhD diss., University of Alabama, 1993.

Moseley, Edward H., and Helen Delpar. "Yucatán's Prelude to Globalization." In *Yucatán in an Era of Globalization,* edited by Eric N. Baklanoff and Edward Moseley, 20–41. Tuscaloosa: University of Alabama Press, 2008.

Nash, Linda. *Inescapable Ecologies: A History of Environment, Disease, and Knowledge.* Berkeley: University of California Press, 2006.

Navarro, Moisés González. *Raza y tierra: La Guerra de Castas y el henequén.* Mexico City: El Colegio de México, 1970.

Needell, Jeffrey D. "The Revolta contra Vacina of 1904: The Revolt against 'Modernization' in Belle-Epoque Rio de Janeiro." *Hispanic American Historical Review* 67, no. 2 (1987): 233–70.

Neil, Dan. "The Road to Ruins: The Internet Leads Our Man Astray on a Trip to See the Mayan Splendors of the Yucatán." *Expedia Travels* (January–February 2001): 90–99.

Nugent, Daniel, ed. *Rural Revolt in Mexico: U.S. Intervention and the Domain of Subaltern Politics.* Durham, NC: Duke University Press, 1998.

Numbers, Ronald, and Todd L. Savitt, eds. *Science and Medicine in the Old South.* Baton Rouge: Louisiana State University Press, 1989.

Olcott, Jocelyn. *Revolutionary Women in Postrevolutionary Mexico.* Durham, NC: Duke University Press, 2005.

Oliver Sánchez, Lilia V. "Una nueva forma de morir en Guadalajara: El cólera de 1833." *El cólera de 1833: Una nueva patología en México causas y efectos*. Colección Divulgación. Mexico City: Instituto Nacional de Antropología y Historia, 1992.

———. *Un verano mortal: Análisis demográfico y social de una epidémica de cólera: Guadalajara, 1833*. Guadalajara, Mexico: Gobierno de Jalisco Secretaria General Unidad Editorial, 1986.

Ong, Walter J. *Orality and Literacy: The Technologizing of the Word*. New York: Methuen, 1982.

Ortega, Enrique Montalvo. "La hacienda henequenera, la transición al capitalismo y la penetración imperialista en Yucatán, 1850–1914." *Revista Mexicana de Ciencias Políticas y Sociales* 24, no. 91 (1978): 137–76.

———. "Revolts and Peasant Mobilizations in Yucatán: Indians, Peóns, and Peasants from the Caste War to the Revolution." In *Riot, Rebellion, and Revolution: Rural Social Conflict in Mexico*, edited by Friedrich Katz, 296–308. Princeton, NJ: Princeton University Press, 1988.

Ortega y Médina, Juan A., ed. *Ensayo político sobre el reino de la Nueva España*. Mexico City: Editorial Porrúa, 1966.

Packard, Randall M. "The Invention of the 'Tropical Worker': Medical Research and the Quest for Central African Labor on the South African Gold Mines, 1903–36." *Journal of African History* 34, no. 2 (1993): 271–92.

Palmer, Steven, and Iván Molina Jiménez. *Educando a Costa Rica: Alfabetización popular, formación docente y género (1880–1950)*. San José, Costa Rica: Editorial Porvenir, 2000.

Parker, David S. "Civilizing the City of Kings: Hygiene and Housing in Lima, Peru." In *Cities of Hope: People, Protests, and Progress in Urbanizing Latin America, 1870–1930*, edited by Ronn Pineo and James A. Baer, 153–78. Boulder, CO: Westview, 1998.

Patch, Robert W. "Decolonization, the Agrarian Problem, and the Origins of the Caste War, 1812–1847." In *Land, Labor, and Capital in Modern Yucatán: Essays in Regional History and Political Economy*, edited by Gilbert Joseph and Jeffery T. Brannon, 51–82. Tuscaloosa: University of Alabama Press, 1991.

———. "Sacraments and Disease in Mérida, México, 1648–1727." *Historian* 58, no. 4 (1996): 732–43.

Patterson, K. David. "Disease Environments of the Antebellum South." In *Science and Medicine in the Old South*, edited by Ronald Numbers and Todd L. Savitt, 152–65. Baton Rouge: Louisiana State University Press, 1989.

Peard, Julyan G. *Race, Place, and Medicine: The Idea of the Tropics in Nineteenth-Century Brazilian Medicine*. Durham, NC: Duke University Press, 1999.

Pelling, Margaret. *Cholera, Fever and English Medicine, 1825–1865*. Oxford: Oxford University Press, 1978.

Pérez de Sarmiento, Marisa. *Historia de una elección: La candidatura de Olegario Molina en 1901*. Mérida, Mexico: Universidad Autónoma de Yucatán, 2002.

Piccato, Pablo. *City of Suspects: Crime in Mexico City, 1900–1931*. Durham, NC: Duke University Press, 2001.

Pineo, Ronn. "Public Health Care in Valparaíso, Chile." In *Cities of Hope: People, Protests, and Progress in Urbanizing Latin America, 1870–1930*, edited by Ronn Pineo and James A. Baer, 179–217. Boulder, CO: Westview, 1998.

———, and James A. Baer, eds. *Cities of Hope: People, Protests, and Progress in Urbanizing Latin America, 1870–1930*. Boulder, CO: Westview, 1998.

Platt, Tristan. "Liberalism and Ethnocide in the Southern Andes." *History Workshop Journal* 17 (Spring 1984): 3–18.

Plesset, Isabel. *Noguchi and His Patrons*. London: Associated University Presses, 1980.

Pomeranz, Kenneth, and Steven Topik. *The World That Trade Created: Society, Culture, and the World Economy 1400 to the Present*. New York: M. E. Sharpe, 1999.

Powers, Ramon, and James N. Leiker. "Cholera among the Plains Indians: Perceptions, Causes, Consequences." *Western Historical Quarterly* 29, no. 3 (Autumn 1998): 317–40.

Quintal Martín, Fidelio. *Correspondencia de la Guerra de Castas: Epistolario documental, 1843–1866*. Mérida, Mexico: Universidad Autónoma de Yucatán, 1992.

Radding, Cynthia. *Wandering Peoples: Colonialism, Ethnic Spaces, and Ecological Frontiers in Northwestern Mexico, 1700–1850*. Durham, NC: Duke University Press, 1997.

Ramírez, José Fernando. *Viaje a Yucatan: 1865*. Edited by Carlos R. Menéndez. Guadalajara, Mexico: Ediciones Et Caetera, 1971.

Ramos, J. L., J. Chávez, A. Escobar, C. Sheriday, R. Tranquilino, and T. Rojas, coord. *El Indio en la prensa nacional mexicana del siglo XIX: Catálogo de noticias*. Vol. 2. Mexico City: Centro de Investigaciones y Estudios Superiores en Antropología, Cuadernos de la Casa Chata, 1987.

Redfield, Robert. *The Little Community and Peasant Society and Culture*. Chicago: University of Chicago Press, 1960.

———. *A Village That Chose Progress: Chan Kom Revisited*. Chicago: University of Chicago Press, 1950.

Reed, John. *Insurgent Mexico*. New York: International, 1969. First published 1914.

Reed, Nelson. *The Caste War of Yucatan*. Stanford, CA: Stanford University Press, 1964.

Reff, Daniel T. *Disease, Depopulation, and Culture Change in Northwestern New Spain, 1518–1764*. Salt Lake City: University of Utah Press, 1991.

Remmers, Lawrence. "Henequén, the Caste War and Economy of Yucatan, 1846–1883: The Roots of Dependence in a Mexican Region." PhD diss., University of California, Los Angeles, 1981.

Restall, Matthew. *Maya Conquistador*. Boston: Beacon, 1998.

Richard, Carlos Macías. *Nueva frontera mexicana: Milicia, burocracia y ocupación territorial en Quintana Roo (1902–1927)*. Chetumal, Mexico: Universidad de Quintana Roo, 1997.

Rigau-Pérez, José G. "The Introduction of Smallpox Vaccine in 1803 and the Adoption of Immunization as a Government Function in Puerto Rico." *Hispanic American Historical Review* 69, no. 3 (1989): 393–423.

Rivero, Piedad Peniche, and Kathleen R. Martin. *Dos mujeres fera de serie: Elvia Carrillo Puerto y Felipa Poot*. Mérida, Mexico: Instituto de Cultura de Yucatán, 2007.

Roberts, Donald. "DDT Risk Assessments." *Environmental Health Perspectives* 109, no. 7 (July 2001): a302.

Roberts, Jennifer L. "Landscapes of Indifference: Robert Smithson and John Lloyd Stephens in Yucatán." *Art Bulletin* 82, no. 3 (September 2000): 544–67.

Rodríguez, Hernán Menéndez. *Iglesia y poder: Proyectos sociales, alianzas políticas y económicas en Yucatán (1857–1917)*. Mexico City: Consejo Nacional para la Cultura y las Artes, 1995.

Rodriguez Losa, Salvador. *Geografía política de Yucatán*. Vol. 1: *Tomo I censo inédito de 1821 año de independencia*. Mérida, Mexico: Universidad Autónoma de Yucatán, 1985.

———. *Geografía política de Yucatán*. Vol. 2: *División territorial, gobierno de los pueblos y población 1821–1900*. Mérida, Mexico: Universidad Autónoma de Yucatán, 1989.

———. *Geografía política de Yucatán*. Vol. 3: *División territorial, categorías políticas y población 1900–1990*. Mérida, Mexico: Universidad Autónoma de Yucatán, 1991.

Roediger, David R. "And Die in Dixie: Funerals, Death, and Heaven in the Slave Community, 1700–1865." *Massachusetts Review* 12 (Spring 1981): 163–83.

Rosenberg, Charles E. *The Cholera Years: The United States in 1832, 1849, and 1866*. Chicago: University of Chicago Press, 1987.

Roth, Mitchel. "Cholera, Community, and Public Health in Gold Rush Sacramento and San Francisco." *Pacific Historical Review* 66, no. 4 (November 1997): 527–51.

Rotz, Lisa D., MD, and William L. Atkinson, MD, MPH. "Clinical Features." Electronic document, www2.cdc.gov/nip/spoxclincian/contents/video01_transcript.htm (accessed December 10, 2009).

Roys, Ralph L., ed. *The Book of Chilam Balam of Chumayel*. Norman: University of Oklahoma Press, 1967.

———. *The Ethno-Botany of the Maya*. New Orleans, LA: Department of Middle American Research, Tulane University, 1931.

———. *The Indian Background of Colonial Yucatán*. The Civilization of the American Indian 118. Norman: University of Oklahoma Press, 1972.

———, ed. *The Ritual of the Bacabs*. Norman: University of Oklahoma Press, 1965.

Rugeley, Terry. "The Maya Elites of Nineteenth-Century Yucatán." *Ethnohistory* 42, no. 3 (1995): 477–93.

———, ed. *Maya Wars: Ethnographic Accounts from Nineteenth-Century Yucatán*. Norman: University of Oklahoma Press, 2001.

———. *Of Wonders and Wise Men: Religion and Popular Cultures in Southeast Mexico, 1800–1876*. Austin: University of Texas Press, 2001.

———. *Rebellion Now and Forever: Mayas, Hispanics, and Caste War Violence in Yucatán, 1800–1880*. Stanford, CA: Stanford University Press, 2009.

———. *Yucatán's Maya Peasantry and the Origins of the Caste War*. Symposia on Latin America. Austin: University of Texas Press, 1996.

Salazar-García, Félix, and Esperanza Gallardo-Díaz. "Reproductive Effects of Occupational DDT Exposure among Male Malaria Control Workers." *Environmental Health Perspectives* 112, no. 5 (April 2004): 542–47.

Sánchez Novelo, Faulo M. *La rebelión delahuertista en Yucatán*. Mérida, Mexico: Diario del Sureste, 1991.

Sandos, James A. "Pancho Villa and American Security: Woodrow Wilson's Mexican Diplomacy Reconsidered." *Journal of Latin American Studies* 13, no. 2 (November 1981): 293–311.

Savage, Melissa. "Ecological Disturbance and Nature Tourism." *Geographical Review* 83, no. 3 (July 1993): 290–300.

Schwarz, Maureen. "The Explanatory and Predictive Power of History: Coping with the Mystery Illness." *Ethnohistory* 42, no. 3 (Summer 1995): 375–401.

Scott, James C. *Domination and the Arts of Resistance: Hidden Transcripts*. New Haven, CT: Yale University Press, 1990.

———. *The Moral Economy of the Peasant: Rebellion and Subsistence in Southeast Asia*. New Haven, CT: Yale University Press, 1976.

———. *Weapons of the Weak: Everyday Forms of Peasant Resistance*. New Haven, CT: Yale University Press, 1985.

Sellers, Christopher. "Thoreau's Body: Towards an Embodied Environmental History." *Environmental History* 4, no. 4 (1999): 486–514.

Servín Massieu, Manuel. *Microbiología, vacunas y el rezago científico de México a partir del siglo XIX*. Mexico City: Centro Interdisciplinario de Investigaciones y Estudios sobre Medio Ambiente y Desarrollo CIIEMAD, 2000.

Seymour, Ralph Fletcher. *Across the Gulf: A Narration of a Short Journey through Parts of Yucatan, with a Brief Account of the Ancient Maya Civilization*. Chicago: Alderbrink, 1928.

Shattuck, George Cheever. *The Peninsula of Yucatan: Medical, Biological, Meteorological and Sociological Studies*. Washington, D.C.: Carnegie Institute, 1933.

Slater, Candace. "Amazonia as Edenic Narrative." In *Uncommon Ground: Toward Reinventing Nature*, edited by William Cronon, 114–31. New York: W. W. Norton, 1995.

Smith, Michael M. "Carrancista Propaganda and the Print Media in the United States: An Overview of Institutions." *Americas* 52, no. 2 (1995): 155–74.

———. "The 'Real Expedicion Maritima de la Vacuna' in New Spain and Guatemala." *Transactions of the American Philosophical Society, New Series* 64, no. 1 (1974): 1–74.

Smith, Robert Freeman. "The United States and the Mexican Revolution, 1921–1950." In *Myths, Misdeeds, and Misunderstandings: The Roots of Conflict in U.S.-Mexican Relations*, edited by Jaime E. Rodríguez O. and Kathryn Vincent, 181–98. Wilmington, DE: Scholarly Resources, 1997.

Snook, Laura K. "Sustaining Harvests of Mahogany (*Swietenia macrophylla* King) from Mexico's Yucatán Forests: Past, Present, and Future." In *Timber, Tourists, and Temples: Conservation and Development in the Maya Forest of Belize, Guatemala, and Mexico*, edited by Richard B. Primack, David Bray, Hugo A. Galletti, and Ismael Ponciano, 61–80. Washington, D.C.: Island, 1998.

Snow, John. *Snow on Cholera; Being a Reprint of Two Papers. Together with a biographical memoir by B. W. Richardson and an introduction by Wade Hampton Frost*. Johns Hopkins School of Hygiene and Public Health, facsimile of 1936 edition. New York: Hafner, 1965.

Solomon, Susan Gross. "Knowing the 'Local': Rockefeller Foundation Officers' Site Visits to Russia in the 1920s." In "Tourism and Travel in Russia and the Soviet Union," special issue, *Slavic Review* 62, no. 4 (Winter 2003): 710–32.

Solorzano, Armando. *Fiebre dorada o fiebre amarilla?: La Fundación Rockefeller en México, 1911–1924*. Guadalajara, Mexico: Universidad de Guadalajara, 1997.

———. "The Rockefeller Foundation in Revolutionary Mexico: Yellow Fever in Yucatán and Vera Cruz." In *Missionaries of Science: The Rockefeller Foundation and Latin America*, edited by Marcos Cueto, 52–71. Bloomington: Indiana University Press, 1994.

Soluri, John. *Banana Cultures: Agriculture, Consumption, and Environmental Change in Honduras and the United States*. Austin: University of Texas Press, 2006.

Soto, Shirlene. "Women in the Revolution." In *Twentieth-Century Mexico*, edited by W. Dirk Raat and William H. Beezley, 17–28. Lincoln: University of Nebraska Press, 1986.

Sowell, David. *The Tale of Healer Miguel Perdomo Neira: Medicine, Ideologies, and Power in the Nineteenth-Century Andes.* Wilmington, DE: Scholarly Resources, 2001.

Spenser, Daniela. "Workers against Socialism? Reassessing the Role of Urban Labor in Yucatecan Revolutionary Politics." In *New Approaches to Mexican Regional Historiography: Land, Labor, and Capital in Modern Yucatán*, edited by Jeffrey Brannon and Gilbert Joseph, 220–42. Tuscaloosa: University of Alabama Press, 1991.

Spielman, Andrew, and Michael D'Antonio. *Mosquito: The Story of Man's Deadliest Foe.* New York: Hyperion, 2002.

Spinden, Herbert Joseph. *A Study of Maya Art, Its Subject Matter and Historical Development.* New York: Dover, 1975. First published 1913.

Staples, Anne. "La lucha por los muertos." *Dialógos* 13, no. 5 (1977): 15–20.

———. "Policía y Buen Gobierno: Municipal Efforts to Regulate Public Behavior, 1821–1857." In *Rituals of Rule, Rituals of Resistance: Public Celebrations and Popular Culture in Mexico*, edited by William Beezley, Cheryl English Martin, and William E. French, 115–26. Wilmington, DE: Scholarly Resources, 1994.

Stepan, Nancy Leys. *"The Hour of Eugenics": Race, Gender and Nation in Latin America.* Ithaca, NY: Cornell University Press, 1996.

———. *Picturing Tropical Nature.* Ithaca, NY: Cornell University Press, 2001.

Stephens, John Lloyd. *Incidents of Travel in Yucatan.* 2 vols. New York: Harper, 1843. Reprint, Washington, D.C.: Smithsonian Institution Press, 1996.

Stern, Steve J., ed. *Resistance, Rebellion, and Consciousness in the Andean Peasant World 18th to 20th Centuries.* Madison: University of Wisconsin Press, 1987.

Stevens, Donald F. "Eating, Drinking, and Being Married: Epidemic Cholera and the Celebration of Marriage in Montreal and Mexico City, 1832–1833." *Catholic Historical Review* 92, no. 1 (January 2006): 74–94.

Stronza, Armanda. "Anthropology of Tourism: Forging New Ground for Ecotourism and Other Alternatives." *Annual Review of Anthropology* 30 (2001): 261–83.

Sullivan, Paul. *Unfinished Conversations: Mayas and Foreigners between Two Wars.* New York: Alfred A. Knopf, 1989.

Sutton, Ann, and Myron Sutton. *Among the Maya Ruins: The Adventures of John Lloyd Stephens and Frederick Catherwood.* New York: Rand McNally, 1967.

Swadesh, Mauricio, María Cristina Álvarez, and Juan Ramón Bastarrachea Manzano, eds. *Diccionario de elementos del Maya yucateco colonial.* Vol. 3. Mexico City: UNAM, Centro de Estudios Mayas, 1970.

Swann, Michael M. "The Demographic Impact of Disease and Famine in Late Colonial Northern Mexico." In *Geoscience and Man: Historical Geography of Latin America: Papers in Honor of Robert C. West*, edited by William V. Davidson and James J. Parsons, 97–109. Baton Rouge: School of Geoscience, Louisiana State University, 1980.

Tannenbaum, Frank. *The Mexican Agrarian Revolution.* Hamdem, CT: Archon Books, 1929.

Taubenberger, Jeffery K., and David M. Morens. "1918 Influenza: The Mother of All Pandemics." *Emerging Infectious Diseases.* Internet serial published by the CDC, 2006. Electronic document, www.cdc.gov/ncidod/eid/vol12no01/05-0979-htm (accessed July 10, 2010).

Taussig, Michael. "Peasant Economics and the Development of Capitalist Agriculture in the Cauca Valley, Colombia." In "Peasants, Capital Accumulation and Rural Underdevelopment," special issue, *Latin American Perspectives* 5, no. 3 (Summer 1978): 62–91.

Taylor, William B. *Drinking, Homicide and Rebellion in Colonial Mexican Villages*. Stanford, CA: Stanford University Press, 1979.

Tenenbaum, Barbara A. "Streetwise History: The Paseo de la Reforma and the Porfirian State, 1876–1910." In *Rituals of Rule, Rituals of Resistance*, edited by William H. Beezley, Cheryl English Martin, and William E. French, 127–50. Wilmington, DE: Scholarly Resources, 1994.

Tenenbaum, David J. "Trampling Paradise: Dream Vacation—Environmental Nightmare?" *Environmental Health Perspectives* 108, no. 5 (May 2000): A214–19.

Thompson, Angela T. "To Save the Children: Smallpox Inoculation, Vaccination, and Public Health in Guanajuato, Mexico, 1797–1840." *Americas* 49, no. 4 (1993): 431–55.

Thompson, Edward Herbert. *People of the Serpent: Life and Adventure among the Mayas*. Boston: Houghton Mifflin, 1932.

Thomson, James C., Jr. *While China Faced West: American Reformers in Nationalist China 1928–1937*. Cambridge, MA: Harvard University Press, 1980.

Tibbetts, John. "Toxic Tides." *Environmental Health Perspectives* 106, no. 7 (July 1998): A326–31.

Tomes, Nancy. *The Gospel of Germs: Men, Women and the Microbe in American Life*. Cambridge, MA: Harvard University Press, 1998.

Torre, Josefina Muriel de la. *Hospitales de la Nueva España fundaciones de los siglos XVI, XVII y XVIII*. Mexico City: Editorial Jus, S.A, 1956/1960.

Trennert, Robert A. *White Man's Medicine: Government Doctors and the Navajo, 1863–1955*. Albuquerque: University of New Mexico Press, 1998.

Turner, Frederick C. *The Dynamic of Mexican Nationalism*. Chapel Hill: University of North Carolina Press, 1968.

Turner, John Kenneth. *Barbarous Mexico*. 3rd printing. Austin: University of Texas Press, 1990.

Tutino, John. *From Insurrection to Revolution in Mexico: Social Bases of Agrarian Violence, 1750–1940*. Princeton, NJ: Princeton University Press, 1986.

Urrea, Luis Alberto. *Across the Wire: Life and Hard Times on the Mexican Border*. New York: Anchor Books, 1993.

Valadés, Diego. "Salvador Alvarado, Un precursor de la Constitución de 1917." In *Estudios jurídicos en homenaje a don Santiago Barajas Montes de Oca*, edited by Santiago Barajas, 417–44. Mexico City: Universidad Nacional Autónoma de México, 1995.

Vanderwood, Paul J. *The Power of God against the Guns of Government: Religious Upheaval in Mexico at the Turn of the Nineteenth Century*. Stanford, CA: Stanford University Press, 1998.

van Heyningen, W. E., and John R. Seal. *Cholera: The American Scientific Experience, 1947–1980*. Boulder, CO: Westview, 1983.

Van Young, Eric. *Hacienda and Market in Eighteenth-Century Mexico: The Rural Economy of the Guadalajara Region, 1675–1820*. Berkeley: University of California Press, 1981.

———. "The New Cultural History Comes to Old Mexico." In "Mexico's New Cultural History: Una Lucha Libre," special issue, *Hispanic American Historical Review* 79, no. 2 (May 1999): 211–47.

———. "To See Someone Not Seeing: Historical Studies of Peasants and Politics in Mexico." *Mexican Studies/Estudios Mexicanos* 6, no. 1 (Winter 1990): 133–59.

Vaughan, Megan. *Curing Their Ills: Colonial Power and African Illness*. Stanford, CA: Stanford University Press, 1991.

Vega, E., H. Ruiz, G. Martínez-Villa, G. Sosa, E. Gonzalez-Avalos, and E. Reyes. "Fine and Coarse Particulate Matter Chemical Characterization in a Heavily Industrialized City in Central Mexico during Winter 2003." *Journal of Air Waste Management Association* 57, no. 5 (May 2007): 620–33.

Villa Rojas, Alfonso. *The Maya of East Central Quintana Roo*. Washington, D.C.: Carnegie Institute, 1944.

Voekel, Pamela. *Alone before God: The Religious Origins of Modernity in Mexico*. Durham, NC: Duke University Press, 2002.

———. "Piety and Public Space: The Cemetery Campaign in Veracruz, 1789–1810." In *Latin American Popular Culture: An Introduction*, edited by William H. Beezley and Linda A. Curcio-Nagy, 1–25. Wilmington, DE: Scholarly Resources, 2000.

Wachtel, Nathan. *Gods and Vampires: Return to Chipaya*. Translated by Carol Volk. Chicago: University of Chicago Press, 1994.

Walton, John, Paul B. Beeson, and Ronal Bodley Scott, eds. *The Oxford Companion to Medicine*. 2 vols. New York: Oxford University Press, 1986.

Warner, Margaret H. "Public Health in the Old South." In *Science and Medicine in the Old South*, edited by Ronald Numbers and Todd L. Savitt, 226–75. Baton Rouge: Louisiana State University Press, 1989.

Warren, Adam. "Piety and Danger: Popular Ritual, Epidemics, and Medical Reform in Lima, Peru, 1750–1860." PhD diss., University of California, San Diego, 2004.

Watanabe, John M. "Unimagining the Maya: Anthropologists, Others, and the Inescapable Hubris of Authorship." In "Shifting Frontiers: Historical Transformations and Identities in Latin America," special issue, *Bulletin of Latin American Research* 14, no. 1 (January 1995): 25–45.

Watts, Sheldon. "Cholera Politics in Britain in 1879." *Journal of the Historical Society* 7, no. 3 (2007): 291–347.

———. *Epidemics and History: Disease, Power and Imperialism*. New Haven, CT: Yale University Press, 1997.

———. "Yellow Fever Immunities in West Africa and the Americas in the Age of Slavery and Beyond: A Reappraisal." *Journal of Social History* 34, no. 4 (Summer 2001): 955–67.

Wedeen, Lisa. "Seeing Like a Citizen, Acting like a State." *Comparative Studies in Society and History* 45, no. 4 (2003): 680–713.

Wells, Allen. "All in the Family: Railroads and Henequen Monoculture in Porfirian Yucatán." *Hispanic American Historical Review* 72, no. 2 (May 1992): 159–209.

———. "Family Elites in a Boom and Bust Economy: The Molinas and Peóns of Porfirian Yucatán." *Hispanic American Historical Review* 62, no. 2 (May 1982): 224–53.

———. "Forgotten Chapters of Yucatán's Past: Nineteenth-Century Politics in Historiographical Perspective." *Mexican Studies/Estudios Mexicanos* 12, no. 2 (1996): 195–229.

———. *Yucatán's Gilded Age: Haciendas, Henequen, and International Harvester, 1860–1915*. Albuquerque: University of New Mexico Press, 1985.

———, and Gilbert M. Joseph. *Summer of Discontent, Seasons of Upheaval: Elite Politics and Rural Insurgency in Yucatán, 1876–1915*. Stanford, CA: Stanford University Press, 1996.

Williams, David. "The Bureau of Investigation and Its Critics, 1919–1921: The Origins of Federal Political Surveillance." *Journal of American History* 68, no. 3 (December 1981): 560–79.

Williams, Edward J. "The Resurgent North and Contemporary Mexican Regionalism." *Mexican Studies/Estudios Mexicanos* 6, no. 2 (Summer 1990): 299–323.

Winberry, John J. "Development of the Mexican Railroad System." In *Geoscience and Man: Historical Geography of Latin America; Papers in Honor of Robert C. West*, vol. 21, edited by William V. Davidson and James J. Parsons, 111–19. Baton Rouge: School of Geoscience, Louisiana State University, 1980.

Wolf, Eric R. *Peasant Wars of the Twentieth Century.* Norman: University of Oklahoma Press, 1999.

Wright, Angus. *The Death of Ramón González: The Modern Agricultural Dilemma.* Rev. ed. Austin: University of Texas Press, 2005.

Yoder, Michael S. "Globalization and the Evolving Port Landscape of Progreso." In *Yucatán in an Era of Globalization*, edited by Eric N. Baklanoff and Edward Moseley, 42–68. Tuscaloosa: University of Alabama Press, 2008.

Zapata, Dorothy Andrews Heath de, ed. *El libro del Judío ó medicina doméstica: Descripción de los nombres de las yerbas de Yucatán y las enfermedades a que se aplican, siglo XVII.* Mérida, Mexico: Oficina del Copiador, 1979.

Zeger, Scott L. Francesca Dominnici, Aidan McDermott, and Jonathan M. Samet. "Mortality in the Medicare Population and Chronic Fine Particulate Air Pollution in Urban Centers (2000–2005)." *Environmental Health Perspectives* 116, no. 12 (December 2008): 1614–19.

Zulawski, Ann. *Unequal Cures: Public Health and Political Change in Bolivia, 1900–1950.* Durham, NC: Duke University Press, 2007.

INDEX